Doctors at the Borders

DOCTORS AT THE BORDERS

Immigration and the Rise of Public Health

Michael C. LeMay

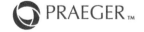

PRAEGER™

An Imprint of ABC-CLIO, LLC

Santa Barbara, California • Denver, Colorado

Library of Congress Cataloging-in-Publication Data

LeMay, Michael C., 1941–
   Doctors at the borders : immigration and the rise of public health / Michael C. LeMay.
     Pages cm
   Includes bibliographical references.
   ISBN 978-1-4408-4024-1 (hardback) — ISBN 978-1-4408-4025-8 (e-book)
1. Medical assistance.   2. Communicable diseases—Transmission.   3. Emigration and immigration—Health aspects.   I. Title.
   RA643.L45 2015
   362.1969—dc23   2015012766

ISBN: 978-1-4408-4024-1
EISBN: 978-1-4408-4025-8

19 18 17 16 15   1 2 3 4 5

This book is also available on the World Wide Web as an eBook.
Visit www.abc-clio.com for details.

Praeger
An Imprint of ABC-CLIO, LLC

ABC-CLIO, LLC
130 Cremona Drive, P.O. Box 1911
Santa Barbara, California 93116-1911

This book is printed on acid-free paper ∞

Manufactured in the United States of America

CONTENTS

LIST OF TABLES

PREFACE

The recent outbreak of an Ebola pandemic in Africa and the first cases discovered in the United States demonstrate that the world is once again facing a pandemic disease outbreak and the threat of more and newer pandemics, both naturally produced and, possibly, manufactured by bioterrorists bent on mass murder for political purposes. As the first decade of the twenty-first century closed, we witnessed an old threat of human disease— a new variant of the H1N1 type A influenza virus, more popularly known as the swine flu. It spread amazingly quickly. In one month's time, nearly 17,000 cases were confirmed in fifty countries around the globe, resulting in 117 deaths. Within the first month of the epidemic, forty-nine of the fifty American states reported nearly 9,000 cases resulting in fifteen deaths. That pandemic began in Mexico in April 2009. Its fatality rate was less than 0.1, mild in comparison to the Great Influenza pandemic of 1918–1919, which was also a variant of Type A, H1N1. The 1918–1919 pandemic infected an estimated 1 billion people worldwide and caused more than 50 million deaths. The 1918 outbreak of the virus had a fatality rate of 2.5. The 2009 outbreak of the H1N1 flu virus raised anew concerns over how to cope with pandemics that arise during a period of mass migration (Time, 2014: 80–82). Those concerns are enhanced by the very speed with which humankind can transverse the globe, as well as the sheer volume of worldwide migration. Air flights from virtually anywhere in the world to the United States routinely take far less time than the incubation stage of many epidemic viral diseases and thus their apparent manifestation of symptoms.

Then, in March 2014, the United States experienced an epidemic outbreak of a new mutation of the Enterovirus-D68. As of this writing, it has struck over 500 primary school–aged children in dozens of states, having killed four children and one adult by October 1, 2014. It seems to be a new variant of the enterovirus, easily transmissible as well as more pathogenic (CDC, 2015).

Fears of pandemic disease outbreaks influence the debate over reforming immigration policy. Having previously written several books on U.S. immigration policy, I realized that the experiences of coping with pandemics over a century ago, during the last era of mass migration, provided useful and timely insight for today.

The swine flu and now Ebola pandemics raise some compelling questions. How did the quarantine officials working at the U.S. quarantine/immigration stations at the nation's borders at the turn of the twentieth century come up with devices and procedures to guard against highly contagious diseases while processing the tens to even hundreds of thousands of immigrants who annually immigrated to America? Can we learn any important lessons from that last era of massive immigration? As we debate health care and what opponents of health care reform label "the government takeover of health care," can we learn from the past about how successful, or not, a government-run program of public health and disease prevention worked? Does the past have any lessons for us about the **appropriateness** and the **effectiveness** of a **federal** program of preventive public health? Can we learn anything about the relative efficiencies or problems of state and local public health approaches to what is undoubtedly a national threat of another massive pandemic? Is this one area in which **only** a federal program makes sense in facing a national problem?

During my research for prior books, one photograph I had occasion to see showed an autoclave, a small steam chamber used for the sterilization of surgical equipment. It suggested a question to me: How did they go from the concept of that small, countertop-sized device for the sterilization of surgical instruments to the huge steam chambers I knew were used to disinfect large cartloads of baggage and similar personal belongings of entire shiploads of immigrant passengers arriving daily at U.S. shores by the many hundreds or even thousands? I remembered photographs of similar, yet huge, chambers that had once been used on Angel Island in San Francisco Bay. My curiosity aroused, I wanted to know how such an innovation in processing large numbers of immigrants while guarding against highly contagious and often deadly disease came to be spread. Did they go, for example, from the huge station at Ellis Island to the more moderately sized station at Angel Island to a relatively tiny station such as that at New Orleans?

The late nineteenth and early twentieth centuries saw unprecedented global mass migrations. The United States was the major immigration-receiving nation of this vast migration of literally tens of millions of persons who permanently migrated from their nation of origin to their new homes in North America—to both Canada and the United States. Millions came from many of the same countries of origin and, proportionally, in similar waves. Truly they made the United States a nation of nations. The size, scope, diversity, and duration of the massive migration at the close of the nineteenth century and the beginning decades of the twentieth century posed enormous public policy problems for the receiving country. Development of the bureaucracies and of the facilities to process annually the immigration of tens to even hundreds of thousands of persons at dozens of stations of entry was no simple task. Unprecedented levels of immigration required innovations to cope with what has been quite accurately called a flood of immigration.

It is significant that more than people participated in this era of mass migration. The tale of how governments sought to cope with problems of microscopic "fellow travelers"—germ and viral pathogens causing outbreaks of epidemic diseases—is of compelling human interest, offering lessons for today if we are attentive. Some outbreaks became pandemics—global in scope and with morbidity rates in the hundreds of millions and with mortality rates in the tens of millions. Today, these epidemic outbreaks seem to be things of the distant past, so we tend to forget about them. But it is precisely because they took place long ago that they are again so potentially dangerous. Immunities built up in the population against these microbes—old enemies of mankind—have disappeared from within our population. The United States is, essentially, once more nearly virgin territory for an invasion of microbial and viral threats, especially from old diseases that may have mutated so that they are unrecognized by our immune system.

The late nineteenth century saw revolutions in medicine, in agricultural production, in industrialization, and in urbanization that enabled a population explosion that compelled mass migration. Scientific medicine and the germ theory of disease developed in the late decades of the nineteenth century and provided a basic understanding of disease and how it spread among humankind. These developments contributed to public policy to cope with processing millions of immigrants in their movement and resettlement while preventing or mitigating outbreaks of epidemics and curtailing their pandemic scope—what came to be known as public health.

Doctors at the Borders relates the story of those developments: of the era of mass migration, of the period of epidemics and pandemics, and of innovations in methods for coping with mass migration as seen at three reception stations that became the most important ones in America for the development of national public health programs. It tells how developments in scientific medicine and public health are inextricably intertwined with immigration and procedures to cope with mass migration. It is the tale of some of the medical officers posted at those quarantine stations and their respective hospitals and labs who struggled daily with fighting disease while screening a vast multitude of immigrants—truly heroic "doctors at the borders." A few of the medical researchers of the era are well known, but most are unsung heroes. And calling them heroes is not hyperbole. We call heroic persons who save lives. We call heroic persons who put their lives on the line for their fellow humans, sometimes paying the ultimate price. Without question, the doctors working at these quarantine stations saved many lives—collectively, many tens of thousands of lives. Quite possibly, their preventive efforts saved millions of lives. Some gave their lives combating epidemics. Some innovated apparatus and procedures that applied insights from germ theory to practical methods to extend barriers against disease outbreaks from the laboratory to the quarantine stations processing hundreds to even thousands of persons daily and hundreds of thousands annually. They advanced the field of public health and shaped its practice for the twentieth century—spreading their innovations to major cities across the nation and to doctors at state and local boards of public health that developed as a result of their pioneering efforts.

The story of these three stations offer lessons for today as the United States once again copes with legal and illegal immigration in excess of 1 million a year (Passel, 2014). In the nineteenth century, the development in transportation from sailing vessels to steamship transports posed new problems for those coping with the spread of disease. People migrated farther than ever before. They traveled to locations where the population had little natural immunity to new disease-causing microbes. They migrated faster than before, sometimes in less time than the incubation periods of the communicable diseases traveling with them. Today, air transportation presents a similar case. The turn of the century from the nineteenth to the twentieth came with wondrous breakthroughs in medical knowledge. What we know of as modern medicine emerged. Medical research became scientific. The processes of quarantine—inspection, disinfection, and detention—became more scientific. Coping with viral disease is equally challenging in the twenty-first century. Disease-causing germs and viruses are mutating to more drug-resistant forms that increasingly defy the efforts of bacteriological treatments or require medical scientists to develop new germicides, vaccines, and sera. The experiences of these three immigration stations are more than just interesting stories of the distant past. They offer relevant lessons for us and for policy makers today.

This book is divided into six chapters. Chapter 1 discusses the age of mass migration, focusing on the period 1820 to 1920. It analyzes how and why millions of people chose to emigrate. It explains push factors compelling millions to emigrate and the pull factors drawing those millions to the United States. It discusses exemplary trends in that flow, as well as how the population in the receiving nation reacted to the millions of newcomers and the perceived threat of epidemic diseases entering with them. It describes public policy developments designed to cope with the flood of immigration. It explains the use of quarantine stations to process mass migration given the state of medical knowledge at the time.

Chapter 2 discusses the nineteenth century as a period of epidemic and pandemic diseases. It describes the major epidemic outbreaks that threatened and that on occasion became pandemics. It discusses the development of the germ theory of disease and how modern medicine developed to prevent or to treat epidemics of contagious and often deadly maladies. Medical science contributed to public policy, to the emergence of public health as a field of practice in medicine, and to the development of public health bureaucracies. The story of how those medical practices emerged and were innovated at three particularly important immigration stations then follows.

Chapter 3 presents the story of Angel Island in San Francisco Bay. It is not as well-known as Ellis Island and has been called the Ellis Island of the west coast. It may surprise readers to learn that it developed important innovations in apparatus and in public hygiene procedures that spread to other immigration stations and other quarantine hospitals, including Ellis Island. The "rat campaign" to combat bubonic plague developed by the doctors at the quarantine station at Angel Island in San Francisco Bay wrote the book on how to effectively conduct a massive public health effort. The extensive eradication campaign, for the first time in history, stopped a bubonic plague outbreak instead of merely isolating people from spreading the contagion while waiting for the disease to spend itself. Because of their efforts, the plague epidemic took only a few hundred lives, rather than the thousands of lives lost in typical plague outbreaks before San Francisco's experience. It was the first and, in no small measure because of their efforts, the only severe case of a bubonic plague epidemic in the United States. One of the doctors innovated important changes in the design of the steam apparatus used for large-scale disinfection of baggage—the Kinyoun–Francis decontamination tubes.

Chapter 3 presents a brief history of Angel Island, including how the medical staff there dealt with epidemics and pandemics, among them the 1900–1908 outbreak of bubonic plague. Two of the doctors stationed there were especially important in developing innovations to cope with epidemic disease and with plague in particular. One went on to become surgeon general of the United States, heading the newly named U.S. Public Health Service and achieving, in effect, the status of being the nation's "top doc."

Chapter 4 tells the tale of Ellis Island, New York, unquestionably the largest and best known of the quarantine and immigration stations in the United States and thus in the world. It presents a brief history of the island and its quarantine station, discussing how Ellis Island coped with unprecedented numbers of immigrants while containing epidemics and pandemics. It suffered an outbreak of the Spanish Influenza of 1918–1919, the greatest killing pandemic in the world and in the United States. The chapter covers the contributions Ellis Island made toward spreading procedures to cope with epidemic and pandemic diseases while processing immigrants on an unprecedented scale.

Chapter 5 relates the story of the New Orleans station. Perhaps precisely because it was the smallest of the three immigration reception stations, it was the most innovative with regard to testing and developing germicides to combat diseases after European medical researchers had proven the validity of the germ theory of disease. The doctors there battled somewhat different pandemic threats—tropical diseases such as yellow fever, malaria, and typhoid fever. But it was also the site of frequent battles with smallpox epidemics that so plagued the U.S. South in the nineteenth century. New Orleans was in many ways a proving ground for the concept of vector control. It demonstrated the effectiveness of mosquito control as organized public health campaigns combating the spread of yellow fever and malaria. It was one of the major sites to demonstrate the effectiveness of compulsory vaccination to cope with smallpox. One of its U.S. M.H.S. medical officers became the leading authority on coping with smallpox.

Chapter 6 offers ten insights, lessons learned from these three immigration stations teaching us how better to cope with epidemic and pandemic outbreaks. These lessons infused the practices of the Public Health Service and from there spread to the practice of medicine more generally and to a consortium for public health organized in Canada, the United States, and Mexico. From that consortium it spread, ultimately, to the world. These lessons contributed to the development of bureaucratic agencies in the United States: the Food and Drug Administration, the National Institute of Health, and, particularly, the national and now international system of Centers for Disease Control. They offer insight into how better to cope with the threat from the new viruses of the twenty-first century—from natural outbreaks to the spread of new hot viral diseases. They suggest better ways to cope with the threat of bioterrorism—the intentional spread of epidemic disease used as a bioterrorist weapon of mass murder.

ACKNOWLEDGMENTS

This volume synthesizes the work of many who preceded me in analyzing these topics. They are cited in its extensive bibliography. Unfortunately, major fires during the history of operation of the stations destroyed many files and records that would have been a primary source of invaluable information to the historian or public policy analyst examining immigration. Serious gaps in the records mean that sketchy data must sometimes be used to infer what was taking place at these three stations or exemplify longer trends. But many records are available in some key archives, and today some scholars are mining them as new caches of data not previously researched. In addition to the information provided by many government reports and secondary sources, I would be remiss if I did not acknowledge the assistance of the wonderful staff at several of the archives of primary source documents used and noted in chapter parentheses and in chapter endnotes as well as in the bibliography. I researched at the Library of Congress, the National Archives and Records Administration (at both Washington, D.C., and College Park, Maryland); the National Library of Medicine; the National Museum of Health and Medicine in Washington, D.C.; the United States Navy Memorial and the Naval Heritage Center in Washington, D.C.; and the Angel Island Immigration Station Foundation in San Francisco. In particular, I wish to acknowledge the assistance of Marjorie H. Ciarlante of NARA's College Park archives. She was a helpful guide to the Public Health Service Records, Record Group 90, Central Files 1897–1923, so often cited throughout this volume. In addition, Holly Reed, a still pictures archivist at NARA, College Park, was very helpful in my obtaining several of the photographs for illustration herein. Similarly, Crystal Smith, the reference librarian at the History of Medicine Division of the National Library of Medicine, helped me find important information on key medical staff, as well as some of the biographies of several of the important doctors discussed herein.

I received invaluable assistance from the historian/archivists at Parks Canada, especially Madame Christine Chartré, historienne; Andre Charbonneau, Conseiller Services historiques; and architectural historian Yvan Fortier. They shared important insights with me, as well as the Chamberland photographs and exhibition slide that illuminated the development of the steam chamber apparatus and the procedures and processes employed that spread to stations in Canada and the United States.

I wish to acknowledge the assistance of Erika Lee, director of education, Angel Island Immigration Station Foundation, for her assistance and for referring me to two researchers who did groundbreaking work on Angel Island—Bob Barde and Maria Sakovich. They very kindly shared information from their research and provided me with useful insights. Likewise, I was assisted in my contacts with them by Dayle Reilly, coordinator of the North Bay Regional and Special Collections at the Sonoma State University Library. What is especially worthy in this volume is the result of their input. Any errors or mistakes in judgment are solely my responsibility.

Chapter 1

THE AGE OF MASS MIGRATION, 1820–1920

Imagine if *you* were responsible for developing policy and procedures to process the immigration of 40 million people! What would you do? Where would you begin? These are not far-fetched questions. As the twenty-first century reaches the midpoint of its second decade, the United States is again experiencing mass migration. Legal and illegal immigrants are entering at a rate of about 1 million a year, a scale echoing the turn of the nineteenth to the twentieth century. Immigration policy reform is again a major topic of American politics, on the agenda of governments at both the national and state levels. It was a key issue early on in the 2008 presidential election campaigns and remained a timely policy issue revisited in political debates leading up to the 2012 primary and general presidential elections, as well as in Congressional debates after the 2012 elections. The United States absorbed more than 70 million legal immigrants since 1820, and current estimates of illegal immigrants put them at 10–11 million. In numbers, the United States is the world's leading immigrant-receiving nation (Department of Homeland Security, 2010). Their arrival has a profound effect on American culture, economy, politics, and society. Understanding the magnitude and the effects of mass migration in the past has important lessons for today. Regardless of whether we face the issue, this renewed wave of legal and illegal immigration will affect our policy and politics in future decades.

The immigration process and flow are inherently interesting subjects. How the Unites States became "a nation of immigrants" is a story rich in human interest. The vast diversity of groups who intermingled to make America home compels our focus, as does how immigration bureaucracies coped with the process. Of special concern is how those agencies dealt with absorbing millions of immigrants without experiencing deadly outbreaks of epidemic diseases that came with surges of immigrants. Notable lessons from the past can inform policy to better cope with epidemic and pandemic diseases. Such lessons are timely when international terrorism threatens the use of bioterrorism. New diseases and natural mutations in virus strains threaten to break out into epidemics that may become pandemics (see, for example, Barry, 2005; Davies, 2000; Drexler, 2002; LeMay, 2006; and Walters, 2004). How past pandemics were dealt with offers lessons for today's policymakers and for informed citizens.

Historian Edwin Guillet called the nineteenth century the "Great Migration." It experienced a vast global movement from northwestern Europe, from south/central/eastern Europe, and from Asia (China, Japan and Korea particularly), to Australia, Canada, and the United States. From 1820 to 1920, nearly 35 million immigrants came to the United States. According to U.S. Immigration and Naturalization Service data, the official count of legal immigrants to the United States from 1820, when the country first began keeping count, until 1920 exceeded 33,600,000 persons (LeMay, ed. 2013, vol. 1, table 1.1: 3; and LeMay, ed. 2013, vol. 2, table 1.1: 3–4). That official count is undoubtedly less than the actual numbers of immigrants, for it does not include many thousands who went uncounted for various reasons. From 1820 until after the Civil War, for example, official figures represent simply alien passengers arriving at U.S. seaports. From 1892 until 1903, aliens entering by cabin class were not counted as immigrants. Significant levels of land arrivals (those coming across the borders with Mexico and Canada) were not completely enumerated until 1908. Often as many as 25 percent of immigrants entering Canada proceeded on to the United States (LeMay, 2006: 30–31; table 1.2) They responded to inducements such as the Homestead Act, drawing settlers to the Midwestern states, and the fact that the Canadian government supported the migrants by subsidizing their railroad fares through Canada.

The United States developed policy and procedures to process annually literally tens of thousands to hundreds of thousands of persons seeking entrance as permanent resident aliens. It did so at thirty-two seaports, for in the nineteenth century most international migration was by ship—first by sailing vessels, and later by steamship transport. Seaport cities became the sites of reception stations. By the late 1890s, New York alone (at Ellis Island) processed 700,000 immigrants each year. As one scholar notes: "Twenty-four million people migrated to the United States between 1880 and 1924, two thirds of them entering through the Port of New York" (Willrich, 2011: 217; see also Nugent: 27–33).

During the sailing era of "packet" ships, they came by the tens of thousands despite horrendous and dangerous conditions. Stephen Fox describes the dangers:

> At their worst, the emigrant ships ran aground, or sank in storms, or caught fire, or just vanished. In 1847 the *Exmouth*, a tiny vessel of only 320 tons, was blown by a storm onto a rocky Scottish coast, killing 240 emigrants; the *Carrick* after six weeks at sea hit a shoal and broke up off Newfoundland, with about 180 deaths, the *Canton* ran onto rocks near Durness, Scotland, leaving no survivors among the three hundred on board. On the *Ocean Monarch* in August 1848, only a few hours from Liverpool, someone lit an illegal fire below deck, the ship burned to the water line, killing over four hundred emigrants bound for Boston. In 1849, the *Maria*, heading from Limerick to Quebec, ran into an ice field in a storm, could not get free, collided with an iceberg, and went down with 109 people. Together these five shipwrecks caused well over 1,200 deaths, and during the first six years of the famine, in all about fifty ships foundered on their way to North America. So it went, year after year, a steady drumbeat of disasters with no evident remedy. (Fox, 2004: 170–71)

This global movement, moreover, occurred at an unprecedented scale. It was, simply put, an age of mass migration. It raises important questions. How and why did so many leave their homelands for America? What were the major trends in the flow of immigration? What were the reactions of the native stock to this vast influx of strangers? Who favored or opposed open immigration? Depressions (called panics until 1930) and recessions periodically developed as the economy of the nation adjusted to the millions of new arrivals. Economic upheavals fueled political movements among natives who called for restriction and even a total ban on immigration. Mixed public policy reactions to massive immigration both promoted and attempted to restrict it.

The movement of tens of millions for permanent resettlement entails a complex process. To grasp the complexity of this massive migration historians have distinguished two major eras: the old immigrant wave, from 1820 to 1880, and the new immigrant wave, from 1880 to 1920. They distinguish "push" and "pull" factors contributing to these waves.

Push factors are events that compel large numbers to emigrate, to permanently leave their nation of birth. They include floods, typhoons, massive earthquakes, volcanic eruptions, or similar natural disasters devastating homeland communities. They include outbreaks of epidemic diseases such as smallpox, typhus, yellow fever, bubonic plague, and cholera that scourge the human population, or crop diseases such as the potato blight and phylloxera that attack and destroy the leaves and roots of certain plants, including grain and tuber crops and grapevines. They include the urbanization and industrialization revolutions that spread across Europe, causing severe economic, political, and social disruptions. Horrendous economic conditions and chronic poverty resulted from overpopulation. Others were pushed out by the decline of feudalism and resulting political, religious, and ethnic persecutions, such as the pogroms of Eastern Europe—government-sponsored campaigns of violence begun in 1881 and continuing for some thirty years thereafter—forcing millions of Jews to flee the brutal outbreaks of beatings, killings, and lootings. The vast majority of them—well over 1 million—fled to the United States.

Pull factors draw immigrants to particular nations for resettlement. For the United States, these include the ease of transatlantic travel afforded by the steamship lines which cut the journey from months to days. Letters from friends and relatives in America induced others in Europe or Asia to join them in the lands of opportunity—called "chain migration." The gold rush drew millions to the United State. Government policy, such as the Homestead Act, which promised free or cheap land, drew millions from land-starved Europe. The richness of the natural resources in America was another pull. European farmers marveled when hearing that topsoil in the American Midwest was measured in feet, not millimeters. Mining abundant ores attracted thousands. The vast forests of Michigan, Minnesota, and Wisconsin drew thousands from northern Europe and from Canada. Whole new industries were being created, drawing those who had the necessary skills or the entrepreneurial spirit to carve out a niche in the new American economy. The culture of America, with its freedom of religion, speech, and political assembly, as well as the openness of a political system with near universal suffrage, attracted those fleeing political, religious, or ethnic persecution. Tens of millions, often coming in groups, occasionally in large surges of refugees, came to the United States.

THE OLD IMMIGRANT WAVE, 1820–1880

The initial policy of the United States was to open its doors—to actively seek immigrants for permanent resettlement. Both government and private enterprises reached out to attract northwestern European immigrants in a policy period characterized as the Open Door Era (LeMay, 1987: 20–37). The national interest, its very security, was viewed as needing population to fill the frontiers, to guard against invasion from colonial Europe, and to push back the American Indians to enable Euro-American settlement of frontier lands (LeMay, 2006: 16).

The U.S. Constitution was silent on the issue of immigration, but the necessary and proper clause was interpreted expansively by the U.S. Supreme Court as granting Congress wide latitude in regulating immigration. The court was restrictive with regard to state governments' enacting laws to limit immigration or the rights of permanent resident aliens. Among the first acts of the new Congress in 1790 was to pass law regulating the naturalization of citizens by requiring merely a two-year period of residency and a renunciation of former allegiances. In 1795, Congress amended that law by increasing the period of residency to five years but retained a very liberal approach to immigration and naturalization. In 1798, fear aroused by the French Revolution led Congress to pass the Alien and Sedition Acts. These acts gave the president sweeping powers to deport aliens found guilty of seditious acts. The law, permitted to expire in 1800, had little effect on actual immigration during the early years of the open-door era (LeMay and Barkan, 1999: 13–16).

The old immigrants came overwhelmingly from northern and western Europe, mostly from Germany, Ireland, and Scandinavia. The old immigrants arrived in two great surges: from 1845 to 1854, dominated by the Irish and the Germans; and from 1865 to 1875, when the British and Scandinavians figured in heavily, along with continued, though lessened, flows from Germany and Ireland.

Germans

German immigration tops the list of those settling in the United States. In the 2000 U.S. census, about 46.5 million persons reported German ancestry (in the 2010 census, the bureau no longer asked about claimed ancestry). Germans rank first among all Euro-American ancestry groups, comprising about 2 percent of the foreign-born persons reporting in the 2000 census. More than 10 percent of all persons legally entering the United States from 1990 to 2000 came from Germany. Total legal immigration from Germany exceeds 7 million. Germans came in heavy, steady numbers throughout the period, but three major currents can be distinguished: (1) the colonial era, when they came mostly for religious freedom or for economic opportunity; (2) from 1848 to the Civil War, when they came for political freedom as well as economic opportunity; and (3) the post–Civil War period, when they came mostly for greater economic opportunity, often having been actively recruited by various frontier-area state governments, several major industries, the railroads, and steamship lines or by friends and relatives already living here (i.e., chain migration).

German immigrants were never one nationality. Their distinctive German identity developed in the United States based on their common treatment. Until 1870, Germany was but a loose federation of many German states. They came from German-speaking states in central Europe and Austria, Hungary, Luxembourg, Switzerland, Poland, Czechoslovakia, and Russia. In North America, they were categorized for immigration purposes based on their common language. Although viewed as a single people, they were diverse, splintered by regional strife and religious lines.

Colonial-era German immigration saw movements of entire communities bound by religious creeds, often persecuted in their homeland: Mennonites, Dunkers, Lutherans (from Catholic-dominated states in what became modern southern Germany), Catholics (from Lutheran-dominated states in what became modern northern Germany, for example, from Prussia), Calvinites, and Jews. They came from Palatine, Salzburg, Wurttenburg, and Hanover. They settled on farmlands in colonial America that served as the breadbasket of the American Revolution. United by language and culture, they were politically inactive until the Revolutionary War, being more interested in local and private affairs (LeMay, 2006: 42).

Widely scattered, they were the largest single nationality group after the British. They felt no loyalty to the crown and were often unfriendly toward Tories, who advocated continued union with England. German immigrants became easy converts to the cause of independence. Several German regiments fought prominently and well in the Revolutionary War, gaining wide recognition that aided their assimilation. As their social and economic conditions improved, they increased their political activity. Reflecting their small-farmer backgrounds, they mostly affiliated with Jeffersonian-Democrats.

In the 1830s and 1840s, Germans began coming for different reasons. The agricultural revolution reached central Europe, especially the southeastern area of Germany, and changes in inheritance law forced the division of agricultural lands. A population explosion and economic change led many to leave when their plots became too small for even subsistence farming. Some turned to manufacturing work—of clocks, tools, and so on. But even these occupations left many vulnerable to economic shifts. When the potato famine hit Germany in the late 1840s, the choice for many Germans— like the Irish—was emigration or starvation.

These events coincided with the opening of the American Midwest. New state governments, along with railroads, shipping lines, and manufacturers, enticed immigrants. Texas, the Great Lakes, and the Ohio River Valley became home to new German-immigrant settlements. Canada, too, sent agents trying to attract German settlers to western Canada. Many settled for but a few years in Canada before migrating to the United States. In the United States, Midwestern cities exploded with the new settlers as cities such as Chicago, Detroit, Milwaukee, Cincinnati, and St. Louis developed in a region stretching from New York to Maryland to the Mississippi River that came to be called "the German belt" (LeMay, 1987: 24).

In Germany, political turmoil resulted in an attempted revolution in 1848, and pushed by that event, thousands of German immigrants, known as the Forty-Eighters, came to the United States and soon dominated German American communities. They began German-language newspapers, reading societies, theatres and other cultural activities. The full extent of their political influence is debated, but they undoubtedly played important leadership roles in the labor movement and the nation's conservation movement, exemplified by Carl Schurz, who became the first secretary of the interior, in 1877. The Forty-Eighters were active in the anti-slavery movement and prominent in the founding of the Republican Party—even taking credit for the election of Abraham Lincoln, who had invested in a German American newspaper.[1]

During and after the Civil War, German immigrants occupied industrial labor positions in the north opened up by war. A booming postwar economy drew labor to high-demand areas, and a large influx of German immigrants came after the war, drawn by the Homestead Act of 1862, which offered free or cheap land. Western states advertised for German farmers. State governments and the railroads sent agents to Germany to entice immigrants to settle and develop the abundant railroad lands. The U.S. became a haven from military conscription during the years of the German wars of unification (1848–1870). Bremen and Hamburg became major ports of embarkation and New York, Philadelphia, and Baltimore major ports of debarkation (LeMay, ed., 2013, vol. 1: 14).

The most notable opposition to German immigration came from the Know-Nothing Party of the 1850s (see Beals, 1960; Billington, 1974; Higham, 1955; Michael Holt, 1973). German immigrants clashed with the Irish for influence in the Catholic Church. Irish immigrants largely dominated the church hierarchy until the early 1900s, when clergy of German American heritage finally filled some leadership roles. World War I resulted in a temporary setback in their assimilation. They initially opposed the war. After the United States entered, however, opposition among German Americans ceased, and the German American community gave its support to the war effort. In 1916, Congress established the Council of National Defense to speed up assimilation of German and other non–English-speaking nationality groups. Midwestern state legislatures passed laws granting state and local governments sweeping powers to investigate and punish for contempt. These councils forbade the use of the German language in schools, churches, over the telephone, and in semi-public places. Xenophobic postwar isolationism was strongest in those states having heavy German American populations.

Irish

More than 33 million residents claimed Irish American heritage in the 2000 U.S. census, second only to German Americans in number and percentage of the total population. Today, they are somewhat evenly balanced in regional distribution: 24 percent in the Northeast, 25 percent in the Midwest, 33 percent in the South, and 17 percent in the West. Among them, less than 200,000 are foreign-born, comprising less than 1.2 percent of the foreign-born population, with only 18 percent coming to the United States since 1980. Since 2000, conditions in Ireland have no longer propelled large-scale emigration (U.S. Bureau of the Census, 2001).

Their 1847–1852 "flood" of immigration has been described as follows:

> Yet despite all these dangers and difficulties, the annual totals of Irish emigration to the United States kept rising: 68,000 in 1846, then 118,000 and 151,000 and 180,000, and over 184,000 by 1850. From America, newly prospering recent Irish arrivals—who had made the ocean trip and so well knew its hardships—still sent home to relatives in Ireland more than a million pounds a year, "passage money," to bring them over as well. This swelling traffic, against the many known perils and burdens of crossing the North Atlantic, by itself suggests just how truly desperate these emigrants were to escape the famine, and to try out what they had heard about the distant dream and reality of America. (Fox: 171)

Irish immigrants trickled in during the colonial and early years of the United States, settling mostly in Pennsylvania and Maryland. By 1790 they made up roughly 2 percent of the country's population of just more than 3 million. After 1830, they began arriving in larger numbers, fleeing political and religious persecution under British rule, the ravages of a potato blight, and smallpox and cholera outbreaks. The trickle became a flood by in the 1840s. Between 1842 and 1854 an estimated 1.2 million Irish immigrants came, peaking in 1851, when nearly a quarter-million arrived (LeMay, 1987: 25). At first, they settled in such northeastern cities as New York and Boston, moving to the Midwest only as they worked on railroad construction during the Civil War. A second Great Irish Potato Famine–induced emigration emptied the island of half its population, with large numbers going to Australia and Canada as well as to the United States. As one scholar notes:

> The line of demarcation between philanthropy and self-interest is sometimes hardly distinguishable, and never was it less so than in assisted emigration from the United Kingdom. In several instances the state aided the migration of those who were not entirely destitute, but others were transported overseas as the easiest means to be rid of them. Emigration arranged by parish or landlord were even more objectionable, and in Ireland particularly, every imaginable fraud was perpetrated upon the defenseless tenantry whose eviction and enforced emigration it was the landlord's interest to effect. (Guillet: 20)

In the United States, their arrival in deluge numbers and their Catholicism activated existing prejudice. Their sheer numbers, dire poverty, and openly anti-British feelings fueled antagonism. Their poverty trapped them in the nation's major eastern seaboard cities. High rates of illiteracy and few marketable job skills forced them into unskilled labor—they took on lower-class status just when class-consciousness was developing. By 1860, some two-thirds of domestics working in Boston were Irish.

They became the first immigrant group to face overt job discrimination. Advertisements in Boston, New York, and other eastern cities included for some time the line "No Irish Need Apply" (LeMay, 1987: 25). Irish took what work was open to them—unskilled jobs as ditch diggers, dock workers, stevedores, and teamsters. They filled construction gangs that razed or erected buildings in the explosively expanding cities. They built the roads, dug the canals, and laid the railroads from the east westward to the Midwest and beyond. Much to their dismay, not only were the streets of America not paved with gold, as they had heard, but they discovered that the streets were unpaved—and they would be doing the paving! Such work was seasonal, low-paying, back-breaking, and subject to the constant threat of job-competition. Labor competition led to problematic race relations among Irish, blacks, and Chinese.

The Irish used politics and the labor movement to climb the socioeconomic ladder. Their unstable working conditions attracted them to the labor movement, where they became early leaders in unions from New York to San Francisco, encompassing the gamut of skilled craftsmen from tailors to bricklayers, shoemakers to carpenters, teamsters to longshoremen. By the 1860s they began showing up in leadership roles at the national level: In 1861, Martin Burke helped form the American Miners Association; by the 1870s, Terrance Powderly gained control of the Knights of Labor, and

Peter McGuire, the "Father of Labor Day," led the formation of the American Federation of Labor in 1886 (O'Grady: 163).

The massive flood of Irish immigrants helped fill burgeoning cities, as rapid urbanization required an ever-expansive local government workforce. The Irish were quick to join, soon dominating bureaucracies such as local police departments. By 1863, a John Kennedy led New York City's police force. In the 1870s, a New York City police detective of Irish descent, Michael Kerwin, became police commissioner. By 1900, Irish Americans dominated big-city politics from Boston and New York to Chicago. The steady employment and the status of city politics and city bureaucracies attracted the Irish immigrant, as did the potential power of the police position. In Ireland they had been oppressed by the police—evicted, taxed, seized for questioning, imprisoned, and even killed. In America, they exercised such power.

Irish politics became a model for later immigrant groups. In vast numbers, the Irish settled within ethnic enclaves, where ethnic voting blocs formed. These provided the margin of victory in city elections. Ward leaders and precinct captains in a growing number of urban machines were Irish immigrants or their children. They used church and related ethnic organizations, such as the Knights of Columbus, the Sons of Ireland, and the Irish Catholic Benevolent Union (ICBU), to help establish the machine-like apparatus that gradually controlled the electoral process. By the 1870s, they gained control of the Democratic machine in Brooklyn. Irish Americans served as mayors in Richmond, Memphis, Baltimore, Wilmington, and Scranton. In 1871, an Irishman entered Congress as a representative from New York City; in 1876, another won a seat from Pennsylvania.

The highly influential ICBU sent several of its members to seats on the Philadelphia city council. William Harrity served as chairman of the Philadelphia Democratic City Committee and later served as chairman of the Democratic National Committee during President Cleveland's 1892 campaign. This set the precedent for a string of Irish American chairmen of the Democratic National Committee. Other ICBU members served as local judges, beginning in the 1870s, and by 1880, its founder, Dennis Dwyer, won a seat on New York State's Supreme Court. The zenith of Irish machine political power was their domination of Tammany Hall in New York City, the prototypical classic urban political machine. As the late Senator Daniel Patrick Moynihan so aptly put it:

"Dick" Connolly and "Brains" Sweeny had shared power and office with Tweed, as had any number of their followers, but with few exceptions the pre-1870s Irish had represented the canaille. With the dawning of the Gilded Age, however, middle-class and upper-class Irish began to appear; thus ranging across the spectrum, the Irish appeared to dominate a good part of the city's life for half a century. They came to run the police force and the underworld; they were as evident on Wall Street as on the Bowery; Irish contractors laid out the subways and Irish laborers dug them. The city entered the era of Boss Croker of Tammany Hall and Judge Goff of the Lexow Committee, which investigated him; of business leader Thomas Fortune and labor leader Peter J. McQuire; of reform mayor John Purroy Mitchel and Tammany Mayor "Red Mike" Hylan. It was a stimulating miscellany, reaching its height in the Roaring Twenties with Al Smith and Jimmy Walker. (cited in Fuchs, 1968: 79–80)

Successive waves filled cities that exploded upward and outward. By 1920, immigrants comprised 44 percent of New York, 41 percent of Cleveland, 39 percent of Newark, and 24 percent of Pittsburgh, Detroit, Boston, Buffalo, and Philadelphia (LeMay, ed., 2013, vol. 2: 125–141). The waves coming after 1880—the "new" immigrants—had low job skills and resources similar to those that characterized the Irish peasants. Like them, the newcomers tried to employ politics to cope with their minority status, but they never used it as well as did the Irish who had arrived before them, and they were more reluctant to budge from their newly acquired middle-class status than were the Yankees who were replaced by the Irish.

Irish immigrants continued to dominate those arriving into Canada through Quebec during the years 1852 to 1867, when they comprised over 28 percent of all arriving immigrants there. At more than 112,000, they exceeded those from Scandinavian countries (at just over 84,000 and 21 percent), the English (just over 76,000 and 19 percent), the Germans (just under 57,000 and 14 percent), and the Welch (just under 55,000 and 14 percent) (Sevigny, 1995a).

Scandinavians

Another old immigrant group, the Scandinavians, came from Denmark, Norway, and Sweden. According to the 2000 U.S. census, 1,505,450 identify themselves as Danish, 4,524,953 as Norwegians, and 4,342,150 as Swedish. Nearly 10.5 million Americans claim Scandinavian background.

Among the first European peoples to explore the New World, Viking explorations and tiny settlements have been traced to about 1050. In the mid-1600s, several settlements from the region were established in what is now the state of Delaware. They were few in numbers prior to the Civil War. After the 1870s, they began arriving in significant numbers, driven by push factors such as religious dissension, voting disenfranchisement, crop failures, and related economic dislocations. Scandinavians came in large numbers given the populations of their sending countries. Total Scandinavian immigration to the United States exceeds 2.5 million. The Swedes hit their peak in 1910 and the Norwegians in the 1920s (LeMay, 1987: 26). Although Danes, Norwegians, and Swedes came from countries having diverse governments, traditions, and languages, their physical characteristics and tendency to settle together in the United States led to the use of the term "Scandinavian" to refer to people of all three groups (as well as the much smaller group from Finland).

Remarkably successful, they came willing to work hard and arrived in better financial shape than did most other immigrant groups. They escaped the poverty, slums, and resulting stereotyping and social stigma of the eastern seaboard cities teeming with immigrants. By 1880, the average Swedish immigrant arrived with $60 to $70, sums allowing them to reach the Midwest and its abundant and cheap land, on which their farming skills were put to good use (LeMay, 1987: 26–27). In the then frontier settlements, they went into business, commerce, manufacturing, finance, and the professions. They set up their own shops, stores, factories, and banks. By 1890 they were concentrated in the Midwest, whose soil and climate reminded them of their homelands, and where their successful settlements attracted others. Minnesota, Wisconsin, Iowa, Illinois, and the Dakotas all saw dramatic increases in population resulting from their influx. By the 1890s, they were attracted to the Northwest. By 1920, Chicago had the largest number of Swedes of any city but Stockholm (Sweden's capital city), and more Norwegians resided in Chicago than any city but Oslo (Norway's capital).

Scandinavians assimilated quickly. They incorporated into majority society mostly through an economic path. Their political involvement followed economic and social success. Several factors account for their ease of incorporation. They did not have to overcome the stigma of some undesirable trait. They were Caucasian and escaped racial prejudice. They were ardent Protestants, avoiding the strong anti-Catholic sentiment. They came in smaller but steady numbers over a longer period than the huge waves of Irish and Italians, who were feared as job competitors driving down wages and working conditions and who were disliked as "papists." Arriving with desired skills and sufficient money to reach the Midwest, they bolstered the labor force in a nonthreatening way. They sought to assimilate and mastered English quickly. Schools were important in their settlements. They insisted on schools that taught English.

Overwhelmingly Protestant, religion gave them a common bond with majority society. They were predominantly Lutherans and were considered devout and strait-laced. Their stern religion and culture frowned on drinking, dancing, and levity and stressed piety and the work ethic. Many were avid anti-Catholics, accepted readily by the native stock, with whom they shared a common enemy. Unlike the Irish and Italian groups, whose loyalty to a unified Catholic Church retained ties to the old country and its customs, earning them the suspicion and enmity of Protestants, Scandinavians formed numerous new churches based on American ideas and customs, easing incorporation.

Financial success eased social acceptance. The Homestead Act provided cheap land, and they became established without incurring heavy debt. Their standard of living was soon comparable to that of the dominant society located in frontier settlements. "Most of them came with just enough money to buy government land and build a shack. Now they loan money to their neighbors . . . every county has Norwegians worth $25,000 to $50,000, all made since settling in Dakota" (Dinnerstein and Reimers, 1975: 87–98; see also 37–44, 172–174).

By the turn of the century, they had a solid understanding of American-style politics that afforded points of access: elections, representation, constitutions (city charters), and fragmented political power distributed among many local governments. They were patriotic. They organized political groups to get information on laws and elections and learned American-style politics by organizing new townships, working on town government, levying and collecting taxes, and laying new roads. In the early stages of their political development, often more than a fifth of the men participated in town affairs. In many locations in the Midwest, they voted in local affairs even before they were naturalized.

The first Scandinavian-born politician to enter statewide politics was a Norwegian, James Reymert, who in 1847 represented Racine County in the second constitutional convention of Wisconsin. After the Civil War, they became more visible. Norwegian-born Knute Nelson was the first Scandinavian to become a state governor. He was elected in succession to the legislatures of Wisconsin and then of Minnesota, to the U.S. Congress, and as governor of Minnesota on the Republican ticket in 1892. By the turn of the century, many served in the state legislatures of Wisconsin, Minnesota, and the Dakotas. They tended to be Republicans, attracted by the party's stand against slavery and the "moral ideas" espoused by the party (LeMay, 2006: 49–51).

THE NEW IMMIGRANT WAVE, 1880–1920

Nearly 25 million immigrants arrived in the United States during the four decades of the era of new immigrants (Department of Justice, 2001). Immigrants from southern/central/eastern Europe dominated the new immigrant wave. Immigrants from the region had entered during colonial times and during the 1820 to 1880 era, but their numbers and influence were small until after 1880. The turning point between northwestern and southern/central/eastern Europe was 1896, the year in which the numbers from southern/central/eastern Europe exceeded those from northwestern Europe for the first time. They were noticeably different physically and culturally from both the old immigrants and the original Euro-American settlers, the British Isle–dominated native stock. Southern/central/eastern European immigrants arrived in great surges and settled in ethnic enclaves in burgeoning cities. They retained their customs and languages longer than did the old immigrants. These factors contributed to increased prejudice and discrimination. As Lieberson puts it:

> What accounted for the exceptionally unfavorable response to the newcomers from these more distant parts of Europe? Several new forces were operating: religious issues; concentration in urban centers; implicit and often explicit racial notions; anxiety about assimilation; and the threats to existing institutions posed by the enormous numbers arriving. These concerns, later aggravated by domestic issues during World War I as well as the social and political tumult that followed, eventually led to the end of an unrestricted migration policy in the 1920s. (21)

New immigrants included millions of Catholics, Greek and Russian Orthodox, and Jewish adherents. More than 2 million Eastern European Jews fled the pogroms and related persecution of Europe during this era, about 90 percent of whom came to the United States. Jewish population in the United States rose from about 250,000 in 1877 to over four million in 1927 (Dinnestein and Reimers: 37–38).

Several push and pull factors were at work in the vast migration of 1880–1920. The urbanization and industrialization revolutions spreading across Europe reached southern/central/eastern European nations, bringing severe cultural, economic, political, and social disruptions. Several great epidemics broke out, from which millions fled. Overpopulation and chronic poverty fed unsuccessful attempts at revolution, and eventually the successful Bolshevik Revolution in Russia in 1917. The decline in feudalism and its resulting social and economic dislocations and the shift from agrarian to industrial concerns all contributed to the governments of southern/central/eastern Europe viewing emigration as expedient. They encouraged waves of emigrants bound for North America. Czarist Russia exemplifies the governments of the region using minorities as scapegoats for the country's ills. Pogroms against Jews began in 1881 with the assassination of Czar Alexander II. For three decades thereafter, periodic outbreaks of violence against Jews forced millions to leave the region (Irving Howe, 1976; Samuel, 1969).

Pull factors were at work as well. Transatlantic travel by steamship lines replaced the slower and more dangerous sailing vessels. As Fox noted, steamships were able to transport vastly larger numbers of immigrants (Fox: 105).

Southern/central/eastern Europeans were pulled here by the promise of economic opportunity in the land "where the streets were paved with gold," by the freedom of religion, by democracy and a lack of ethnic strife, at least in comparison to that which they experienced at home.

On arrival, they found themselves trapped in teeming urban centers. Many were peasants from small villages, making more difficult the adjustment to urban tenement neighborhoods. Disproportionately, they faced outbreaks of epidemic diseases. A slum-bred cholera epidemic, for example, caused the general mortality rate of the city of New York to rise dramatically. The slums of New York's East Side then comprised the world's most densely populated district. At 290,000 persons per square mile, their density far exceeded the 175,000 persons per square mile of Old London. Cities in America virtually exploded in population. Chicago, for instance, grew from a population of about 5,000 in 1848 to 1,690,000 in 1900. Immigrants accounted for a significant portion of that explosive growth rate (LeMay, 2006: 71).

Italians

Italian immigration was a massive, mostly post-1870 phenomenon. More than 5 million Italians immigrated during the four-decade era. A few arrived during the colonial and Revolutionary War period. Italians were scattered lightly throughout Virginia, Georgia, the Carolinas, New York, and Florida. Political repressions in Italy during the 1780s induced some intellectuals and revolutionaries to immigrate. Pre-1880 immigrants were mostly from northern Italy and were not peasants in background. Many were successful and prominent in the areas in which they resettled. Two Italian immigrants were elected to the Texas state legislature in 1848. In 1849, Secchi de Casali began a prominent Italian-language newspaper in New York City (*L' Eco d' Italia*). It supported the Whig Party and, later, the Republican Party. There was a significant pre–Civil War Italian settle-ment in Chicago, where Italians were saloonkeepers, restaurateurs, fruit venders, and confectioners, commissioned artists, and unskilled ditchdig-gers. The California gold rush drew many to the west coast. Often, how-ever, instead of mining, they grew grapes and began the wine industry there, grew vegetables, and became merchants. This gave rise to the Italian American folk saying that "the miners mined the mines, and the Italians mined the miners" (LeMay, 1987: 41). Many northern Italian immigrants were skilled craftsmen seeking better economic opportunity. That pattern changed dramatically after 1870.

The turmoil associated with the unification of Italy in the 1870s induced a mass exodus. Nearly 9 million Italians crossed the Atlantic to both North and South America seeking opportunity denied them by the very move-ment they had supported at home. From 1880 to 1910, more than 3 million came to the United States, most from southern Italy. They settled in the cit-ies of the industrial northeast. By 1930, Italian residents in New York City exceeded 1 million and made up 15.5 percent of the city's total population (Federal Writers Program, 1969: viii).

In the 2000 census, nearly 16 million persons claim Italian ancestry. Today they are concentrated in the east, where over half reside. About 17 percent reside in both the Midwest and the south, and about 15 percent live in the west.

Italians arriving in the 1880s and 1890s were hardly a static bloc. They moved back and forth between Italy and the United States and among ethnic enclaves, "Little Italy" settlements. Many who arrived returned to Italy in the winter, working the remainder of the year in the United States. Several push factors influenced their migration. Southern Italy was impoverished. During the 1890s, agricultural workers in Italy earned only 10–20 cents a day, and miners only 30–56 cents per day. General laborers earned only $3.50 for a six-day, 60 hour workweek, compared to $9.50 for a 56-hour workweek in the United States. Skilled carpenters earned 30 cents to $1.40 a day, or $1.80–$8.40 for a six-day workweek. That same worker in the states earned an average $18 for a 50-hour work-week (Ibid.: 36–49). Floods, volcanic eruptions, and earthquakes plagued Italy and contributed to its bleak agricultural outlook. The region was also hit by phylloxera, which struck on a scale akin to the potato blight of the 1840s. Southern Italy also suffered frequent and severe epidemics of malaria. Others fled compulsory military service required during the unification effort. In the 1890s Italian immigrants were especially feared as a threat for bringing along smallpox, cholera, plague, typhus, or yellow fever (Willrich: 223).

Pull factors drawing them were the development of the steamship lines which made the journey cheaper, faster, and easier. Chain migration drew others. Returning "Americani," who made the trip back and forth seeking brides or wintering at home in Italy, attracted others to emulate their success. State governments, such as Illinois, New York, Pennsylvania, California, and Louisiana, sent agents to contract for laborers. And come they did. From 1890 to 1914, they arrived in excess of 100,000 per year. Between 1900 and 1914, nearly 3 million came. Immigrants from Italy exceeded those of all other nations of origin entering through Ellis Island (LeMay, 2006: 74).

The southern Italian peasants were oppressed and exploited at home, despised as *cafoni* (boors). Typically illiterate, unschooled, and preindustrial in custom and mentality, they were hardly suitable to occupy the teeming neighborhoods of crowded Boston, Chicago, or New York City. They exhibited a sojourner attitude, motivated to escape the grinding poverty by coming to North America to work a few years, save enough money to return for their brides, and ultimately to be able to buy land at home. Of the millions who came, about half returned to their villages having accomplished their mission or having met with defeat. Those who remained often harbored a desire to return, and that persistent mentality influenced their slower rate of incorporation. Why learn English, why become a citizen, if one were going back to the old country—if not this year, then next?

They filled cities, finding jobs as common laborers, digging canals, waterways, and laying pipes for the sewer systems and water supply. Many took up vending and vegetable farming. Match and shoe factories recruited them and soon found that chain migration worked so well that employers no longer needed agents to recruit laborers. In San Francisco, they dominated the fruit and vegetable truck farming business. In California, "Del Monte" became a household word. By 1881, the Italian colony at Asti in Sonoma County began the valley's wine industry. They played a similar role in upstate New York, in New Jersey, and in Geneva, Wisconsin. In 1850, Louisiana had Italians working the cotton fields and New Orleans had a larger population of Italians than any other city in the states. By 1920, however, New York City led the nation with more than a half-million Italian-born residents (LeMay, 2006: 76).

The fact that Italians arrived in large numbers during an economic upheaval, such as the Depression of 1873, spurred animosity, led by the Ku Klux Klan. Italians were seen as radicals and criminals who filled the ever-growing slums, fueled class conflict, and supported the blatantly corrupt big-city urban political machines. The 1910 census found that Italian immigrants accounted for 77 percent of Chicago's foreign-born population,

78 percent of New York's, and 74 percent of Boston's, Cleveland's and Detroit's. They lived in Little Italys, neighborhoods, where conditions were grim. Muck-raking journalist Jacob Riis described New York City's Little Italy as follows:

> Half a dozen blocks on Mulberry Street there is a rag-pickers settlement, a sort of overflow from "the Bend," that exists today in all its pristine nastiness. Something like forty families are packed into old two-story and attic houses that were built to hold five, and out in the yards additional crowds are, or were until very recently, accommodated in shacks built of all sorts of old boards and used as drying racks by the Italian stock (Riis: 49).

Such conditions were typical of Italian ethnic enclaves in other major cities, such as Boston, Chicago, and Philadelphia (LeMay, ed. 2013, vol. 2: 121–136).

Concentrated settlements afforded benefits in coping. A *padroni*, or "boss" system, exploited them economically but served as an important coping mechanism. The *padroni* had contacts with employers and helped their compatriots find and keep jobs. They spoke English and translated and provided intermediary services with the majority society, especially for political, police, and labor–management interactions. They organized labor gangs. They collected wages, wrote letters, acted as bankers, and supplied room and board to youth. The Foran Act of 1885 banned contract labor, but the golden era of the *padroni* system was from 1890 to 1900 (LeMay and Barkan, 1999: 56–60). In 1897 an estimated two-thirds of the Italian workers in New York City were controlled by *padroni*. This system declined rapidly after 1900.

Another coping mechanism was the labor movement. By the 1890s, Italian immigrants ranked second only to Poles in percentage of white ethnics belonging to blue-collar, working-class, organized labor unions. They used the church as an aid to assimilation. Churches were often the base for such "self-help" associations as the Italian Mutual Aid Society, the Italian Union and Fraternity, and the Sons of Italy. By 1912, New York City had 212 such societies, and Chicago had eighty. They started as burial societies but soon helped members find jobs, housing, insurance, and a host of social services and were the base of much of the social life of the immigrant community (LeMay, 2006: 77–79).

Mafia and crime-related organizations emerged in a similar fashion and served, in part, as self-protective associations. Careers in crime became "a curious ladder of social mobility" (Vecoli and Lintelman: 205) and, when linked with the urban political machine, led to political clubs and party activity. In politics, Italians followed the Irish American model, although less successfully. They supported machine politicians. The first state-level Italian American politician in Illinois was a Democrat, Charles Cois, elected to the state house in 1918. In New York City, Republican Fiorello LaGuardia emerged as a political leader. LaGuardia served as an interpreter at Ellis Island. He was admitted to the bar in New York in 1910 and was elected to the U.S. House of Representatives in 1916. After service in the war, he was again elected to Congress in 1918. In 1932, he cosponsored the Norris–LaGuardia Act, which restricted the court's power to ban strikes. In 1933, he was elected mayor of New York and during the next decade developed a reputation as an honest and efficient "reform" mayor (LeMay, 2006: 80).

Greeks

Some Greeks came to America during colonial times. An ill-fated settlement in Florida, the Smyrna colony, began in 1768. Greek explorers, sailors, cotton merchants, and even gold miners were scattered throughout the colonies. Greeks arrived in truly significant numbers between 1900 and 1920, when 350,000 arrived, from all parts of the homeland. Most were young, unskilled males from small villages in southern Greece. Americans claiming Greek ancestry numbered 1,175,591 in the 2000 census, nearly a quarter of them born in Greece (U.S. Bureau of the Census, 2001).

Their push factors are similar to those of other southern/central/eastern European groups: political persecution, overpopulation, a troubled economy, an ongoing war (with Turkey). Their peak year of immigration, 1912–1913, coincided with the Balkan war.

They were pulled here by economic opportunity. Many came intending to stay a short while and earn enough to provide a dowry for prospective brides in their families. About 95 percent of Greek immigrants were young males, so many returned home for brides (LeMay, 1987: 45).

They settled in the west, where they worked on railroad gangs; in New England, where they worked in shoe and textile factories; and in New York City and Chicago, as well as other large cities, where they worked in factories, as busboys, dishwashers, bootblacks, and peddlers. Greek immigrants used a *padrone system*, a modernized version of the late seventeenth-century indentured servant system. The *padrone* found jobs, settled disputes, assisted with language problems, and arranged for room and board. Clients were often young boys sent directly to him by their parents. The parents were usually unaware of the conditions under which their sons lived—squalid and crowded basement rooms in the heart of tenement slum neighborhoods. Greek young men worked twelve-hour days with no time set aside for lunch. The *padrone* received from $100 to $500 per year per boy. The boys themselves earned $100 to $180 annually in wages (Soloutos, 1964; LeMay, 2006: 81).

Greek professionals emigrated, although Greek lawyers and doctors could only practice after studying in American schools for at least a year and passing qualifying exams in English. Many tended to have practices serving their ethnic community. A sizable number of Greek immigrants began their own businesses, concentrating on confectionaries, candy stores, and restaurants. By World War I, there were more than 500 Greek restaurants in San Francisco and more than 450 Greek American confectionary shops in Chicago, which also had ten candy manufacturing concerns (LeMay, 2006: 82).

Greek immigrants were used as strikebreakers. This aroused severe anti-Greek sentiment in the union movement, occasionally leading to riots. There was also an active campaign against them led by the Ku Klux Klan.

The Greek Orthodox Church played a prominent role, as did notable Greek societies, such as the American Hellenic Educational Progressive Association (AHEPA), founded in 1922 to preserve Greek heritage and help immigrants adjust to life in America. Greek churches taught the Greek language to the children of immigrants, preserving their culture and relations to the church, ensuring the church's lifelong influence on the new generation. Their political involvement parallels that of other southern/central/eastern European groups, especially Italians. Most Greek Americans supported the Democratic Party. By the 1970s, AHEPA emerged as a strong lobbying organization, influencing Congress on foreign policy matters (Dinnerstein and Reimers: 54).

Russians/Slavs

The Slavic peoples are grouped into three regional groups: the eastern, western, and southern Slavs. Eastern Slavs include Russians, White Ruthenians, and Ukrainians. Western Slavs include Poles, Czechs, Slovaks, and Lusatin Serbs. Southern Slavs, primarily in the Balkans, include Slovenians, Croatians, Montenegrins, Serbs, Macedonians, and Bulgarians (LeMay, 2006: 84). They are exemplified in the United States by the Russians and Poles, and their migration has been mostly post-1870s. During colonial times there were a few Slavic settlers in the New Amsterdam and New Sweden colonies, as well as some Moravians in the Quaker colony in Pennsylvania. The earliest Russian colonists date back to 1747, in Alaska's Kodiak Island. Some colonial-period Ukrainians settled in California, and

Polish Americans proudly emphasize the role of Generals Pulaski and Kosciusko as heroes of the American Revolutionary War. Those arriving after 1880 settled in the industrial centers of the northeast, with sizable numbers in Illinois and Ohio. Major cities in which they settled in large numbers include New York, Chicago, Detroit, Cleveland, Boston, Philadelphia, Milwaukee, Buffalo, Baltimore, Pittsburgh, Providence, San Francisco, and Los Angeles. In the 2000 census, more than 9 million claimed Polish ancestry, and 3 million identified themselves as of Russian ancestry (LeMay, 2006: 84).

Slavs tended to replace German and Irish immigrants in the mines and factories of Pennsylvania and the Midwest and in the slaughterhouses of Chicago. They were sojourners. An estimated 2 million returned to Europe between 1908 and 1914. They faced severe segregation in ethnic ghettos, as well as extreme economic hardship. An estimated 2 million Hungarians came between 1871 and 1920, but half returned before World War I. New York City had some 76,000 Hungarians in 1920, and Cleveland had such a large Hungarian enclave that it was referred to as "an American Debucan," growing in twenty years from 8 percent to 18 percent of Cleveland's foreign-born population (Weinberg: 174–175).

In the early 1870s, Mennonites from Russia fled persecution to the Great Plains and numbered over 40,000. Hundreds of thousands of Russian Jews fled pogroms in 1880s and 1890s. From 1900 to 1913, more than 51,000 Russians arrived, peaking between 1880 and 1914. Although many fled political and religious oppression, most were simply peasants seeking economic opportunity. The Russian Revolution in 1917 largely much stopped emigration until about 1970. Their official count puts them at just over 3.33 million (Dinnerstein and Reimers, 1975: 172–174).

Russian immigrants worked in coal and other mines, the iron and steel mills of Pennsylvania, and the slaughterhouses of Chicago. In New York City, they were heavily involved in the clothing industry and in cigar and tobacco manufacturing. They held unskilled jobs in construction and with the railroads and were mostly nonunionized, except for the United Mine Workers and the Industrial Workers of the World. Their pay was low. In 1909, they averaged just over $2 for a twelve-hour day. Coal mine workers earned $15 for a sixty-hour work week. As late as 1919, Russian immigrants in Chicago earned only $12–$30 per week (Dinnerstein and Reimers, 1975: 177). In tenement slums of big cities, they lived in ethnic enclaves of substandard housing. Conditions for construction crews typically had thirty-six men sharing three-tiered bunkhouses.

They sought refuge in church and ethnic mutual-aid societies. By 1916 the Russian Orthodox Church in the United States numbered some

100,000, with nearly 7,000 students in church schools. The Russian Orthodox Society of Mutual Aid, founded in 1895, grew to more than 7,000
members. The Russian Brotherhood Society, begun in 1900, had 3,000
members by 1917 (Dinnerstein and Reimers, 1975: 44; Leventman: 40).
These mutual-aid societies provided health insurance, death benefits, and
helped members find jobs. After the 1917 Bolshevik revolution, they took
on avowedly political aims and formed the anti-Bolshevik Society to Help
Free Russia.

Russian workers joined several unions, notably the clockworkers and
the men and women's garmentworkers unions. There was also a Society of
Russian Bookmakers and the Society of Russian Mechanics. At the other
end of the political spectrum, some 200 Russian socialistic, anarchistic,
and radical clubs were started as of 1917, the largest of which was the
Union of Russian Workers. These groups inflamed anti-Russian and anti-
Bolshevik attitudes and contributed to a wave of prejudice, discrimination
and anti-Russian violence. The 1919 formation of the American Communist Party and the American Communist Labor Party set off a hysterical
reaction that culminated in the infamous Palmer Raids and the Red Scare
of 1919, which saw the arrest of thousands and the deportations of some
500, as well as the suppression of the Russian-language press. From 1900
to 1920, a total of fifty-two Russian-language papers were published. By
1921 there were only five, and the fifth daily, the radical *Novi Mir* (The
New World), was suppressed by the U.S. government in 1921 (LeMay,
2006: 88).

Poles

Because official numbers did not enumerate them directly during all the
years of 1820–1920, estimates of the number of Polish immigrants vary
widely, from about 875,000 to more than 1.5 million. At various times,
they were counted among the Germans, the Austro-Hungarians, and the
Russians (Iorrizo and Mondello: 13–26; see also LeMay, 1987: 41). The
official number of Polish immigrants is just more than 500,000.[2]

Polish immigrants came as farm laborers, unskilled workers, and
domestic servants. Less than 12 percent were skilled workers, and about
25 percent were illiterate. They tended to be young male sojourners. Their
strong attachment to the homeland reflected that the ills of life in Poland
were blamed on foreign occupations. Resentment of the Polish upper class
seemed less pronounced than was typical among other Slavic groups. Polish immigrants worked on farms in the northeast and Midwest, concentrating on truck farming in Long Island and the Connecticut Valley and on

corn and wheat farming in the north-central Midwest. The Panna Maria settlement in Texas, founded in 1854, was entirely of Polish immigrant families. Poles concentrated in Buffalo, Chicago, Milwaukee, Pittsburgh, Detroit, and New York City. Chicago ranks as the third largest Polish city in the world, after Warsaw and Lodz (LeMay, 2006: 86).

Young Poles shared common labor jobs in the coal mines, earning less than $15 per week for six ten-hour days. Poles were slower in upward mobility than many other immigrant groups—even today about 40 percent are blue-collar workers.

The most influential institution in the Polish American community is the church, unrivaled for unification of the Polish American community (called Polonia) (Ibid.: 87). Tension with a hierarchy dominated by Irish Americans manifested itself in parish mutual-aid societies joining the Polish Roman Catholic Union (PRCU), organized in 1873; the Polish National Alliance, begun in 1880; and the Polish National Catholic Church (PNCC), founded in 1897 and re-formed in 1904.[3] A number of isolated parishes have split from Rome but are not yet in the PNCC. Most Polish Americans, however, remain loyally Roman Catholic, and today there are many Polish American bishops in the hierarchy—and, of course, the late Roman Pontiff John Paul was a Pole. As with the Italians and Russians, Polish mutual-aid societies link Polonia to the homeland. Politically, they lobbied American immigration policy and tried to affect Poland's emigration laws and U.S. foreign policy related to Poland and eastern Europe. More than 10,000 such societies were organized. They were especially active in the American Liberty Loan fund drives before World War I, raising over $20 million for the Polish cause. They purchased $67 million in U.S. Liberty Bonds during World War I and sent 28,000 volunteers to fight in the war. Polish Americans invested more than $18 million in Polish government bonds between 1914 and 1918 (LeMay, 1987: 49).

Eastern European Jews

Data regarding eastern European Jews is even sketchier than for other southern/central/eastern European groups. Perhaps half of immigrants from southern/central/eastern Europe who came between 1870 and 1920 were Jewish, and Dinnerstein and Reimers estimates their immigration from 1899 to 1973 at nearly 2.5 million (172–174). They came for many of the same push and pull reasons as did other Slavic groups. By 1860, the serfs or peasant class in Russia were attaining a degree of freedom and slowly began to develop a middle class. At that time, about 5 percent of Russia's labor force was Jewish. About 11 percent were employed in industry, and 36 percent in commerce. By law, they were forbidden to own land, so they became merchants, tailors, administrators, and other commerce-oriented businessmen. European Jews were urbanites. Ultimately, the most compelling push factor for Jews was religious/political persecution. The czarist government used Jews as scapegoats for long-festering economic, political, and social grievances and openly encouraged ethnic minorities to emigrate. Jewish immigration to the United States can be directly correlated with historical events in Russia, particularly the pogroms that swept the nation during the 1880s up to World War I. In the Pale of Settlement area of Russia, the land between the Baltic and the Black seas, pogroms were especially violent, with looting, pillaging, riots, murders, and even total destruction of Jewish ghettos. Government troops sat idly by or even joined in these periodic venting of frustrations taken out upon hapless Jews. Jewish emigrants fleeing such persecution came in family groups intending to stay here. No sojourner attitude among them! To remain in Russia was to risk life and limb, to remain rigidly confined within legal limitations on education and occupational opportunities, and to suffer conscription to years of compulsory military service.

Eastern European Jews settled in ports of entry such as New York, Philadelphia, and Baltimore. They lived in low-rent sections near business districts, which quickly developed into ghetto-like areas. Jewish enclaves in the United States were neither as uniform nor oppressed as were the ghettos of Europe (LeMay, 2006: 91).

Jewish immigrants were better suited to the environment they found in the United States than were many of the southern/central/eastern European peasants among whom they arrived. They generally had more urban backgrounds and better job skills that fit the needs of the expanding American urban economy and that eased their incorporation into American life. Sixty-seven percent of Jewish male immigrants were classified as skilled workers, compared to an average 20 percent for all other immigrant groups (Dinnerstein and Reimers, 1975: 44).

They were active in the union movement, especially in the garment industry, where the Amalgamated Clothing Workers (ILGWU) was dominated by Italians and Jews. By World War II, 60 percent of ILGWU members were Jewish, and an estimated half of the city's Jewish labor force worked in the industry. They also worked prominently in cigar manufacturing, bookmaking, distilling, printing, and skilled carpentry. In the unskilled category, they tended toward peddling and sales. A 1900 census study found numbers of Jewish immigrants in the professions to be the highest of all non–English-speaking immigrant groups.[4]

Anti-Semitism was evident in the United States, although less pronounced than the pogroms from which they fled. Jewish immigrants were small in numbers and mostly from Germany prior to 1880. Anti-Semitism was generally mild. Most Jewish immigrants were middle-class and skilled or professionals. When large-scale immigration from eastern Europe reached vast proportions, and when more lower-class immigrants (peasants) were prominent among them, prejudice against them escalated. By the 1870s, latent anti-Semitism broke into the open in New York, where they were blackballed from the Bar Association and prestigious college fraternities and were barred from private clubs, resorts, and private schools. The Ku Klux Klan, revived during the early 1900s, became a leading anti-Semitic force.

Pogroms broke out in Russia in 1903 and 1906, inspiring the American Jewish community to organize to help their brethren. The American Jewish Committee was formed and raised millions for those suffering in Europe. In 1909, some 2,000 Jewish American charities raised and spent more than $10 million. They organized orphanages, educational institutions, homes for unwed mothers and delinquent children. They set up hospitals and recreational facilities, supported the Jewish Theological Seminary, and began a host of Yiddish language newspapers. Between 1885 and 1915, 150 such papers were begun, including the highly influential *Daily Forward*. In 1913, B'nai B'rith's Anti-Defamation League (ADL) was formed (LeMay, 2006: 91).

In religious and family life, Jews stressed formal education. Advanced learning was highly valued for males, and professional occupations were held as the ideal for their secure incomes and social prestige. Education became the tool to secure a future and a path to higher occupational and economic status and incorporation. According to Dinnerstein and Reimers, by 1915, Jews made up 85 percent of the student body of New York City's free but renowned City College, a fifth of those attending New York University, and a sixth of the students at Columbia (53).

Politics followed economic gains. They were slow to enter and use the classic urban machines, though a few played prominent roles in city politics. This slowness in political involvement reflected a lack of political experience in their homelands. The more prominent Jewish immigrants were uncomfortable with big-city machine politicians with their strange skills, codes, vulgarities, and often blatant corruption. But politics was key to power, and power was needed to protect their economic gains and to influence U.S. foreign policy, so in the post-1920s they became active in American politics, mostly affiliated with the Democratic Party.

REACTION TO CHANGE—THE NATIVIST MOVEMENT AND GROWING RESTRICTIONISM

The waves of old and new immigrants stirred reactions among white Anglo-Saxon Protestants (WASPs). Some WASPs accepted immigrants as necessary sources of population to fill the land, develop the railroads, and provide cheap labor for the budding manufacturing industry. The politically powerful steamship industry of transatlantic shipping lines actively recruited immigrants, as did the railroads and many manufacturing concerns. Others reacted far less favorably. The first wave precipitated the American Party, founded on July 4, 1845. It was a specifically anti-immigrant political party whose main platform was a total rejection of the foreigner.

The most prominent nativist movement that developed before the Civil War became known as the Know-Nothing Party. Originally called the Order of the Star Spangled Banner, it began as a secret patriotic society in New York in 1849, reacting to the sudden influx of Irish immigrants fleeing the Great Potato Famine. It quickly spread and achieved success in Rhode Island, New Hampshire, Connecticut, Delaware, Maryland, Kentucky, and Texas. It wielded strong influence in Virginia, Georgia, Alabama, Mississippi, and Louisiana as well (LeMay, 2006: 57–58).

An elder in the Order of the Star Spangled Banner vividly described the sentiments of the new political party in an article published in his *Tennessee Baptist*:

Nothing is more evident than that our political parties have become sadly, deplorably corrupt. . . . Congress has become a most shameful and disgraceful scene of drunkenness, riot, and caucusing for the Presidency, and the minor offices of government. The foreign element is increasing in fearful ratio. Nearly one million per annum of foreign Catholics and German infidels—who, though opposed in all else, are agreed in the subversion of our free institutions—are pouring in upon us, and the tide is increasing. These foreigners have already commenced their warfare upon the use of the Bible in our public schools—against our free school system—against our Sabbath—against our laws. They boldly threaten to overthrow our constitution, through profligacy of our politicians; and we see our candidates for political preferment pandering more and more to Catholics and foreign influence. We see from the last census that the majority of the civil and municipal offices of this government are today in the hands of Catholics and foreigners: an over-whelming majority of our army and navy are foreign Catholics. They hear the editors of Catholic papers, . . . endorsed by their Archbishops, threatening. . . . "If Catholics ever gain an immense numerical majority, religious freedom in this country is at end." So say our enemies. So we believe. (cited in Overdyke: 68)

The party ran a presidential candidate, former President Millard Fillmore, in 1856. Its anti-immigrant, anti-Catholic stance was too narrow a platform to succeed nationally. Silent on the prevailing issue of the day—slavery—it played a spoiler role in the election, carrying only the state of Maryland, where it was strongest in Baltimore. The slavery issue led to its demise, but in 1856 many voters loosened their ties with either the pro-slavery Democrats or the anti-slavery Republicans, finding a temporary home in the Know-Nothing Party (Higham, 1955: 4; LeMay, 2006: 58).

Only native-born and Protestant Americans were allowed to join, swearing an oath to vote for whomever the party endorsed. If asked their goals or stands on an issue, they were told to reply, "I know nothing," giving rise to its popular name. The movement attracted the working class, who feared their jobs would be taken and their society undermined. Movement adherents feared the increasing electoral clout of the immigrant voting bloc evident with the rise of urban political machines. Others attracted to the movement joined out of a deep-seated fear of Catholicism. As Beals showed, the movement "rose up to burn Catholic convents, churches, and homes, assault nuns, and murder Irishmen, Germans and Negroes" (9). It unleashed a hate campaign in cities where immigrants were concentrated. In New York, mobs of Irish and Know-Nothings clashed (as depicted in the movie *The Streets of New York)*, leaving two dead. In Newark, an estimated 2,000 Protestants and Catholics squared off, leaving one dead, many wounded, and a Catholic church burned down. In 1855, Know-Nothings and Germans clashed in Louisville in a riot that left twenty dead and hundreds wounded. In Baltimore, clashes and a riot in 1854 led to eight dead. A spinoff group, the "Plug Uglies," was responsible for much of the physical violence of the period (Hofstadter and Wallace: 93, 113).

Rapid in rise, the party experienced an equally fast demise when its convention in 1855 split over the slavery issue. Its northern members were largely anti-slavery, but its southern wing would not budge from its pro-slavery stand. After the 1856 election, the party disintegrated, its southern wing going Democratic and later secessionist and its northern members joining the Republican Party.

Nativism declined during the Civil War and the immediate postwar period. Economic troubles, such as the Panic of 1873, led to labor unrest and a resurgence of restrictionism. The immigrant flow from southern/central/eastern Europe rekindled anti-Catholicism and sparked nativist fear of "Rum, Romanism, and Rebellion." Catholics had only made up 7 percent of the population in 1850, but by 1900, the 12 million Catholics were 16 percent of the population (Department of Commerce, 2002). Nativists viewed them as growing at an alarming rate. The corruption of the urban machine, exemplified by Boss Tweed and Tammany Hall, which plundered the city of millions of dollars between 1865 and 1871, led anti-machine reformers to call for restrictions on immigration. During the mid-1880s, radical labor agitation by groups such as the Molly McGuires, who engaged in a violent campaign against the mine owners in Pennsylvania, and the Haymarket Riot in Chicago in 1886 sparked formation of a new nativist political party, the American Party, in California. On the west coast, a virulent anti-Chinese and then anti-Asian movement ensued. The Chinese Exclusion League soon expanded to a Japanese and then a Korean Exclusion League, then to the Asian Exclusion League. These groups reflected and promoted a developing racism that exhorted against the "Yellow Peril."

The movement was joined by the growing forces of organized labor. They blamed the Depression of 1893 on immigrants. Nationally, groups such as the Knights of Labor and, in the west, the Workingman's Party, agitated for a complete ban on immigration, or as a reluctant compromise, halving the flow.

The movement was aided in the 1890s by the development of "scholarly" studies supporting the need for restriction and developing and popularizing the concept of racism. Eastern intellectuals joined the movement. In 1890, for instance, General Francis A. Walker, president of MIT and incoming president of the American Economic Association, called for sharp reductions in immigration. John Fiske, Nathaniel Shaler, Prescott Hall, Robert DeCourcey Ward, and Senator Henry Cabot Lodge organized and led the Immigration Restriction League in 1894 (Divine: 3; LeMay, 1987: 59). The league spearheaded the restrictionist movement for the next twenty-five years, advocating a literacy test for immigrants and stressing the differences between the "old" and the "new" immigrants in their capacity to assimilate.

The mid-1890s saw a rapid growth in strength of the American Protective Association. It called for all manner of immigration reforms designed to restrict the flow and change the nature of its composition from the new back to the old immigrants. Violent outbreaks against Italians and eastern European immigrants became almost commonplace from the mid-1890s to the early 1900s and prepared the way for the National Origin laws passed in the 1920s. Bernard notes well that their virulent anti-immigration and racist rhetoric proved useful to the propaganda of the leaders of Nazi Germany in later years (16).

Opposing the league and the American Protective Association was a coalition of business groups that favored an open-door policy to ensure the continued supply of cheap labor. The National Union of Manufacturers and the National Association of Manufacturers helped defeat the literacy bills in 1898, 1902, and 1906, with the aid of a coalition of some southern senators wanting to continue the influx of cheap labor. Their work was aided by some pro-immigrant ethnic associations, such as the German–American Alliance, the Ancient Order of Hibernians, the B'nai B'rith, the Hebrew Immigrant Aid Society, and the Council of the Union of American Hebrew Congregations, all of whom opposed a literacy test.

From 1900 to 1910, the largest-ever surge of immigrants arrived. Nearly 9 million entered during those years, and that massive influx, coupled with the Panic of 1907, and an economic depression that followed in its wake, fed renewed restrictionism.

The Japanese and Korean Exclusion Leagues, formed in 1905, grew to the Asiatic Exclusion League, which by 1907 claimed over 100,000 members in 231 affiliated groups (Ringer: 688). By 1906, the American Federation of Labor (AFL) endorsed enactment of the literacy test at its Nashville Convention by a vote of 1,852–352.

The Immigration Restriction League, accepting social Darwinism theories from the writings of John Commons, and Edward Ross, and in such books as William Ripley's *The Races of Europe* (1899), influenced the Dillingham Commission (1907–1911). It favored the adoption of a literacy test. Racial overtones of the Dillingham Commission's Report were augmented by a popular and influential work, Madison Grant's *The Passing of the Great Race in America* (1916).

The commission's report and restrictionists' racist literature did not go unchallenged. Scholars and social workers disputed the findings of the Commission, particularly Jane Addams of the Hull House movement in Chicago and Grace Abbott of the Immigrants' Protective League and head of the Children's Bureau. Jacob Riis, a muckraking journalist, influenced President Theodore Roosevelt's administration. Other pro-immigration scholars and books were Mary Antin's *The Promised Land*, Carl Schurz's *Reminiscences*, Edward Steiner's *On the Trail of the Immigrant*, and Louis Adamic's *Two-Way Passages*.

The 1917 Russian Bolshevik Revolution aroused fear of radicalism and renewed restrictionists who proved more effective in influencing national immigration policy in the post–World War I years. The American Legion, the National Grange, and the American Federation of Labor supported the literacy bill, passed in 1917 despite President Woodrow Wilson's veto. The 1917 law enacted an Asiatic-Barred Zone that virtually excluded all Asian immigration. The Japanese Exclusion League succeeded in getting a series of alien land acts, first in 1913, then amended and spread beyond California in 1920 and 1923. In 1922, the 1913 and 1920 laws were upheld as constitutional by the Supreme Court in the *Ozawa* case. The Red Scare of 1919 attacked Wobblies, socialists, anarchists and anyone suspected of holding such views. Many were tarred and feathered, jailed—a few were even lynched. The Ku Klux Klan revived and grew, taking on an anti-Catholic, anti-Jew, and increasingly anti-foreign perspective. The Klan, the American Protective League, and the True Americans launched a "100 Percent Americanism" campaign that became the order of the day. Racist ideas provided a rationale for the restrictive immigration laws passed in the 1920s. "Eugenics," a pseudo-science that supposedly "proved" that certain races were endowed with a hereditary superiority or inferiority, provided the basis for the quota system. Campaigning on the theme "A Return to Normalcy," the Republicans elected President Warren Harding with the avowed purpose of returning to conservatism, traditionalism, and a closed society. That climate of opinion signaled the reversal of the open door policy on immigration.

PUBLIC POLICY REACTIONS TO MASS MIGRATION

Laws implementing immigration policy moved gradually from 1820 to 1920 from an Open Door Era, with essentially no restrictions, to a Pet Door Era ushered in by the quota acts of the 1920s that strictly limited total immigration to the United States and tilted the composition of the flow from southern/central/eastern Europe back to northwestern Europe.

When the new nation took its first census in 1790, it enumerated a population of 3,227,000. Most were descendants of seventeenth- and eighteenth-century arrivals or were recent immigrants themselves. More than 75 percent were of British origin, and about 8 percent of German. The rest were Dutch, French, or Spanish in origin. There were about a half-million black slaves and a comparable number of Native Americans (LeMay, ed., 2013, vol. 1: 27). As the flow of immigrants increased from a trickle to a flood, and as its source shifted increasingly from the British Isles and northwestern Europe to southern/central/eastern Europe, sentiment shifted regarding the openness of immigration law.

Immigration law was amended as nativist and restrictionist groups increasingly and with gradually greater effectiveness reacted to the changing scope and composition of the flood of immigration and demanded ever-more stringent restrictions. This section briefly highlights the major laws passed during the century of mass migration that determined the immigration policy of the United States.[5]

The first national law concerning immigration was the act of March 2, 1819, the Manifest of Immigrants Act (3 Stat. 489). It stipulated that captains or masters of ships provide a list of names and the particulars concerning all passengers to be delivered to the United States, establishing for the first time the collection of data on immigration and immigrants to the United States.

Among the most important incentives designed to attract immigrants to the United States was its abundant land, granted through the famous act of May 20, 1862, the Act to Secure Homesteads. The law specified that any person who was the head of a family, or who arrived at age 21 and was a citizen or had filed to become such, was entitled to one quarter section of unclaimed public lands with the filing of a preemption claim at $1.25 cents or less per acre, or eighty acres at $2.50 per acre, not to exceed in aggregate 160 acres.

By the 1870s, concern about immigration from China and Japan in California and on the west coast led to formation of the Chinese Exclusion League, whose members advocated restrictions. In 1875 the first federal anti-Chinese legislation aimed at the immigration of women from China and Japan "for immoral purposes" was enacted. Known as the "Page Law," the act of March 3, 1875 was titled: "Re: Exclusion of Certain Asian Women and Other Matters" (18 Stat. 477; 8 U.S.C.) The first attempt to ban outright the immigration of Chinese laborers was passed in March 1879 but was vetoed by President Rutherford B. Hayes. His veto led to the negotiation of the Burlingame Treaty, which was concluded in 1880 and ratified by the Senate in 1881, and proclaimed by President Chester A. Arthur on October 5, 1881.

Congress passed a law stipulating certain prohibitions of Chinese immigration for twenty years. This was vetoed by President Arthur based on provisions of the Burlingame Treaty. In May 1882, Congress passed a new act that came to be known as the Chinese Exclusion Act. The law does not use the term "exclusion," which would go against the Burlingame Treaty, but rather uses the term "suspension." In response to President Arthur's veto, it set a period of ten years rather than the previous bill's twenty-year provision. It was formally titled "Act of May 6, 1882: To Execute Certain Treaty Stipulations Relating to Chinese" (22 Stat. 58; 8 U.S.C.)

That same year, Congress levied a fifty-cent head tax on all immigrants. The act charged the Secretary of the Treasury to establish contracts with each state's commissioner of immigration and banned the immigration of criminals (Act of August 3, 1882, 22 Stat. 214; 8 U.S.C.).

The effect on wages and working conditions attributed to immigrants spurred organized labor to advocate restrictions. Congress responded with the Act of February 26, 1885, on the Prohibition of Contract Labor, more commonly known as the Foran Act (23 Stat. 332; 8 U.S.C.). Congress amended the Foran Act on February 23, 1887, extending it and increasing the authority of the secretary of the treasury to implement and enforce the act (24 Stat. 414: 8 U.S.C.). Policy used health conditions to begin restricting immigration. Immigration stations began working with the office of the surgeon general of the United States to begin screening immigrants to ensure that they were healthy. Mullan characterizes his important role:

> Surgeon General Wyman enjoyed bureaucracy and he built his very effectively. The fifty-four medical officers and $600,000 budget over which he took command in 1891 grew to 135 officers and a budget of $1,750,000 by 1911. Under his careful political guidance, the Congress enlarged the name of the service in 1902 to the Public Health and Marine Hospital Service and formally eliminated the "Supervising" in the title, Surgeon General. Not only was his meticulous management and penchant for public administration ideally suited to the expansion of his program, but it typified the commitment to bureaucracy that was common to the Progressive era institutions. (35)

In 1888 Congress amended the Chinese Exclusion Act. Known as the "Scott Act," it extended the ban on Chinese laborers and rescinded the right of Chinese immigrants to return to the United States unless they had obtained in advance a certificate of reentry (25 Stat. 476; 8 U.S.C., 261–299). Then, in October of 1888, Congress passed another act barring Chinese laborers, rescinding—ex post facto—the validity of any certificates of reentry previously granted (25 Stat. 540; 8 U.S.C. 270). This ex post facto repeal of the certificates of reentry was challenged in the courts. In *Chae Chan Ping v. United States, 1889*, the Supreme Court ruled against the plaintiff. The court based its decision on the concept of sovereignty. The majority opinion revealed the racial attitudes of the justices, who referenced the "vast hordes" and "different races who will not assimilate with us" (130 U.S. 581–611).

Generally offset by a few years, Canadian immigration law closely paralleled that enacted by the United States. In 1891, Congress passed an immigration act that expanded the classes of individuals excluded from admission, forbade the advertisement for and soliciting of immigrants, increased the penalties for landing an illegal alien, required the shipping lines to defray the costs of detention and pay the costs of deportation of persons they transported, created the position of superintendent of immigration, and generally strengthened or specified enforcement processes. This act was a crucial one in establishing the decisive role of the national government and the new position of superintendent of immigration over immigration affairs, overriding state immigration laws or policies. Its exclusion provisions included a ban on "all idiots, insane persons, paupers or persons likely to become public charges" and excluded, for the first time, "persons suffering from a loathsome or a dangerous contagious disease" (26 Stat. 1084; U.S.C. 101.). The act was quickly challenged in the courts, but the U.S. Supreme Court upheld its constitutionality in *Nishimura Ekiu v. United States, 1892* (142 U.S. 651, January 18, 1892). The court again stressed issues of sovereignty, the power of Congress both to set immigration policy and to delegate such powers to service officers.

In 1892, Congress amended the Chinese Exclusion Act by extending it another ten years and increasing some of its penalties and tightening its procedures. The amendment was commonly known as the Geary Act (27 Stat. 25; 8 U.S.C.). In the Act of November 3, 1893: Re: Amending the Chinese Exclusion Act (28 Stat. 7), Congress extended the period of suspension and increased the restrictions imposed. The act elaborated on the terms "laborer" or "laborers." It excluded both skilled and unskilled manual laborers, Chinese employed in mining, huckstering, peddling, laundrymen, or those engaged in taking, drying, or otherwise preserving shell or other fish for home consumption or exportation, and expanded the definition of the term "merchant." In 1894, Congress again amended the Exclusion act and established a Bureau of Immigration (28 Stat. 390; 8 U.S.C. 174).

In 1896, President Grover Cleveland vetoed the first of several attempts by the Congress to enact a literacy test as a means to control immigration. His was the first of several presidential vetoes of literacy bills.

On April 29, 1902, Congress reenacted and extended the Chinese Exclusion Act. This latest of the exclusion laws remained in effect until its repeal in 1943 (32 Stat. 176; U.S.C.). In 1903, Congress moved immigration policy control from the Department of the Treasury to the newly established Department of Commerce and Labor (32 Stat. 825; 8 U.S.C.). On March 3, 1903, as part of its major codification of immigration laws, Congress increased the head tax on immigrants and prohibited entry to and the naturalization of anarchists—the first such ban on the entry or naturalization of persons based on their political or ideological beliefs. It established provisions for extensive and detailed records on all immigrants arriving in the United States (32 Stat. 1213; 8 U.S.C. and 32 Stat. 1222).

On February 20, 1907, Congress amended the immigration act, increasing yet again the head tax, adding to the excluded classes of individuals, but essentially restating the comprehensive act of June 6, 1906. The 1907 act established what became known as the Dillingham Commission to study immigration and to advise Congress on immigration reform (34 Stat. 898; U.S.C.). Congress added important regulations regarding the issuing of passports, and on expatriation and the marriage of American women to foreigners—stipulating that they take on the nationality of their husbands (34 Stat. 1228: 8 U.S.C. 17). Its section 3 (on women marrying foreigners and thereby losing their citizenship) remained controversial until repealed by the act of September 22, 1922 (42 Stat. 1021).

On March 14, 1907, President Theodore Roosevelt issued an executive order that implemented what was known as "the Gentleman's Agreement" between the United States and Japan to control the emigration of persons from Japan and Korea (then under Japanese jurisdiction) (Executive Order 589, March 14, 1907).

In 1910 Congress attempted to crack down on the practice of bringing in women for the purpose of prostitution by enacting the Act of June 25, 1910: The White-Slave Traffic Act (36 Stat. 825; U.S.C. 397–404).

In 1911, the Dillingham Commission issued its report, calling for increased restrictions and enactment of a literacy bill. Congress enacted an immigrant literacy provision on several occasions: 1896, 1913, 1915, and 1917, all of which were vetoed by Presidents Cleveland, Taft, and Wilson, respectively. Finally, on February 5, 1917, Congress overrode President Woodrow Wilson's veto and enacted a comprehensive immigration law. It essentially reenacted the acts of 1903 and 1907 but included a literacy test, resulting in the most restrictive immigration policy to date and codifying seven major ways that immigrants could be denied entry: Asians, criminals, persons who failed to meet certain moral standards, persons having various diseases, paupers, assorted radicals, and illiterates (39 Stat. 874; 8 U.S.C.; 278–279).

In 1917, a joint order of the departments of state and labor required passports and certain other information from all aliens seeking to enter the United States during World War I. The act required the issuing of visas from an American consular officer in the country of origin rather than allowing a person to enter the United States and seek permission to enter having already arrived at the shores or port of entry (Joint Order issued July 26, 1917, Washington, D.C.: 1042–1044).

Wartime exigencies played a role when on August 8, 1918, President Wilson issued executive order 2932. This fourteen-page order detailed rules and regulations to implement a proclamation concerning the exclusion, entrance, and departure of all aliens during war. It contained thirty-six sections specifying how the secretary of state should implement the departure from or entry into the United States. That same wartime sentiment inspired Congress, by the act of October 16, 1918, to spell out provisions dealing with and amending section 3 of the act of February 5, 1917, which added membership in or espousal of communism to the list of excluded classes or those subject to expulsion which previously had stipulated anarchists (40 Stat. 1012; 8 U.S.C. 137).

CONCLUSION: CLOSING THE GOLDEN DOOR

The litany of changing law and court decisions implementing immigration policy from the period of open door policy in 1820 to the dawn of the highly restrictive policy of the Pet Door Era in the 1920s is a tale of increasing fear: from xenophobia, fear of the foreigner, to fear of economic competition in jobs and the driving downward of wages and working conditions as a result of massive immigration. From the fear of immigrants who were so different that they could not (or were not desired to) assimilate to the fear of the spread of "obnoxious or contagious" diseases, people feared the cultural change arising from the introduction of persons of different languages and religions. From fear based on racism to fear that the nation would experience a renewed flood of immigration in response to the post–World War I economic turmoil in Europe, this multiplicity of fears fed a xenophobic demand for increased restrictions. When an economic recession hit in 1920, the House of Representatives voted to end all immigration. The Senate refused to concur in a total ban, but Congress was clearly primed for increased restrictionism and isolationism in U.S. foreign policy. Restrictionist forces gained not only in numbers, but also in their influence within Congress. Senator William P. Dillingham, who had chaired the Immigration Commission of 1907, became chair of the Immigration Committee in the U.S. Senate. Chairing the House Immigration Committee in the Republican-dominated chamber was Representative Albert Johnson (R–WA), a leading voice for restrictionist policy.

In 1919, the Palmer Raids resulted in over 500 immigrants suspected of being radical anarchists being deported on a ship to Russia, nicknamed the "Soviet Ark." Isolationist sentiment led Congress to reject joining the League of Nations. A postwar isolationist mood was easily tapped by forces advocating restrictions. A new nationalism emerged that was distrustful of Europe, disillusioned in the aftermath of the war and with the failure of the Americanization program, committed to isolationism and disdainful of all things foreign. It echoed through the halls of Congress in debates over joining the League of Nations. It rumbled in the "konklaves" of the Ku Klux Klan. It unleashed a torrent of state laws to exclude aliens from many occupations. Licensing acts barred foreigners from practicing architecture, engineering, chiropractic, pharmacy, surgery, and surveying, as well as from executing wills. They were even barred from operating motorbuses.

Congress responded by enacting a series of laws in the 1920s. These ushered in a new era in immigration policy, the Pet Door Era. Restrictionist policy, best exemplified by the quota acts of 1921, 1924, and 1929, dramatically decreased total immigration and shifted the composition of a much smaller wave of quota immigrants from southern/central/eastern Europe to northwestern Europe (LeMay, 1987: 65–72).

Chapter 2

THE PERIOD OF PANDEMICS

The nineteenth century was an age of pandemics as well as one of mass migration. Pandemic diseases hung like a sword over mankind. Sweeping across the globe, plagues of several maladies killed millions, and no one had a clue as to what caused them, how they spread, how they could be cured, nor how they could be prevented. As people traveled in mass movements, they carried with them, unknown to them, infectious diseases that spread worldwide. In previous centuries, diseases most often spread internationally as armies moved, war being the most common cause of large-scale migrations. In the nineteenth century, disease typically killed twice as many soldiers as did combat, and where soldiers went, plagues followed (Willrich: 119). But what was new to the nineteenth century was that tens of millions of ordinary people moved from nations of origin to nations of resettlement. And a host of diseases moved with them. Fear of epidemics was a concern among policymakers coping with immigration. That fear was well founded and increased as epidemics became more frequent and more deadly. Three epidemic diseases caused the greatest fear and most influenced the development of quarantine immigration stations: smallpox, cholera, and typhus.

Fortunately for humankind, for the immigrants, and for the receiving countries, the late nineteenth century was the critical period when medicine became modern. Medical researchers developed a new theory—germ theory—attempting to explain about disease as well as science-based, practical ways to cope with epidemics.

A few key concepts can usefully be defined here. Most diseases are *endemic*—that is, native to a particular area, country, or region: always present, but under control. Endemic diseases are not highly contagious, because so many people in the population have a high degree of immunity to them. As a result, they are far less deadly. Endemic diseases are also called chronic. The distinction between endemic and epidemic disease is sometimes blurred. Some diseases—for example, malaria, syphilis, and tuberculosis—may be both chronic and epidemic. Although endemic to a country, they may break out in places in which they were not previously common or may have rather sudden increases in morbidity and mortality rates. When that happens, they are considered epidemic.

An *epidemic* disease is prevalent among a people or community at a specific time, typically produced by some special causes not generally present in the affected locality, often resulting in morbidity or mortality significantly in excess of normal rates. Epidemic diseases are associated with such words as "contagions," "infections," and "plagues." Today we know that such diseases are the result of an invasion by an infectious agent—a bacteria or virus. Many, but not all, are contagious—that is, spread directly or indirectly from one person to another. Epidemic diseases are typically associated with three terms: "acute," "high morbidity," and "high mortality." Acute diseases are characterized by rapid onsets, severe symptoms, and relatively short durations, in contrast with chronic diseases. Morbidity refers to the rate of incidence of the disease—how many persons in the population contract it. Mortality refers to the death rate of the disease. Epidemic diseases have soaring morbidity and mortality rates (Hayes, 1998: 5–6). Smith notes:

> Epidemics are like waves: they rise and fall. Sometimes they seem to be spaced at fairly regular intervals of time. Measles may rise to a peak every second or third year. . . . Topography and climate seem to have something to do with both epidemics and endemics. . . . Ophthalmia is traditionally associated with Egypt, malaria with the Mediterranean shores, plague with the East, yellow fever with the tropics of America. Moreover[,] some diseases spread and become threatening at one season of the year, some at another. Pneumonia is a winter disease, measles seem to reach its peak in the spring, babies die of diarrhea in the hot summer months, and one fears poliomyelitis most in the late summer. Some diseases, again, fall upon people of all ages, some upon children, some most severely on the old. (1946: 122)

A *pandemic* refers to when an epidemic spreads to entire countries, or regions, and becomes multinational, even global, in scope. Pandemics have been called "plagues," "contagions," and "pestilences." Plague typically refers to conditions causing very high morbidity or mortality and is accompanied by social dislocation. The historic outbreaks of plagues, like the Black Death of the thirteenth and fourteenth centuries in Europe, the recurrences of cholera spreading globally, and the 1918–1919 influenza epidemic (also known as the Spanish flu), are reminders that these periodic outbreaks of horrific disease are akin to nature's holding a sword over the heads of mankind—suggesting a battle or warfare.

Epidemiology is the study of epidemic and pandemic disease, but, as Omran notes:

> Despite its name, epidemiology is not just the study of epidemics, although it has a great deal to do with epidemics and infectious diseases, its province is rather the broad mass phenomena of health and disease: how these are distributed in groups of people, the causes and consequences of diseases, and how they can be prevented and controlled. (3)

As modern medicine developed, medical scientists and then practitioners increasingly understood, controlled, managed, and began to prevent incidences of the most dreaded epidemic diseases. The old world epidemics have come to be replaced by chronic and degenerative diseases, by disease resulting from stress or manmade causes. Typhoid, tuberculosis, cholera, diphtheria, plague, and smallpox declined as the leading diseases and causes of death, replaced by heart diseases, cancer, strokes, diabetes, gastric ulcers, and the like (Omran: 4).

Five exemplary epidemic diseases, each of which caused especially deadly pandemics in the nineteenth and early twentieth centuries, are yellow fever, smallpox, cholera, the bubonic plague, and influenza. Another nondeadly but highly contagious disease was trachoma. In its severe stage, trachoma causes blindness; it still is a leading cause of blindness worldwide. It was considered "loathsome," a leading cause for exclusion from entrance and permanent residence status in the United States, especially at Angel Island and at Ellis Island but also at New Orleans. Several doctors and medical scientists played key roles in discovering the causes of the diseases or in developing important protocols for mitigating their morbidity or mortality rates. These doctors at the borders were instrumental in the development of public health in the United States.

NOTABLE EPIDEMIC/PANDEMIC DISEASES AND NORTH AMERICAN IMMIGRATION

Diseases that were real scourges in the seventeenth and eighteenth centuries are less known today, because they have been eradicated or so reduced in their threat to life as to be considered almost commonplace childhood disease or diseases rarely seen today. Where inoculation against the disease is common, in most developed countries, measles is today seldom life-threatening (Mayo Clinic, 2014). Much of the population alive today is either immune, having contracted mild cases of the disease as young children, or has been immunized by vaccination of an anti-measles serum. In the seventeenth century, however, measles was a major killer. When European settlers brought the disease to the Americas, it spread and killed enormous numbers of Native Americans, who had no immunity to it and among whom it proved especially deadly. Typhoid fever is an acute infectious disease caused by the bacillus *Salmonella typhi*. It is most often acquired by ingesting food or water contaminated by excreta. It is frequently considered a form of typhus and is characterized by high fever and intestinal disorders. Typhoid fever was a deadly killer in Philadelphia in 1837, in many sections of the United States between 1865 and 1873, and finally in another epidemic that struck Pennsylvania in 1885. Today it is easily treated, and in many places where it previously was epidemic, it has now been largely wiped out by improvements in basic hygiene and decontamination treatment of the water supply. Tuberculosis is an infectious disease caused by the tubercle bacillus. It is characterized by the formation of tubercles in various soft tissues of the body, specifically, tuberculosis of the lungs. In the nineteenth century, it was also known as consumption. Since its bacillus was discovered, effective treatment has greatly reduced its morbidity and mortality. In the first half of the nineteenth century, however, it killed at a rate of 300 to 500 per 100,000 in population and was one of the greatest epidemic killers of the early nineteenth century (LeMay, 2006: table 2.1, 41).

Yellow Fever

Yellow fever is sometimes called the American plague. It is a viral disease, a hemorrhagic illness still prevalent in Africa and South America despite the existence of an effective vaccine. It is a tropical disease spread by infected mosquitoes. The disease has dramatically reemerged since the 1980s; as of 2001, the World Health Organization (WHO) estimated that it still caused more than 200,000 illnesses and 30,000 deaths annually among unvaccinated populations.

There are two kinds of yellow fever. Jungle yellow fever is mainly a disease of monkeys spread from infected mosquitoes to monkeys in tropical rainforest areas and to humans caught in the cycle and bitten by infected mosquitoes. Urban yellow fever is a disease of humans spread by *Aedes aegypti* mosquitoes infected by other people. This type of mosquito has adapted to living in human cities, towns, and villages, where it breeds in brackish water found in discarded tires, flower pots, oil drums, and water storage containers located near human dwelling places. Urban yellow fever is the cause of most yellow fever epidemics. These infections are often mild, but the disease can cause severe, life-threatening illness—accompanied by high fever, chills, headaches, vomiting, and backache. The severe type often leads to shock, bleeding, and kidney and liver failure. That latter symptom causes jaundice (a yellowing of the skin and the whites of the eyes) from which the disease acquired its common name. Symptoms start three to six days after being bitten by an infected mosquito.

The mosquito crossed the ocean aboard ships, riding in water casks, and established itself ashore in places where temperatures stayed about 72 °F. Its affinity for water casks enabled mosquitoes carrying yellow fever from sailor to sailor to remain aboard ship for weeks and even months. This distinguished it from most other infections that usually broke out on shipboard, which usually burned themselves out. People tended to get sick pretty much together and recovered about the same time, thereby acquiring immunity. With yellow fever, reinfections could take place, so ships could suffer a seemingly unending chain of attacks, with no one knowing who would get sick next and die. "Yellow jack" was especially dreaded by sailors of the Caribbean and other tropical seas where the temperature-sensitive *Aedes aegypti* flourished. As we will see below, it was a disease especially battled at the New Orleans station (McNeill: 222).

Yellow fever was the source of several devastating epidemics. Havana, Cuba, suffered one in 1762–1763, as did Philadelphia in 1793. In Haiti, in 1802, Napoleon's troops fell victim to an epidemic that wiped out more than half the army—killing far more than enemy combatants and forcing Napoleon to withdraw his army and give up the campaign, thereby ensuring Haiti's independence. There were notable outbreaks in the Western Hemisphere in 1805, 1822, and 1870. In the U.S. South, an epidemic spread in 1820–1823 and another in 1841. A particularly nasty outbreak occurred in New Orleans in 1847, and again in 1852—when 8,000 died in one summer (LeMay, 2006: 41). It struck in the south of the United States again in 1855, centered in Norfolk, Virginia. It devastated American troops in 1871 at Fort Columbus, New York, and in 1873–75 among the troops at Barrancas, Florida. A yellow fever epidemic struck New Orleans again in 1877, in Memphis, Tennessee in 1878, and in Jacksonville, Florida in 1886 (Ibid.) The fear yellow fever instilled in the population led to the quarantine responsibility of the Marine Hospital Service, as described by Mullan:

A yellow fever epidemic in New Orleans in 1877 that spread quickly up the Mississippi valley riveted national attention on quarantine policy and forced congressional action. The Quarantine Act of 1878 was a victory for the Marine Hospital Service, conferring upon it quarantine authority—its first mission beyond the care of merchant seamen in the eighty years of its existence. (25; see also Willrich: 222–223)

Epidemics among troops were so devastating that the United States army established a Yellow Fever Commission, most often known as the Reed Commission after its leader Major Walter Reed. The commission did a vector analysis of the spread of the disease during an outbreak in Havana, Cuba, in 1900, proving that the *Aedes aegypti* mosquito was the true source in the spread of the disease, disproving the then popular notion that it was spread by direct contact with infected people or contaminated objects such as bedding or clothing. The army was an occupation force in Cuba after the Spanish–American War of 1898. During that war, far more American troops died from yellow fever, malaria, and dysentery than were killed by bullets. The American government in Cuba, under Governor-General Leonard Wood, realized that something had to be done if the occupation were to last years. Cuba was a primary breeding ground for yellow fever in the Western Hemisphere, and the military reasoned that it was an excellent base to study and possibly eradicate the disease.

Dr. William Gorgas, later surgeon general of the United States, is world renowned as the conqueror of the mosquito and the malaria and yellow fever it transmits. His pioneering effort in halting epidemics of yellow fever enabled the United States to build the Panama Canal. A Cuban physician, Carlos Juan Finley, first suspected and postulated the mosquito as a carrier of the disease. Havana suffered about 500 deaths per year for a decade preceding his discovery, and the Reed Commission's work confirmed his suspicions and experimentally proved the connection. William Gorgas saw that the way to eradicate the disease was to exterminate the mosquito that carried it. He undertook the task in Havana and later in Panama. Gorgas and his team disinfected gutters and puddles, screened and oiled cisterns and water barrels, and persuaded Cuban housewives to empty jugs and pitchers of water every day. Yellow fever patients were quarantined and put behind screens to prevent fresh infection. "The results were amazing: in 1896 there had been 1,282 deaths from yellow fever; in 1900 there were 310, in 1901 eighteen, in 1902 none. Gorgas had abruptly ended a century and a half of yellow fever in Havana" (Smith, 1946: 17, 186).[1]

Smallpox

Smallpox is a highly contagious viral disease unique to humans and for which there is no known cure. The only way to deal with the disease is through prevention by vaccination. It is a serious, contagious, and deadly infectious disease. Its name came from the "spotted" look of raised bumps that appear on the faces and body of an infected person. It certainly qualified as a "loathsome and contagious" disease as specified in United States immigration law, which banned entry to persons with the disease. "At the end of the nineteenth century, smallpox was still regarded as the most infamous and loathsome infectious diseases . . . . It killed an estimated 300 million people in the 20th century alone" (Willrich: 20–22).

There are two clinical forms. *Variola major* is the severe and unfortunately more common type. Historically, it has a mortality rate of about 20 percent to 40 percent. Victims exhibit an extensive rash covering much of their bodies and suffer high fever. *Variola major* is itself distinguished as having four types. Ordinary is the more frequent type, accounting for about 90 percent of cases of the disease. Modified is typically a more mild type of the *variola major* form, usually occurring in persons having previously been infected.

Flat and hemorrhagic types are rare but are nearly always fatal (96 percent). In the latter form, the skin does not blister. Bleeding occurs under the skin, making the skin look charred and black (thus this type is often called blackpox). The eyes hemorrhage. Death occurs from fatal levels of bleeding, often as brain hemorrhage, but can also result from multi-organ failure. Kolata has shown that this form occurs in 3–25 percent of fatal cases of the disease, depending on the virulence of the strain (Willrich: 4). *Variola minor* is a milder, less serious presentation of the disease, with death rates historically at about 1 percent of cases (Ibid.: 43).

Smallpox became more deadly over three centuries leading up to the 1800s. Smallpox appears to have entered Europe around 581. Details about early epidemics have been lost owing to the scarcity of surviving records of early medieval society. In Italy, an epidemic between 1424 and 1458 killed only 84 persons. In the mid-seventeenth century, an outbreak in London killed about 7 percent of its victims. A famous outbreak in Boston, in 1721, had a mortality rate of 15 percent, and in 1792, another Boston outbreak claimed 30 percent. A Scotland smallpox epidemic in 1787 killed a third of its victims. An isolated Japanese village, "virgin soil to the disease," experienced an epidemic in 1790 that killed 38 percent, and in Madras, India, a similar epidemic claimed 43 percent of its victims (Fenn: 21, 81). Historical studies of smallpox show the disease claims higher mortality rates among the very old and the very young, with the highest rates among those younger than 1 and older than 50. As Willrich notes: "The story of the smallpox epidemics is a history of violence, social conflict, and political contention" (14). And in the

United States, the battle to control it through compulsory vaccination was one of the most important civil liberties struggles of the twentieth century.

Survivors of smallpox infections are often left blind in one or both eyes due to corneal ulcerations. Most surviving victims retain persistent skin scarring—pockmarks. During the twentieth century, the disease killed an estimated 300–500 million people globally. In 1967, the WHO estimated that 2 million people died among the nearly 15 million people who had contracted the disease that year.

In the mid-eighteenth century, outbreaks in Europe occurred in five-year cycles. Exposure in early life left many survivors with a natural immunity. Transmission is generally by direct, sustained contact with infected bodily fluids or contaminated objects such as bedding and clothing. Humans are the only natural hosts of the virus. Persons who have smallpox are sometimes contagious with the onset of fever, but the highly contagious stage comes with the onset of the rash, and the infected person remains contagious until the last smallpox bump (pustules) is gone and all the scabs have fallen off (generally, three weeks after the rash appears). The incubation period is commonly 12 to 14 days, but the range is 7 to 17 days. Fever brought on by the disease ranges from 101 to 105 degrees and lasts until the scabs are gone. The incubation period became more problematic when the speed of ships' travel by the late 1880s greatly increased the latent contagion issue, making it more difficult for the health inspectors of the U.S. M.H.S. to spot carriers or for medical officers, whose presence was required on board ships of the steamship lines according to the law of 1882, to note smallpox among the steerage passengers during the transatlantic crossing trip itself (Willrich: 219–220; Nugent: 27–33).[2]

Native Americans were decimated by diseases brought by settlers from the Old World for which the natives of the New World had no immunity. Smallpox was a chief culprit of that decimation. Fenn counted thirty-three smallpox epidemics (28–29).

Smallpox is transmitted from human to human, and naturally the public health service, when screening immigrants, watched for smallpox symptoms, especially on ships coming from places abroad where an epidemic outbreak had been reported. From 1898 to 1903, a five-year epidemic of smallpox spread across the country, racking up an official count of 164,283 cases, although the actual number might have exceeded five times that figure. Because it was mostly of the milder form of the disease, the epidemic, particularly prevalent in the South, resulted in only 5,627 fatalities. Racial attitudes stymied smallpox control. However, the five-year pandemic launched the first great massive compulsory vaccination campaign.

Opposition to compulsory vaccination spurred litigation that went all the way to the U.S. Supreme Court in 1905 (Willrich: 11–12).

The 1898–1903 series of epidemics was important in expanding the role and work of the U.S. Marine Hospital Service (U.S. M.H.S.). Founded in 1798, it initially served as sentinels at the nation's borders and overseas outposts to assist sailors and to examine immigrants to prevent their bringing diseases to American soil. In 1878, the National Quarantine Act gave the service enforcement power over quarantine regulation. Until 1898, the service's work consisted mostly of running twenty-two hospitals and 107 relief stations for American seamen on the coasts and interior ports, staffing immigration inspection stations, and administering quarantine when yellow fever threatened. During the smallpox epidemic campaign, Surgeon-General Wyman sent service surgeon C. P. Wertenbaker to assist communities throughout the U.S. South to cope with smallpox outbreaks, and Wertenbaker stablished himself as the service's foremost smallpox expert in the field, known to state governors, city mayors, and various state and local health officials as a master diagnostician of the new mild type of smallpox, a man in possession of a proven strategy for stamping out the disease (Willrich: 78–85).

Charles Poindexter Wertenbaker was born in 1860 in Charlottesville, Virginia, and took his medical degree from the University of Virginia in 1882. He assisted and studied with Dr. Henry Long of the North Carolina Board of Health. In 1888, he entered the U.S. M.H.S., remaining with the service until 1915. He exemplified the service surgeon membership as an elite corps of some 200 who became increasingly mobile federal medical men whose transience became part of their job description. Their readiness to move with their federal medical expertise made them a force for the integration and bureaucratic standardization of public health in the United States. Quite literally, Wertenbaker and his colleagues in the U.S. M.H.S. became the vanguard of a modern, national public health system. In 1902, it was renamed the U.S. Public Health and Marine Hospital Service (Willrich: 76).

And in 1913–1914, for example, another series of outbreaks of smallpox occurred on U.S. ships, particularly military ships. A ship traveling the Mississippi River brought the 1913 epidemic to Memphis, Tennessee. In 1914, the battleship *Ohio* had an outbreak of twenty-one cases. In 1915, doctors from Ellis Island were sent north to Maine to deal with problems of continued infections among people migrating by land from Canada. In 1917, an outbreak in Minnesota numbered eleven deaths among the fifty-eight cases reported. On July 28, 1917, an epidemic numbering thirty-eight cases in Worchester, Massachusetts, resulted in nine deaths. The source of that outbreak was traced to a Swedish immigrant coming into the United States from Norway via Ellis Island on the ship *Kristianafjord*. These spurred the surgeon general to call for reports from all stations of the Public Health Service on outbreaks and on methods of vaccination being used to cope with epidemics or to prevent their onset.[3]

The idea of using inoculation to fight smallpox came to Europe in the early 1700s. The practice is now known to have been used as early as 1000 BC. Indians rubbed pus into skin lesions. Chinese blew powdered smallpox scabs up the noses of the healthy. These practices resulted in patients' developing a mild case of the disease, after which they were immune. The process of inoculation spread to Turkey. Lady Mary Wortley Montagu, wife of the British ambassador, learned of it from an Italian doctor, Emmanuel Timoni, attached to the British embassy in Istanbul. She had the procedure performed on her children, aged 5 and 4. They both recovered quickly, and Timoni reported the process to the Royal Society in England, of which he was a member. He published an account in 1713. When the 1721 epidemic hit London, inoculation was tried on prisoners, all of whom recovered in a few weeks. The royal family was then inoculated, reassuring the English that the procedure was safe. That year, an epidemic also broke out in Boston. The famous Reverend Cotton Mather learned of the procedure from one of his slaves and began promoting it. When the population, which had fled the city, returned in 1722, Mather was called a hero. Out of Boston's population who were not inoculated, 7 percent died of the disease, but among 300 persons who had followed his advice and were inoculated, only 2 percent died. Inoculation, however, was far from a perfect process. It caused cases of smallpox, with a death rate of about 2 percent. It was difficult to administer, and infected patients had to be quarantined to prevent its spread. Fenn notes that despite grave misgivings, General Washington ordered inoculation of his troops during the Revolutionary War when a virulent outbreak occurred in 1777 (Fenn: 81).

The process of vaccination provided a far better preventive method. An English doctor, Edward Jenner, as a medical apprentice aged 13, first noticed that people who had caught cowpox while working with cows were known not to catch smallpox. After Jenner returned to London to attend medical school, a smallpox epidemic struck his home town of Berkeley. He advised local cow workers to be inoculated, and they informed him that cowpox prevented smallpox. He studied cowpox further and developed a process, in 1796, when a patient, a local milkmaid, developed cowpox and sought treatment from him. He inoculated the 8-year-old son of his gardener with cowpox taken from the milkmaid. The boy suffered an extremely weak bout of cowpox and then recovered. Jenner then inoculated him with smallpox, but the boy did not develop even a mild case. He was immune. From this insight, Jenner treated twenty-three more cases, including his son, and none suffered from smallpox. In 1798, Jenner's vaccination was used in Boston, and the innovation spread. Jenner published his work in numerous major European languages and the process was performed all over Europe and the United States by the early 1800s. With Jenner's process, which became known as vaccination after the Latin word for cow—*vacca*—the death rate was zero.

Jenner's dream was the eradication of smallpox by vaccination, a dream eventually realized. In the mid-1950s, about 2 million people died annually from the disease. In 1958, the World Health Organization (WHO) began a global campaign of vaccination. Troop movements and crowded encampments had long been associated with spread of disease, including smallpox. WHO teams began vaccinating troops. Then entire civilian populations followed. The last major European outbreak occurred in 1972 in Yugoslavia after a pilgrim returned from the Middle East. That epidemic infected 175 people, with thirty-five deaths. Massive vaccinations halted that epidemic. The last naturally occurring case was diagnosed in Somalia in October 1977. WHO had successfully eradicated the disease. The U.S. had contributed $300 million to the eradication effort.

Today, the disease exists only in viral research laboratories. Post-9/11, fears have been raised that stockpiles of the disease could be stolen and used as a bioterrorist weapon. In March 2003, the accidental discovery of scab tissues of smallpox found tucked in a Civil War medicine book in Santa Fe, New Mexico, raised concern at the Center for Disease Control (CDC) that these and other such scabs could be used to extract smallpox DNA for use in a biological attack (for a broader discussion, see, for example, Oldstone, 1998).

Cholera

Bubonic plague was the pandemic disease of the fourteenth century. Yellow fever and smallpox were the prevalent pandemic diseases of the seventeenth and eighteenth centuries. Cholera was the classic epidemic disease of the nineteenth century, during which time six great pandemic outbreaks occurred. It was also the epidemic disease of the United States during the nineteenth century. Rosenberg notes, "Cholera . . . appeared in almost every part of the country in the course of the century. It flourished in the great cities, New York, Cincinnati, Chicago; it crossed the continent with the forty-niners; its victims included Iowa dirt farmers and New York longshoremen, Wisconsin lead miners, and Negro field hands" (1987: 1).

Global outbreaks of cholera, smallpox, and other diseases kept hygiene central to the immigration administrative processes. In 1891 and 1893, Congress enacted laws giving the U.S. M.H.S. primary responsibility for keeping immigrants infected with contagious diseases from entering the United States, and by 1894, vaccination became a legal prerequisite for entry (Willrich: 222–223).

Cholera, or Asiatic cholera, is a waterborne disease caused by the bacterium *Vibrio cholerae*. Infection comes from drinking contaminated water or eating improperly cooked fish, particularly shellfish. The disease produces potentially lethal secretary diarrhea. Genetic research has shown that an individual's susceptibility to cholera is affected by blood type— type O being the most susceptible, then type B, then type A, and finally, type AB being the most resistant, conferring virtual immunity. As Rosenberg puts it:

> Cholera could not have thrived where filth and want did not already exist; nor could it have traveled so widely without an unprecedented development of trade and transportation. The cholera pandemics were transitory phenomena, destined to occupy the world stage for only a short time—the period during which public health and medical science were catching up with urbanization and the transportation revolution. Indeed, cholera was to play a key role in its own banishment from the Western world; the cholera epidemics of the nineteenth century produced much of the impetus needed to overcome centuries of government inertia and indifference in regard to problems of public health. (2)

Cholera is transmitted through ingestion of fecal matter contaminated with the bacterium. This typically occurs when untreated sewage is released into waterways, affecting the water supply, any foods washed in that water, and shellfish living in the affected waterways. It is rarely spread directly from person to person.

Cholera was originally endemic to the Indian subcontinent, where the Ganges River served as a contamination reservoir. It spread by both land and sea trade routes, first to Russia, then to western Europe, then to North America. Geddes Smith vividly describes its worldwide march:

> The rise and fall of cholera as a world disease belongs to the story of a single century—the nineteenth. Before 1817 . . . it was a local disease in India. In that year, no one knows why, it started a slow march which carried it over most of India in 1917, over the frontier in 1818, and by 1823 eastward to Japan and westward to the threshold of Europe. In 1826 it traveled again with traders and pilgrims, found its way overland to Russia in 1830, to Germany and England in 1831, to Ireland in 1832, took ship that year

with hungry Irish emigrants, crossed to Canada and the eastern states, and pushed into the western states in 1833. This march was over in 1836, and for ten years the disease remained at home. In 1846 it was abroad again, moving more quickly, and for the next sixteen years it was present intermittently in Europe, North America, and part of South America, reaching its height in the United States in 1849 and 1850. In 1865 it crossed by sea from India to Mecca and the Mediterranean, reaching Halifax, New York, and New Orleans the next year, and spreading twice through the Mississippi basin before it retreated in 1874. Cholera never ranged so far again. Between 1884 and 1887 it visited France, Spain, and Italy. In 1892 it swept across Russia and killed eighty-five hundred in Hamburg. Later waves of infection for the most part fell short of western Europe, and except for a few centers of persistent infection, cholera continues to afflict only its Indian homeland. There, however, it killed more than seven million people in twenty years of the [twentieth] century. (Geddes Smith, 1946: 16)

Asiatic cholera first came to North America (to Canada) in June 1832 aboard the vessel *Carricks*, out of Dublin. After embarking, thirty-nine of its 172 passengers developed the violent vomiting, spasms, and severe diarrhea that are its characteristic symptoms. Owing to the apparent symptoms detected on board, the ship and its passengers were quarantined at Grosse Ile, the island quarantine station in the St. Lawrence, below Quebec, Canada. One hundred thirty-three passengers survived their bouts of fever and, after disinfection, were released. Soon after they arrived in Quebec City, a grave epidemic broke out. During the course of the epidemic, it progressed from Quebec to Montreal. Approximately 3,000 succumbed to the disease in Quebec, 4,000 in Montreal, and about 12,000 throughout the rest of Canada (Chartre, 1995: 35–36). It is probably through that outbreak that it spread to New York and Ohio in 1832–1834 (LeMay, 2006: 41).

Before its cause was discovered, the disease struck terror as it spread its rapid and erratic course. It was unmanageable and incurable in nature, dreadful in its fatality, and devastating in its consequences. When it struck New York, it became entrenched in the slums, where the wretched houses north of Canal Street looked out on the dead strewn about like slaughtered victims on a battlefield. Ever a disease of the poor, in New York it killed thousands in the three-month epidemic in 1849. But conditions favorable to its spread were not in city slums alone. Mississippi riverboats in epidemic years became moving "pest-houses," and infection ran riot among poor travelers between decks, driven incessantly to the toilet by the cruel purging which characterizes the disease. The *Peytonia* lost fifty passengers between New Orleans and Louisville on a single trip in 1849 (LeMay, 2006: 45).

The epidemic outbreak in 1832 was severe. The city mayor had proclaimed a blanket quarantine against almost all of Europe and Asia in June 1832 when a steamboat from Albany brought word that cholera had broken out in Quebec and Montreal, showing that the disease had crossed the Atlantic—the nation's last barrier of defense against the disease. The city of New York designated a board of health comprising the health officer of the port, the resident physician, and the city inspector and appropriated $25,000 for them to erect hospitals and take other measures to alleviate and prevent cholera. The Board had the day-to-day responsibility for keeping a city of a quarter-million residents healthy. Rosenberg describes the cholera epidemic that quickly ensued as beyond their capacity to cope. Soon dead bodies lay unburied in the gutters of the city's slum streets. Coffin makers could not keep up with the demand. Churches closed when their ministers fled the city and its epidemic. Physicians and city officials were sometimes attacked and beaten. The cholera epidemic soon spread to other cities. New Orleans lost an estimated 5,000. In Chester, Pennsylvania, persons suspected of carrying the pestilence were murdered, as was the local resident who gave them shelter. Newly arrived immigrants, especially the Irish, were particularly feared. They occupied the foulest slums of the cities and suffered far out of proportion to their numbers. To respectable Americans, their premature deaths seemed inevitable consequences of a misspent life. The disease was viewed as God's vengeance on them for their drunkenness and their lives as paupers and beggars. They were widely perceived as having brought cholera with them (Geddes Smith: 18–20, 63).

The disease disproportionately hit the poor in large cities everywhere it struck. In Hamburg, Germany, in its epidemic in 1892, those whose income was less than a 1,000 marks were nineteen times more likely to fall victim to the disease than those whose income exceeded 50,000 marks. In New York, in the 1832 epidemic, of 100 cholera victims who died in a single day in July, ninety-five were buried in the city's Potter's Field. In Richmond, Virginia, the poorhouse graveyard was used for 90 percent of those who died of cholera. Rosenberg shows that New York's Negro population was especially hard hit (1987: 57).

In the mid-1800s, quarantine was the only known policy for dealing with the spread of infectious diseases like cholera. Unfortunately, it was not effectively enforced. From the early days of the republic until the 1880s, quarantine policy was an issue left to the states. It became a virtual battleground for the contending forces for the expansion of federal public health. Mullan shows that in the 1830s, the enforcement of quarantine regulations was inconsistent from locality to locality and so variable as to be, in effect, almost nonexistent (22).

In 1832, the idea that disease was a specific, well-defined biological entity was controversial and highly suspect. Disease was viewed as being a lack of balance or disorder in the person. Yellow fever and its black vomit seemed noncontagious. Cholera, like yellow fever, seemed to start simultaneously in widely separated parts of the city. Many doctors suspected an atmospheric origin. They noted that cholera could be contracted more than once, whereas a contagious disease, such as smallpox, could not.

Quarantine measures were the most often used practice against cholera in the 1832 pandemic. Troy, New York, along the Erie Canal, was forced to provide quarantine provisions for 700 immigrants. Hospitals, nurses, and doctors were soon overwhelmed. At New York's Greenwich Hospital, fourteen of sixteen nurses died of cholera contracted while caring for patients (Rosenberg: 95). In Philadelphia, Baltimore, Louisville, St. Louis, and Cincinnati, the cholera hospitals were staffed by the Sisters of Charity. The quarantine procedure proved ineffective in treating or containing the epidemic, for the true cause of the disease was unknown and thus was ineffectively addressed. The filth of New York remained unabated when another epidemic broke out in 1848.

On December 2, 1848, the ship *New York* rode anchor off Staten Island with 300 steerage passengers aboard, all of whom had been exposed to cholera below decks. Quarantine was demanded. That raised the question of where to put them. None of America's port cities had facilities adequate to quarantine fifty persons, let alone 300. After fifteen years without cholera or yellow fever, New York's quarantine was no more than a gesture. In less than a month, sixty immigrants had fallen ill, half of whom died. A new cholera epidemic ensued. Cities to the south fared even worse. Vessels from Hamburg and Bremen brought cholera to New Orleans, from which the disease spread as the immigrants carried cholera with them to steamboat landings along the Mississippi, the Arkansas, and the Tennessee rivers.[4] As in 1832, the working class was the most severely affected by the epidemic—which, fortunately, subsided fairly quickly. New York City, however, suffered more than 5,000 deaths from the disease. As Rosenberg shows, by April, cholera spread to dozens of American cities and villages as river and lake streamers sowed cholera at scores of landings and as railroads, which by then crisscrossed the Northwest, discharged cholera-carrying passengers to even remote points. Along the rivers, steamboat passengers who died from cholera were unceremoniously dumped overboard, drifting ominously past river and lake towns. Gold seekers carried cholera with them across the continent, where many a Forty-Eighter died without physician, minister or friend. Newly established cities in the U.S. West, with inadequate water supplies and primitive sanitation, crowded with a transient population, suffered severe outbreaks. St. Louis lost 10 percent of its population to cholera. Cincinnati suffered almost as badly—and Sandusky even worse than St. Louis (Rosenberg: 115). In city after city, the poorest and most wretched were those whom were most often struck down by the disease.

The connection between cholera and vice became a verbal reflex, and the connection was firmly established. The Christian Revivalist movement of the time helped spread the view that cholera was as an exercise of God's will, a chastisement to a nation sunk in materialism and sin. It was retribution. Asiatic cholera was a disease of "filth, of intemperance, and of vice" (Rosenberg: 121). In 1849, as in 1832, cholera was seen as a chronic malady associated with those immigrants who were viewed as a permanent threat to American institutions. The Irish were seen as the greatest menace. German and Scandinavians were viewed positively as thrifty, hard-working, church-going, and an asset to the nation (Ibid.: 183).

In summer 1849, Dr. John Snow, a prominent London physician, published a pamphlet, "On the Mode of Communication of Cholera." In it, he argued that cholera was a contagious disease caused by a poison reproducing itself in the bodies of its victims. This poison was in the excreta and vomit of cholera victims. When the city was struck again, in 1854, Dr. Snow used painstaking correlation of the incidence of cholera to subscribers of the city's two water companies and was able to trace cholera to a specific city water company whose users suffered cholera far more frequently than did the users of the other. That company drew its water from the lower Thames, after it had been contaminated with London sewage. His study was the first that proved a link between the disease and contaminated water supplies, even though his idea of a specific poison was not readily accepted by the medical profession. It represents the first use of epidemiology. It led in part to Robert Koch's discovery of the *Cholera vibrio* in 1883. Snow's work proved the value of the model of waterborne transmission. He is also noted for his development of chloroform anesthesia to replace the use of ether (Bynum and Bynum vol. 4: 1167–1169).

When a cholera epidemic struck New York again in 1866, the leading medical professionals were still unwilling to accept the theory about the specific cause of the disease (germ theory) but were accepting of the practical recommendations of doctors Snow and Pettenkofer, who had shown that boiling water and disinfecting clothing and bedding greatly reduced the incidences of cholera during an outbreak (see, for example, the discussion in Rosenberg, 1992).

On April 18, 1866 the steamship *Virginia* arrived in New York. Thirty-seven of her passengers had succumbed to cholera during the voyage, and another lay dying. There were 1,080 steerage passengers (and four-teen cabin passengers) who were presumed to have been exposed. More infected ships were expected, so the city decided to establish a perma-nent quarantine. The first cholera victims in the city appeared on May 1, 1866. Another was reported on May 2, and four days later a third. By June, scores of others developed. The cases, however, were scattered and rela-tively few—nothing like the explosions of cholera experienced in 1832 and 1849. The mildness of the epidemic was due to careful planning and hard work by the new Health Board, which had done much to clean up the worst sections of filth. The Battery Barracks were used as a hospital, and another barrack to store chemicals to disinfect the excreta and personal effects of cholera victims. City streets, for the first time, were cleaned. Some 160,000 tons of manure were removed from vacant city lots. Thousands of yards were ordered cleaned, more than 700 cisterns were emptied, and 6,500 privies were disinfected. The new Metropolitan Health Board effectively turned away a major cholera epidemic from the largest and most congested city in North America. In cities throughout the country, prominent citizens called for creation of health boards similar to that credited with saving New York City. No other city had a board of health having nearly the pow-ers of New York's, however, and few such cities escaped the 1866 epidemic of cholera so lightly scathed. But New York had demonstrated that a public health campaign could drastically reduce the mortality rate of a cholera outbreak (Rosenberg: 205).

Then, in 1883, German scientist Robert Koch, directing a German sci-entific commission in Egypt, isolated the mechanism that causes cholera—*Vibrio comma*, a mobile comma-shaped bacteria (Magill: 71–78). Upon entering the human intestine, it produced an acute disease that, untreated, killed half those who contracted it. Cholera, like typhoid, could be spread by any pathway leading to the human digestive tract: unwashed hands, uncooked fruit and vegetables, sewage-contaminated water supplies, and so on. More will be discussed in the closing section of this chapter about Koch and other scientists and doctors who led the way in modernizing medicine. The discovery of the bacillus that caused cholera, however, was a medical breakthrough that paved the way for more effective treatment and preventative measures that were used in the United States during the cholera epidemics of the early twentieth century. Although the outbreaks were frequent, none approached the deadly pandemics of the nineteenth century in their severity.[5]

When in 1893 an outbreak in Asia spread to Russia, then to western Europe, Congress passed the Act of February 15, 1893. It authorized the detailing of medical officers to the offices of the United States Consuls to enforce Treasury regulations relating to vessels, their cargoes, passengers, and crews. These medical officers were sent to fourteen principal ports of Europe. The policy was generally credited with having prevented an epidemic in the United States in 1893 (letter from Surgeon-General Walter Wyman, September 5, 1905 to the secretary of the treasury, in NARA, RG90, File 397, Box 053).

After the disease was understood, the public health service (then still called the U.S. Marine Hospital Service) took measures to establish, in effect, an early warning system regarding epidemic outbreaks so that corrective measures could be put in place. Consular clerks in foreign cities from which immigrants came were instructed to alert the secretary of state and the surgeon general's office of any such outbreak or suspected epidemic of cholera. In 1902, for instance, consular clerk George Murphy reported a cholera outbreak in Posen in August, with twenty-four severe cases and spreading rapidly. In August, cholera broke out in Manila. There J. G. Perry, the chief quarantine officer for the islands, noted 143 cases and 122 deaths in Manila—and in provincial towns 2,111 cases and 1,336 deaths. From August 3 to August 9, he reported another 181 cases with 137 deaths in Manila and 2,302 cases and 1,701 deaths in provincial towns (RG 90, File 397, Box 052).

Subsequent reports from Manila put total cases at 3,225, resulting in 1,977 deaths in Manila and 19,444 cases and 11,691 deaths in the provinces. Perry was sent to Hong Kong to monitor reported outbreaks of both cholera and bubonic plague there. His reports led Assistant Surgeon-General J. W. Kerr of the U.S. M.H.S. to order that all vessels headed for the United States be quarantined for 5 days, that all water be boiled, and that crews not be allowed to go ashore—and, moreover, that Chinese food for crews on all such vessels be destroyed and the crew members disinfected, that water in the water tanks be boiled, and that the decks be washed down with a solution of bichloride (RG 90, File 397, Box 053).

In August, cholera outbreaks were reported in Bremen, in Cairo, Egypt (with over 1,800 cases and nearly 1,500 deaths), in Japan (thousands), in China (10,000 victims, with 3,000 dead), and others in Naples, Italy, and Batavia, Java (Ibid.).

In 1904, similar reports were filed from Batum, Russia, and Teheran, Persia, where the American vice consul general noted that death rates were very high. Restrictions on ships from those ports were immediately ordered. In 1904, Egypt suffered an outbreak, as did Baghdad, Iraq, where thousands of cases and hundreds of deaths were reported. In Russia, the epidemic was especially severe. Hamburg ordered the quarantine against all emigrants from Russia in 1905. The Cunard

Steamship Lines wrote a letter to the U.S. Department of State in September, 1905, noting that all Russian emigrants were being detained for five days under strict medical inspection and that such measures were being enforced at Cunard Line operations in the ports of Liverpool, Southampton, Hamburg, Bremen, Antwerp, Rotterdam, and Havre. Passed Assistant Surgeon A. J. McLaughlin, stationed in Naples, was sent to Hamburg to investigate the situation. By June 1906, the special cholera restrictions were removed. In January 1908, the consulate general in Berlin, Germany, lifted the restrictions requiring that all Russian emigrants be disinfected and bathed, and the quarantine restrictions were removed for the ports of Hamburg, Bremen, Rotterdam, Antwerp, Liverpool, Hull, Southampton, Glasgow, and other English ports of embarkation (File 8143, dated January 17, 1908). Despite that lifting of restrictions, the quarantine station at Staten Island, New York, declined to take any steps to remove restrictions it was enforcing against Russian immigrants.

Another outbreak of cholera hit Manila in 1908, but it was quickly eradicated from the lessons learned in how to disinfect for *Cholera bacilli*. The U.S. M.H.S. led a campaign in September to disinfect water closets where the bacilli were spread. Disinfecting squads totaling 600 men were put to work immediately for the exclusive duty of disinfecting closets. They used 150,000 pounds of lime per day and 700 gallons of carbolic acid daily, or its equivalent in creolin, tricresol, or formalin. More than 4,000 gallons of Jeyes fluid secured from Hong Kong and Japan were spread, using ordinary street pumping water wagons converted into disinfecting wagons. A report on the campaign in Manila noted that ordinary chemical fire engines made excellent disinfecting apparatus (Cholera report, J. C. Perry, Folder 397, Box 53). They used eighty-gallon tanks charged by CO_2 to spread a mixture of bicarbonate of soda and sulfuric acid, which made an efficient disinfection solution. The Manila campaign used eleven such wagons. The report noted four things of prime importance for the suppression of cholera:

1. Good water supply for all the people
2. Safe disposal of defecations
3. Prompt discovery of cholera cases, suspects, or bacilli carriers with immediate isolation and disinfection
4. Habits of cleanliness (the report noted related bacilli carriers to be eradicated: flies, cockroaches, and other insects or animals having access to the stools of infected persons, then carrying the infection to food and drink) (File 397, Box 053)

The 1902 cholera outbreak in the Philippines was extensive. Perry noted in a letter dated August 19, 1902, there were 522 cases resulting in 272 deaths, and in the report dated August 2, 1902, wherein the official reported cases totaled 2,545 cases with 1,877 deaths, Perry estimated the total number of cases in the provinces at 15,555 with 11,691 deaths and 3,225 cases in Manila alone.

In October 1909, cholera broke out in Rotterdam. Assistant Surgeon R. A. C. Wollenberg was sent from Naples to Rotterdam to monitor the episode. He cabled New York to alert the city to the vessel *Cheyenne* bound for New York, which had two suspected cases of the disease on board.

In December 1910, H. D. Geddings, posted in Naples, Italy, worked with his British counterpart, Consul Churchill, to monitor the health situation in Italy. They expressed a deep lack of confidence in Italian medical authorities' accurately reporting cases (File 397, Box 053). December 1910 saw outbreaks of cholera in St. Petersburg, Russia, and Yokohama, Japan. By mid-December, the quarantine station at Grosse Isle, received its first suspected cholera carriers from Russia, as well as reports of Asiatic cholera outbreaks in Madeira, and Lisbon, Portugal. These were passed on to the United States. Reports in December were also received regarding outbreaks in Japan and in Turkey.

In 1911, Surgeon Geddings, at Naples, confirmed outbreaks of cholera in Naples and in south Italy more generally. The director of the Municipal Laboratory in Quebec, Canada, Dr. Vallee, reported cholera carrier cases from Russia, as did reports from Norway. In April 1911, the Honolulu station reported cases and some deaths and elaborated on measures being taken to deal with the outbreak (Ibid., Box 955). In May, Honolulu reported on the outbreak in extensive detail in hundreds of pages describing the cases and the disinfecting measures being taken. On May 29, 1911, Dr. Vallee, at Grosse Isle, Quebec, reported that the tenth exam for bacilli among carriers quarantined at the station found no evidence of cholera using refined new tests (Box 055).

September 1911 saw confirmed reports of outbreaks in Naples, Italy, with 664 cases and 280 deaths, as well as cholera in Europe—in Austria/Hungary, Italy, Russia, Rumania, and Turkey. Havana, Cuba, reported cases aboard a ship arriving from Spain with some deaths on board. Egypt reported cases in late September 1911. In August, a full report from Naples noted 1,691 cases and 659 deaths, and from Russia, a report noted eighty-four cases and fifty-four deaths (Box 056).

In 1912, cases were reported in Shanghai, China, with numerous cases and deaths, and the consul's office suspected many more cases and deaths than were being reported. Outbreaks occurred in Tobago, near Trinidad in the British West Indies, and vessels from Messina and Genoa were quarantined in June, 1912. Cagliari and Sardinia, Italy, had outbreaks. By February 1912, ports from which cholera outbreaks requiring passengers from eastern Russia be quarantined included ports in France and Norway (Ibid., Box 057). British ports detained for five days all persons, foodstuffs, and baggage of emigrants from Russia.

In October r 1916, the station at Angel Island in San Francisco sent an elaborate report on the steps being taken to deal with possible cholera carriers from China and Japan.[6] In November, the Surgeon-General received an extensive report from Vancouver, British Columbia, on procedures for inspection, disinfection, and treatment of detainees at the quarantine station at Williamshead, British Columbia (the Canadian Pacific coast equivalent of Angel Island) and emphasizing the ability of the United States to accept their certificates of inspection as being equally as efficient as those used in the United States (File 397, Box 057).

In December 1919, the Department of State posted reports of cholera in Korea, in Vladivostok, in Poland, in China, and in Singapore (Box 057). Similar sporadic reports continued to come in to the surgeon general's office throughout 1921–1923 regarding cholera outbreaks in Italy, Korea, Poland, China, Japan, Baghdad, Teheran, and Russia. These reports served as an early warning system for increased vigilance and inspection of ships, passengers, and crews from any port where cholera was suspected or confirmed. The surgeon general's office stressed the need of screening returning U.S. military servicemen who had been posted in those countries to guard against their bringing in cases of cholera, typhus, and plague.

Plague

Plague was the classic pandemic of the fourteenth century. Its first outbreak has been attributed to 1338 near Genoa, Italy. Others put it in Sicily in October 1347. Nearly all agree the massive pandemic that ensued killed an estimated 30–40 percent of the European population of the time (see Hayes, 1998: 37; Kelly, 2005: 18–19; Nohl, 1960). It was called the Black Death. "[W]ith an estimated mortality rate of 90 percent, the Black Death was the greatest calamity in recorded history" (Nohl, 1960: v). Nohl describes the pandemic in sweeping and stark terms:

No greater calamity has ever fallen on Mankind. In the next fifty years, the Black Death killed more than one-third of the total population of Europe! Outbreaks of the plague were recorded in Russia, Italy, Germany, England and France over five centuries. At the height on one epidemic, more than

200,000 market towns in Europe were completely depopulated. . . . Today the plague is virtually unknown. But for 500 years it stalked the world, and its influence may be seen in politics, religion, folklore, economics, music, and art. (Nohl, 2006: i)

Plague is caused by the microorganism *Yersinia pestis* (formerly known as *Pasteurella pestis*), a parasite found in various burrowing rodents and typically carried from rodent to rodent by fleas, which bite infected rodents and carry the bacteria to other rodents. Plague carriers include marmots, ground squirrels, prairie dogs, and especially the black rat (*Rattus rattus*), the urban rat most at home in human dwellings. A number of diseases are transmitted to humans by vermin: schistosomiasis via snails, typhus by fleas and lice, plague by rats (see, for example, Oldstone, 1998; Rosenberg, 1992).

Plague is among the slowest-moving of wandering diseases. Whereas strains of influenza can travel around the world in a year or two, *Yersinia pestis* can take decades to unfold. The rodent flea is the original host. When the rodent host dies, the flea hops to a new host, transferring the plague bacillus. It infects the new host by a skin bite. Humans get infected by one of many flea species that prey on wild rodents, but most often by the black rat flea, *Xenopsylla cheopis*. Plague jumps from rat to man in desperation. As the plague kills off the local rat community, the flea's alternatives are starvation or *Homo sapiens*. After becoming embedded in a human population, the rat flea becomes a very effective vector. *Xeno-pyslla cheopis* can survive up to six weeks without a host, so it can travel hundreds of miles in grain or cloth shipments—hence the concern over disinfecting shipments of rags so common in the nineteenth century. It is an efficient vector because the infected flea builds up plague bacilli in its foregut, producing a blockage. The blockage slows nutrients to the flea's stomach, making it exceedingly hungry. When the flea finds a new host and bites, the plague in the foregut quickly passes to the new host in large numbers, hastening onset of the disease (Davis: 47). McNeill describes the role of the carriers:

Typhus is a particularly instructive case. The same or closely similar strains of the rickettsial organism responsible for typhus inhabit certain species of ticks in a stable fashion, i.e., pass from generation to generation with no apparent ill effect upon the tick or the parasite. Rats and their fleas, however, react to typhus infection by recovering, i.e., they reject the invading organism from their systems after a period of illness. When, however, typhus parasites transfer their activity to human lice and to human bodies, the result is lethal to the louse and often lethal to the person. Such a pattern suggests successive transfers, from a stable co-existence with ticks to a less stable adjustment to rats and rat fleas, to a highly unstable and presumably, therefore, recent transfer to humans and to human lice. (31)

Yersinia pestis is an effective killer, slaughtering nearly anything put in front of it: humans, rats, gerbils, squirrels, prairie dogs, camels, chickens, pigs, dogs, cats, and so on. It is a major pathogen precisely because it is such an adaptable killer. It can be transmitted by thirty-one different flea species, including *Xenopyslla cheopis*, the most efficient vector in the human plague (Rosenberg, 1992; LeMay, ed., 2013, vol. 2: 62).

Vermin carriers of disease to humans are called vectors. When a flea transmits the microorganism to humans, bubonic plague results. Bubonic plague depends on having a continuing source of infected rodents during which humans accidentally get in the path of the rodent–flea–rodent transmission. Some scholars, therefore, argued that bubonic plague is an unlikely candidate for human epidemics on a pandemic scale. Plague, however, may pass from one human to another by the human flea, *Pulex irritans*. This makes the spread of bubonic plague possible without the constant rodent reservoir. All scholars agree that the pneumonic form of plague requires no vector, which results when the *Yersinia pestis* settles in the lungs, whence it spreads by drops of saliva that enter into the respiratory tracts of others. Pneumonic plague was almost certainly the important element in the great pandemic of 1347–1350. Its very fatality, however, as Hayes (1996) notes, lessens its diffusive power, for so many of its victims perish before they can travel far or contact many others (38).

Bubonic plague takes its name for its manifestation in buboes, the large, hard, painful swellings in the groin, armpit, or neck formed when the infection reached the lymphatic system. Headaches, blackouts, and serious digestive disorders follow. Death typically occurs within a week of onset. When the microorganism causes blood poisoning, it is called septacemic plague. Of those infected with bubonic plague, 60–80 percent died within a month. Pneumonic plague is even more terrifying. When untreated with antibiotics, it is nearly always fatal, with fever, coughing, and progressive asphyxiation following the initial infection and death occurring in two to three days.

Survivors of the plague pandemics of the fourteenth century invented the term Black Death for the epidemic. Historians conjecture they may have had in mind the dark blotches on the skin from hemorrhaging. Others conjecture that a "black death" was the only term adequate to picture so calamitous an event (Moote and Moote: 7, 272–273).

Plague-carrying fleas find ideal conditions in terms of temperature and humidity within the burrows of rodent colonies and in human clothing and bedding. Infected colonies may persist in one territory for years and through all seasons. Whereas rodents transfer from one territory to another very slowly, fleas conveyed by human traffic may transmit the disease over considerable distances. Grain mills probably played an important transmission role, being sites where rats gathered and where human traffic originated. The European black rat, *Rattus rattus*, is exceptionally companionable with humans and their dwellings. During the nineteenth century, the population of black rats exploded, as did that of human cities.

Progress in the battle against the plague leaped forward in the late 1800s when the germ theory of disease was proven and when scientists began to identify the bacilli of various diseases. The first breakthrough came in the mid-1850s when a French professor of chemistry, Louis Pasteur, stumbled upon the realm of bacteriology. From the spoilage of beer and wine, Pasteur was led to disease-producing organisms in animals and humans, including anthrax, chicken cholera, and rabies. In 1885, he produced a preventative vaccine for rabies, and in 1889, he established the Pasteur Institute in Paris.

Robert Koch, a German country doctor two decades younger than Pasteur, set up a laboratory in a friend's garden shed. In 1876, his findings on the life cycle of the anthrax bacillus were published. He refined techniques to identify bacilli and by 1880 was attracting young assistants from around the globe. Koch and his associates identified the bacilli that caused tuberculosis and cholera, and soon medical scientists had identified the pathogens for anthrax, cholera, diphtheria, leprosy, malaria, pneumonia, strep sore throat, tetanus, tuberculosis, and typhoid, leading the way to new therapies and eventually the wonder drugs of the twentieth century. New and refined bacteriological techniques led to the discovery, between 1880 and 1900, of twenty-one organisms that caused specific human diseases: typhoid, typhus, and malaria in 1880, tuberculosis in 1882, cholera in 1883, tetanus and diphtheria in 1884, salmonella in 1885, influenza in 1892, plague in 1894, botulism in 1896, whooping cough in 1896, and dysentery in 1898.

In 1894, during an outbreak of the plague in China, two biologists, one Japanese and one French, studied the disease and identified the plague bacillus. Although little awareness occurred at the time, they noted a suspected linkage to rat fleas. In 1885, the San Francisco Board of Health formed an ad hoc committee of physicians and prominent businessmen to investigate conditions in Chinatown in the wake of a devastating epidemic of smallpox that issued an unequivocally damning report (Craddock: 2, 127; this section is drawn from Craddock). Cultural differences between

Chinese immigrants and the Euro-American native stock contributed to racial attitudes that influenced the report and, as we will see, efforts to deal with epidemic outbreaks (tuberculosis, smallpox, and plague). David Rosner notes: "Disease intensifies the rhetoric of hatred, fear, and blame utilized against undesirable populations" (1995: 4).

Plague arrived in San Francisco in March 1900. The first fatality from it was a Chinese resident of San Francisco, whose corpse was discovered in the basement of the Globe Hotel. The San Francisco city bacteriologist, Dr. Wilfred Kellogg, suspected plague because of the appearance of the corpse. He took samples from the lymph glands and brought them to the laboratory of the U.S. Marine Hospital Service facility located on Angel Island, directed by Dr. Joseph Kinyoun., who confirmed plague. An epidemic ensued that did not end until 1904. The initial outbreak had 124 confirmed cases (there were likely many more unconfirmed) and 112 deaths, most of them among the Chinese.

Dr. Kinyoun had been sent to Angel Island by Dr. Walter Wyman, surgeon general of the Marine Hospital Service. As bacteriology expanded its knowledge of disease, Dr. Wyman and others used medical science and laboratory procedures to manage epidemic outbreaks. Although the plague bacillus had been identified, how it was propagated was little understood. The bacillus was thought to be transmitted through the air into the lungs or into the stomach. Craddock notes that the rat was known to have some connection with plague, but its critical role in harboring plague-infested fleas that in turn bit humans was not known until the research and campaign conducted to cope with the 1900 epidemic in San Francisco (127).

Dr. Kinyoun initially led the campaign against the plague outbreak. He imposed strict quarantines on Chinatown. Moving the residents of Chinatown was seriously considered by Kinyoun, and after exploring several sites, he concluded that Angel Island would likely be best for transporting Chinese having or suspected of having the plague. Kinyoun's worst-case scenario of the epidemic's spread projected the potential movement of thousands of Chinese to be accommodated on the island. Kinyoun's diagnosis of the plague, and especially of the quarantine he imposed, soon raised fears and opposition to his plan. Some said Kinyoun's real plan was to move the Chinese to the island while Chinatown was burned to the ground and rebuilt (McClain: 447–470). As McClain describes it:

> By June, 1900, the board of health was making plans to evacuate fifteen hundred Chinese to Mission Rock, having received permission from the California Dry Dock Company to use its docking facility on the island. Discussions were still underway to get permission from the federal government to vacate a much larger number of Chinese to Angel Island. (135)

Opposition to Dr. Kinyoun soon led his political opponents to pressure for his removal. Surgeon-General Wyman responded and transferred Dr. Kinyoun. He replaced him with Dr. Rupert Blue. Although Blue was not nearly the scientist that Kinyoun was, he was certainly more diplomatic in dealing with the Chinese and with the local business and political community. More important, reports coming in on the suspected role the rat played in transmission of the disease gave Dr. Blue insight that led him to focus on eradication of the rats rather than on an oppressive quarantine of the Chinese. He was helped by the fact that by the time he took over the campaign against the plague epidemic in San Francisco, cases of non-Chinese residents had developed, and its spread convinced all that they were, in fact, dealing with the plague. His efforts to eradicate the rats of the city took a few years but ultimately turned the tide on the outbreak, and he was hailed the hero of the day, going on to become surgeon general. His report on the rat eradication program was published by the service, and his procedures soon spread to other cities (for various but generally favorable views of Blue and his role in the epidemic, see Chase, 2004; Craddock, 2000; Hirst, 1953, and Shah, 2001; and RG 90, File 5608, Box 627).

By 1908–1909, when a severe outbreak struck Honolulu, the Marine Hospital Service contracted to clear rats and mice from various government buildings, and the fumigation contracts killed nearly 1,000 rats (File 544, Box 065). The service soon required reports from many stations, and cables and reports in the hundreds came in detailing rat-proofing and rat destruction in various ports. Numbers of rats trapped, found dead, numbers of traps set daily, the number of rats examined and the numbers infected and the hundreds of extermination efforts filled these reports. All major ports sending ships to the United States from Europe, Asia, Africa, and South America were asked to make such rat reports. Cabled reports from steamship line companies soon became routine as well. They reported on the number of vessels fumigated, especially in rat- and plague-infested ports. By 1912–1914, reports on devices to better trap rats and on more effective trap guards on ships and ship cables (so that rats could not debark into a new port) became routine and were widely circulated by the service. From 1909 to 1923, the service conducted an ongoing warehouse rat control program in port cities (File 544, Boxes 066–067).

Between 1880 and 1900, the mystery of the etiology of such perennial killers as typhoid, tuberculosis, cholera, malaria, leprosy, tetanus, and plague yielded to the probing intelligence of the new science of bacteriology. The recognition of carrier states in cholera, diphtheria, and typhoid as well as the discovery of insect and animal vectors in plague, malaria, and yellow fever rounded out the germ theory of disease and gave physicians and public health workers a vastly improved position in the battle against disease. (Mullan: 32)

It made lesser strides, however, in understanding the etiology of virus-caused disease, such as influenza.

Influenza

The pandemic disease of the twentieth century was influenza, its status confirmed by one pandemic outbreak of the disease—the 1918–1919 pandemic commonly, though erroneously, known as the Spanish flu. In the succinct words of Kolata:

> The 1918 flu epidemic puts every other epidemic of the century to shame. It was a plague so deadly that if a similar virus were to strike today it would kill more people in a single year than heart disease, cancer, strokes, chronic pulmonary disease, AIDS, and Alzheimer's disease combined. The epidemic affected the course of history and was a terrifying presence at the end of World War I, killing more Americans in a single year than died in battle in W. W. I, W.W. II, the Korean War, and the Vietnam War. (ix–x; see also 38)

The pandemic struck in three waves. The first, a less deadly outbreak, occurred in spring 1918 and spread mostly among military camps. It was not immediately identified as a deadly epidemic, seeming like just another outbreak of the flu. The second wave was the truly devastating one, occurring in fall 1918. The third assault broke out in spring 1919. This last wave was more severe than the first, but not as deadly as the second (Davies: 47). This particular pandemic is officially estimated to have claimed 20–50 million lives worldwide, and some scholars believe that it may have killed closer to 100 million (see, for example, Barry: 4; Davies: 48; and Kolata: 7). In the United States alone, 500,000 to 650,000 people perished.[7] It killed more people in one year than have died from the HIV pandemic in two decades. In 1918, in India, perhaps as many as 17 million died. The epidemic in India took more lives in October 1918 (during its second wave) than had been lost to cholera in twenty years' time.

> The virus is the only known life-form that does not eat, drink, breathe, or produce waste. Viruses cannot reproduce or travel by themselves. They must be forcibly sent from one victim to another. . . . The flu virus travels in droplets of mucus that come from the throats and noses of infected people. Influenza

is usually innocuous, coming around every winter, endemic to an area. Most people come down with it and suffer a week or so of misery. Crosby notes that it seems unavoidable. Since it is spread through the air, there is little that can be done to prevent it. Perhaps because the flu is so familiar, its terrors in 1918 were all the more dreadful. It is like a macabre science fiction tale in which the mundane becomes the monstrous. (Kolata: 6)

The 1918 strain was especially mysterious in that it reacted in ways different from previous experiences with the flu virus. Influenza has been around for centuries. In 1580, a pandemic of the disease began in Asia and spread throughout Europe, Africa, and America. It nearly wiped out entire villages in Spain and Italy. Similar outbreaks have occurred in every century since then, though none with as devastating a result as the 1918 strain (Getz: 4). One anomaly of the 1918 strain was that it killed young, healthy adults at far higher rates than ever before (or since) seen. Most influenza viruses are more life-threatening to infants and very old people who are already ill. In the past, and really in outbreaks of influenza since the 1918 strain, young adults and children tended to quickly get over the flu. They are less likely to contract it, and they experience lower mortality rates. By contrast, the 1918 flu's most likely victims to die were young adults aged 20–40 (Dr. Jeffrey Taubenberger, cited in Getz: 4). Kolata documents that the death curve for the second wave outbreak was W-shaped, with peaks for babies and toddlers younger than 5, the elderly aged 70–74, and the largest-middle part of the curve people aged 20–40 (5).

Another anomaly of the 1918 strain was its far higher morbidity rates. In the October 1918, wave an estimated 20–25 percent of the population contracted the disease, and in a third to half of the cases, it was fatal (File 3655, Box 363). In his definitive study of the pandemic, John Barry estimates that 8–10 percent of all young adults than living may have been killed by the virus (4). The 1918 strain was twenty-five times more deadly than ordinary influenzas (Kolata: 7). This strain had a much higher morbidity rate as well. An estimated one-fifth of the world's population contracted the illness during the 1918–1919 pandemic, including 28 percent of Americans. So many lives were taken by the epidemic that the average life-span in the United States fell by twelve years in 1918. "In 1918, there was little anybody could do. There were no medicines and no medical treatments that could stop what many soldiers had begun calling "the Purple Death" (Getz: 7). Barry notes that another anomaly was its ferocity and speed:

Although the influenza pandemic stretched over two years, perhaps two-thirds of the deaths occurred in a period of twenty-four weeks, and more than half of those deaths occurred in even less time, from mid-September to early December 1918. Influenza killed more people in a year than the Black Death of the Middle Ages killed in a century; it killed more people in twenty-four weeks than AIDS has killed in twenty-four years. (5)

In Augusta, Georgia, at Camp Hancock, by early October there were 3,000 cases, and doctors noted incubation rates as short as *six* hours (File 1622, Box 144)! In El Paso, Texas, and Charlotte, North Carolina (Camp Greene), so many cases broke out that temporary hospitals had to be set up in public schools, with school teachers serving as nurses, cooks, and clerks. By October 28, Charlotte reported 2,600 cases and sixty-five deaths. The surgeon general's office sent out letters to army posts to counter rumors that whiskey would prevent influenza. These alerts countered the rumors with the fact that alcohol did not prevent, and might even hasten, suscep-tibility. In a letter dated November 10, 1918, the office had to counter even silly reports—e.g. the "Connection of Epidemic of Influenza with the Motion of the Planet Jupiter" or that the epidemic was the work of "Huns" (i.e., Germans spreading the disease).[8]

In mid-November 1918, the Metropolitan Life Insurance Company sent letters to the surgeon general's office offering to support a national confer-ence of statisticians (which it did) to develop methods to establish uniform reports on the vital statistics (age, sex, race, etc.) of persons who were taken ill, of mortality rates, and so on. Surgeon-General Rupert Blue issued a report dated November 8, 1918, stating that the influenza outset had been in Europe (hence "the Spanish flu") and noting that pandemic procedures were being put in place to guard against its spread. These procedures were those used against cholera, the plague, yellow fever, and typhus fever. The first recognized outbreaks of what was by then actually the second wave in the United States were in Boston and Philadelphia, and from there it spread throughout Massachusetts, then along the Atlantic seaboard. It quickly threatened war production of munitions, the mining of war-related ores, and shipbuilding.

On October 1, 1918, Congress granted $1,000,000 to the Public Health Service to combat "the Spanish Influenza" after it spread to New York, New Orleans, and Mobile. In the ensuring months, the service assigned a third of its commissioned officers to the battle and hired more than 2,000 doctors, nurses, and clerks to influenza duty. But the disease seemed impervious to their efforts. According to Mullan, the epidemic struck an estimated 5 million Americans, leaving 500,000 dead (74–75).

Epidemiologists now believe the disease actually began in Haskell County, Kansas. It traveled east to a huge army base, and from there to Europe. The first epidemic-level outbreak of the disease struck Camp

Funston in March 1918, whence it quickly spread to military camps all over (Getz: 14; Barry: 92). Some of the military camps, assembling soldiers to be sent to Europe to fight in World War I, had morbidity rates as high as 90 percent (File 1622, Box 144). Infected American troops brought it to Europe. It was called the Spanish flu because in the United States, France, Great Britain, and Germany, strict censorship was imposed during World War I, and the outbreak of the disease among troops and then civilian populations in those countries was censored. Spain was officially neutral and had no censorship. When the epidemic broke out there (brought in by U.S. military troops in transit to the front), Spanish newspapers reported widely on the strange new disease that seemed like no other flu before in its swift spread and high mortality rate. Because Spanish newspapers were the first to report on it, it became known as the Spanish flu.

In Europe the disease had been labeled the Spanish Influenza, and from that beleaguered continent the germ spread to every part of the world. In a short period of time, twenty million people succumbed to the dread disease. . . . By the time peace negotiations commenced in November 1918, every state in the U.S. had been invaded by the epidemic. In fact, more than ten times as many Americans were killed by the disease as were killed by German bombs and bullets during World War I. In the nation's cities, the disease struck quickly. In a week in October, 4,500 died in Philadelphia, and 3,200 died in Chicago. (Luckingham: 1; Surgeon-General Rupert Blue Report, November 8, 1918, File 1622, Box 144)

From Europe it spread eastward and westward until it covered the globe. By October 1918, it was everywhere in Europe and North America, as well as in many parts of South America. By November it was in India, China, Persia, and South Africa. By late November, it ravaged the islands of the South Sea and pierced deep into the heart of Africa. By January, it invaded Australia.

The disease was mysterious and dreadful in its virulence. At the time, nobody knew where it came from or how it was communicated. In Nashville, Tennessee, 40,000 people contracted it between late September and the end of October, of whom 15,000 died. In New York City, in the 1918 outbreak, 800 people a day were dying, and the city lost more than 19,000 to the disease from October to December. In its initial month of outbreak in New York (October), 4,925 cases were reported, and 200 died. In Philadelphia that month, it killed 700 in the first week, 2,600 in the second week, and 4,500 in the third (Luckingham: 3–5; Getz: 17–20). During the second wave outbreak in the United States, in fall 1918, an estimated third of the population was infected. There were massive shortages of medical care of all kinds, of coffins, undertakers, and gravediggers. In Philadelphia, 200 bodies were crowded into a morgue built for thirty-six. A street railway repair shops was turned into a coffin manufactory. In New York, street cleaners were assigned to the city's cemeteries to help dig graves (Geddes Smith: 28–29).

The second wave in the United States saw it move from east to west in a pattern akin to the pioneers. Although the disease arrived later and ended later in the cities of the U.S. West, it was no less devastating. In Denver and Seattle, Los Angeles and San Francisco, city officials tried every technique, procedure, and remedy that had been used in eastern cities (and recommended in the Rupert Blue Report of November 8) in a futile effort to slow the advance of the deadly malady. In San Francisco, for example, there were 50,000 reported cases and 3,500 deaths from the disease. It seemed to move from the east coast to the west coast, spreading first to military camps and then to cities near them. In West Point, the college and army barracks reported that 90 percent of the troops contracted it and 19 percent died; in the civilian population, 20 percent had influenza, and about half of cases proved fatal (report of October 22, 1918, File 1622, Box 144).

What accounts for the extraordinarily high rates of morbidity and mortality of the influenza pandemic of 1918–1919? Two variables seem critical, one natural, one manmade. The natural variable has to do with the adaptability of the flu virus and its capacity and tendency to mutate. The manmade variable has to do with the policies and procedures associated with the exigencies of a global war and the lack of understanding, at the time, of the nature of viruses.

Among infectious diseases, influenza seems special for causing pandemics because it is transmitted so effectively that it spreads virtually unabated until it exhausts the supply of susceptible hosts. Influenza viruses, moreover, mutate constantly. There are three basic types of viruses: A, B, and C. Only influenza virus A causes epidemics and pandemics (Barry: 101–102). Most mutations are minor, and the immune system recognizes the invading virus, bonds to them, and overcomes them before they become lethal. Sometimes, the mutation causes what is known as antigen drift. When this happens, the mutated virus is not quickly recognized by the immune system. The invading virus can take a foothold even in people whose immune systems are loaded with antibodies for flu but whose antibodies are shaped to bind with older version of the virus. Antigen drift can create epidemics, Barry notes:

One study found nineteen discrete, identifiable epidemics in the United States in a thirty-three year period—more than one every other year. Each one caused between ten thousand and forty thousand "excess deaths" in the United States alone—an excess over and above the death toll usually caused by the disease. As a result, influenza kills more people in the United States than any other infectious disease, including AIDS. (110)

Pandemics develop when the mutation involves an antigen change so radical that the shape of the new antigen bears little resemblance to the old. This is called "antigen shift." With antigen shift, the immune system does not recognize the virus at all. The human population is essentially "virgin territory" to the newly mutated virus. In 1847–1848 in London, more people died from influenza than during the great cholera epidemic of 1832. In 1889–1890, influenza struck again, although not as deadly as it did in 1918. We now understand that each of these was caused by an antigen shift.

> When even normally mild diseases such as whooping cough, chicken pox, and mumps invade a "virgin" human population, a population not previously exposed to them, they often kill in large numbers, and young adults are especially vulnerable. In the Franco–Prussian War in 1871, 40 percent of those who contracted measles died. . . . in 1911 a measles epidemic in the U.S. army killed 5 percent of all the men who caught it. (Barry: 136)

Measles became deadly because of a complication of the disease—pneumonia. From September 1917 to March 1918, as the country built up for war, 30,784 soldiers became ill of measles at Camp Shelby, and 5,741 of them died of pneumonia subsequent to measles. A staggering 46.5 percent of *all deaths* at the camp—those from all diseases, car wrecks, work accidents, and so on—were from pneumonia brought on by measles. In 1918, pneumonia was the leading cause of death around the world—greater than tuberculosis, greater than cancer, greater than heart disease, greater than the plague. Like measles, when influenza kills, it usually does so through pneumonia (Barry: 151). In 1918, when the swine flu jumped from animals to humans and then mutated to infecting its new hosts, it turned lethal. The large army encampments became virtual "killing fields" for the disease. As soldiers spread from camp to camp, from America to France, the mutated flu virus kept finding virgin hosts, and pandemic ensued.

The second variable—the exigencies of a worldwide war—enabled that spread. During the first wave of the disease, its lethal nature was not recognized. War policy dictated sending millions of men to military camps, even after epidemic disease broke out, because of the need for troops to be trained for war and pressure to send more and more troops to the battlefields. The truly global scope of the war and the transportation of troops and supplies spread the infection on an unprecedented scale and speed.

The state of war necessitated and justified censorship of the press as never before, something condoned or supported by the population and the media itself. News of the disease and the extensiveness of its outbreak were suppressed. The wartime administration, the medical profession, and even the military medical profession simply did not understand the nature of the medical threat, so they were slow to respond. The lack of knowledge about viral disease and how it spread (by air) contributed to the slowness in developing protocols. The medical weapons that worked against bacterial diseases, serums and vaccines, were powerless against the new virus (the best discussion is in Barry, 2005; and Crosby, 1989 and, for the failure of sera tried unsuccessfully, RG 90, File 3655, Box 363).

The American Expeditionary Force jammed millions of men into extraordinarily tight quarters. War production needs drew millions to the factories in cities where density increased the pool of virgin hosts. They worked in shifts, for long hours, where people shared beds, cups, knives, forks, and the like with strangers. This wartime effect enabled the pandemic to develop and spread on an unprecedented scale. The very regimentation of society (in America, in Britain, in Canada, in France, in Germany) meant that the populace bore the hardships of war—including epidemic disease outbreaks—with astounding stoicism. When in June 1918 the British freighter *City of Exeter* docked in Philadelphia, the U.S. Public Health Service issued no orders to maritime service to hold the influenza-ridden ship in quarantine, and she was released, the troops and passengers fanning out to return home. As Barry so aptly describes it, soon from Boston to San Francisco, the lethal virus exploded with a killing rate more than double that of the serious epidemic of bubonic plague that struck San Francisco in 1900 (193).

The war made President Wilson decide to militarize the Public Health Service. Wartime needs trumped policy dictated by a medical profession researching the disease in peacetime. Supplies, troops, and people continued to be shifted about the world even after the lethal nature of the pandemic became apparent. The U.S. Public Health Service (formerly the U.S. M.H.S.) entered into contracts with a host of companies and laboratories to develop and supply various serums. The U.S. Army even developed its own manufacturing capability for diphtheria antitoxin, for typhoid serum, for smallpox vaccines, for meningitis serum, for tetanus serum, for tuberculosis serum, and for salvarsan (a treatment for syphilis). The service inspected horses and barns used in the manufacturing of virosi serums and bacterial toxins and sent these various sera in large quantities to the various army camps throughout the 1918–1919 pandemic, largely to no avail. In 1917–1920 it developed and supplied huge quantities of anti-pneumonococcus serum, anti-rabies treatments, anti-smallpox and anti-typhoid vaccines, and so on (Barry: 86; Duffy, 1974; Fee, 1987; Hirst, 1953; Ravenel, 1921; and Winslow, 1923).

Trachoma

The final disease to be discussed here is one that pales in comparison to the deadly influenza pandemic. Trachoma is non-deadly, but it is a highly contagious infection of the conjunctiva and cornea. Caused by the bacterium *chlamydia trachomatis*, if untreated, trachoma results in chronic scarring and blindness. It has an incubation period of five to twelve days. It begins slowly as conjunctivitis (an irritation near the eye, also known as pink-eye). As it advances, the eyelids are severely irritated and the eyelashes may turn in and rub against the cornea, causing eye ulcers, further scarring, and visual loss.

The disease is one of the earliest recorded eye diseases, identified as early as the twenty-seventh century B.C. It is the leading cause of blindness worldwide, having afflicted over 400 million people in mostly underdeveloped countries in Africa, the Middle East, and Asia. It is still endemic in Africa and among aboriginal communities in Australia. The WHO estimates 84 million people in 55 countries have active trachoma.

Trachoma is preventable by adequate diet, proper sanitation, and education. It progresses through four stages: The conjunctival tissues become follicular, heal, and finally scar. The glands and ducts of the eye become affected. The upper lid turns inward, and the lashes then abrade the cornea. If untreated, corneal ulceration becomes infected and scars. Blindness results when scarring is extensive. The disease is spread by contact, often from children to the women who care for them. Women are two to four times as likely as men to contract the disease and suffer blindness as a result. Repeated episodes of reinfection within a family can cause chronic follicular or intense conjunctivitis. It can also be transmitted by flies and gnats.

The disease was once endemic in North America and Europe but has disappeared there with improvements in living standards and basic hygiene. The scarring process can be treated surgically to prevent the progression to blindness. If treated early with antibiotics (usually tetracycline drugs or sulfonamides), the prognosis is excellent. Trachoma became one of the leading diseases characterized as "loathsome and contagious" used as the medical basis to bar entrance to immigrants. This designation was frequently used at Angel Island, at Ellis Island, and at New Orleans during the period 1900–1920. In the United States, 1–4 percent of immigrants were debarred from entering for any reason. Medical reasons were the basis used to debar entrance between 1898 and 1924 8–58 percent of the time. Among those debarred for a "dangerous and loathsome disease" between 1898 and 1924, trachoma was the basis from 6 percent to as high as 86 percent of the time (LeMay, ed., 2013, vol. 2: 66; Mullan, 1989; 64–65; Parascondola, 1998: 2; RG 90, File 219, Box 38). Combating trachoma was a near crusade of the Public Health Service, particularly at Ellis Island, as Mullan notes:

> The conquest of trachoma, a chronic, debilitating and, ultimately, blinding infection of the eyes, was the chosen cause of John McMullen. A large and affable man reared in the South, McMullen was schooled in trachoma surgery— the only curative treatment at the time—on Ellis Island where he served from 1904 to 1911. McMullen began his twelve-year war on trachoma when he was sent to Kentucky in 1912 to conduct a trachoma survey in response to a request for assistance from the state. The survey showed some 8 percent of the 18,000 people examined to be infected—figures dramatic enough to warrant special language in the 1913 Federal Appropriations Act authorizing the Public Health Service to treat trachoma patients. (65)

GERM THEORY AND MEDICAL SCIENCE DEVELOPMENTS TO COPE WITH PANDEMICS

The nineteenth century was one of pandemics because the mass movement of people spread them, and medical science and public health had to catch up with the capabilities of disease to become pandemic. This closing section discusses six persons who made truly significant contributions to that catching-up. A couple of these pioneers are well known, but all played heroic roles in the war against pandemic diseases. Subsequent chapters will describe others who made their contributions in battles against particular epidemics at their quarantine stations.

The first breakthrough involved the very concept of disease—germ theory. Until late in the nineteenth century, most people, including those in the medical profession, thought of disease as an imbalance in the individual, as resulting from "miasma," a sort of putrefaction in the atmosphere, as resulting from some sort of chemical process, or simply as the effect of "filth." Many thought pandemics were the retribution of God for sin and vice and lives of debauchery. As one scholar notes:

> The idea of specific disease entities played a relatively small role in this system of ideas and behavior. Neither learned physicians nor educated laymen saw most illness as having a discrete cause and characteristic course. Not surprisingly, early nineteenth century hospital case records often failed to record a

diagnosis, for disease was seen as a general state of the organism in relation to its environment—as a disordered individual adjustment, not as a patterned and predictable response to a particular cause. (Rosenberg, 1987: 72)

Germ theory conceived of disease as an *invasion* of the body by a foreign substance:

> Simply put, the germ theory said that minute living organisms invaded the body, multiplied, and caused disease, and that a specific germ caused a specific disease. There was need for a new theory of disease as the Nineteenth Century progressed, as autopsy findings were correlated with symptoms reported during life, as organs from animals and cadavers were put under a microscope, as normal organs were compared to diseased ones, as diseases became more defined, localized and specific, scientists finally discarded the ideas of systems of illness and the humors of Hippocrates and Galen and began looking for better explanations. (Barry: 49–50)

Once proven, germ theory demonstrated a specific connection between infectious ills and particular microorganisms. It explained disease patterns already demonstrated, but little understood, by several generations of clinicians and pathologists. Germ theory changed public perceptions and attitudes toward disease and toward the medical profession. It raised expectations that laboratories could transform the shape of the everyday practice of medicine.

The "Father of Germ Theory," of bacteriology, is the French chemist Louis Pasteur. Born in 1822, Pasteur proved that most infectious diseases are caused by germs. It was among the most important breakthroughs in medical history, and his work became the foundation of microbiology and a cornerstone of modern medicine. Pasteur began his work studying diseases in silkworm, beer and wine diseases, and problems they caused in fermentation—why alcohol became contaminated during fermentation. He found each sort of fermentation is linked to a specific microorganism or ferment and that these could be studied by cultivation in a specific medium. This led to the basis of microbiology. He moved from diseases of the crops used in beer and wine processes to study diseases of animals and then man. His first breakthrough was in discovering the cause of rabies. He championed changes in hospital practices to minimize the spread of disease by microbes. Pasteur was the first to prove that weakened forms of a microbe could be used to immunize individuals against more virulent forms. He proved that rabies was transmitted by agents so small that they could not be seen even under a microscope (a virus). He developed a serum to vaccinate dogs against rabies and to treat humans bitten by rabid dogs.

Pasteur developed a process, "pasteurization," by which harmful microbes in perishable foods could be destroyed using heat, without destroying the food. He discovered that germs could live without air, leading the way to the study of germs that cause septicemia and gangrene and similar infections. He devised techniques to kill microbes and control contamination. In demonstrating how to prevent contagion and infection, his method of sterilization revolutionized surgery and obstetrics (LeMay 2013, v. 2: 54).

One of his disciples, Charles Chamberland, a French physician and bacteriologist working in the Pasteur laboratory between 1875 and 1879, demonstrated the effectiveness of an idea of British doctor Charles Bastian—sterilization. In his 1879 doctoral thesis, Chamberland researched and provided detailed diagrams for a device for the steam sterilization of surgical instruments, the steam chamber or autoclave (in French, *etuve*) which would efficiently and effectively kill microorganisms. This concept was later developed by others to engineer large steam chambers to quickly and effectively disinfect the baggage of entire shiploads of passengers.

In March 1886, Pasteur founded his institute, which became a clinic for rabies treatment, a research center for infectious diseases, and a teaching center drawing brilliant young scientists from around the world. He went on to discover three bacteria responsible for human illnesses: staphylococcus, streptococcus, and pneumonococcus. He developed vaccines against chicken cholera, anthrax, and swine erysipelas. His research techniques revolutionized medicine by using the scientific methodology of experimentation to prove concepts, ideas, and theories of disease and of medical therapies to treat them (Bynum and Bynum: 978–998).

Another pioneer of microbiology was Robert Koch, born in 1843 in Germany. He studied medicine at the University of Gottingen, where he was influenced by a professor of anatomy, Jacob Henie, who taught that infectious diseases were caused by living parasitic organisms. Koch then studied chemistry in Berlin and began practicing medicine in Hamburg, and then in Posen. He volunteered for service in the Franco–Prussian War and from 1872 to 1880 served as district medical officer for Wollstein, in which role he began his epoch-making research in scientific medicine that ultimately led to a Nobel Prize for medicine (Magill: 71–78; Fox, Maldrum, and Rezak: 312–315).

At the time of his research, anthrax was prevalent among farm animals in the region, so he began to study the disease. He made his own laboratory in his tiny four-room rented flat, where he worked using a microscope given him by his wife. The anthrax bacillus had been discovered earlier by Pollender, Rayer, and Davaine, and Koch set out to prove scientifically that the bacillus caused the disease. Using homemade slivers of wood, he inoculated mice with anthrax bacilli taken from the spleens of farm animals that had died of anthrax and found that all the inoculated mice died from the disease, whereas mice inoculated with blood from the spleen of healthy animals did not suffer from the disease. His experiments confirmed that the disease could be transmitted by means of the blood of animals suffering from it. He obtained pure cultures of the bacilli. He examined, drew, and even photographed them. He experimented to find out conditions that promoted their multiplication and conditions that were unfavorable to them. He found that they resisted certain conditions by forming spores. The spores survived the lack of oxygen, and when put in suitable conditions, the spores gave rise to the bacilli again.

His work was published in 1876 and brought him immediate fame. He refined his techniques for fixing, staining, and photographing bacteria and did other important work on the study of bacterial infections. He went on to be called "the most notable medical scientist of his time, and the Father of the Science of Bacteriology" (Fox et al: 313).

Moving to Berlin and a better laboratory, he refined his bacteriological methods and cultivated cultures on the potato and on agar kept on a flat dish invented by his colleague Petri—still in use today. He laid down the conditions for obtaining pure cultures, known as Koch's postulates. These must be satisfied before it can be accepted that a particular bacteria cause a particular disease. He identified the complete life cycle of the anthrax bacillus. As Barry notes, his 1882 discovery of the tubercle bacillus confirmed germ theory (51; see also Fox et al: 314).

Two years after arriving in Berlin, Koch discovered the tubercle bacillus, published his work on the subject in 1882. In 1883 he was sent to Egypt to lead the German Cholera Commission and discovered the cholera bacillus, a vaccine against which was developed by 1893 (Barry: 53; McNeill: 278). He proved that cholera bacteria lived in human intestines and that they were transmitted in water. He did pioneering work on immunology of diphtheria, studied malaria, blackwater fever, surra of cattle and horses, and plague. He did useful work on the control of malaria with quinine. He showed that human and bovine tuberculosis are different diseases. His discovery of the tuberculosis bacilli won him instant fame in 1882, and by 1921 an effective vaccine against it was developed, after which deaths from the disease declined dramatically. His work on typhus led to the idea—then a new one—that the disease was spread from drinking water more often than from person to person. This insight led to new control measures (decontamination). His work helped develop a vaccine against typhoid by 1896, and mass inoculation against typhoid was proven capable of checking the disease in epidemics during 1900–1910 (McNeill: 279). As

Kolata notes, his pioneering work led to dramatic drops in mortality rates of tuberculosis and measles (47). He was awarded the Nobel Prize for Medicine in 1905. He died in 1910 (http://nobelprize.org/medicine/laureates/1906/koch-bio.html; see also LeMay 2013, v. 2: 55),

Another doctor who made important contributions to modern medicine and the fight against epidemic and pandemic diseases was Edward Jenner, born in 1749 in England. His important contribution was the development of the smallpox vaccine. At age 13, Jenner was apprenticed to a doctor Daniel Ludlow, a surgeon. He overheard a young girl claim to the doctor that she could not get the dreaded disease of smallpox because she had already had another disease known as cowpox, a nondeadly disease that affected cows and the hands of the milk maids. Cowpox caused a fever and other discomforts, but its victims recovered quickly. That set Jenner on the path to study the disease. In 1770, he went to London to study medicine with an eminent surgeon, John Hunter. Dr. Jenner returned to his hometown of Berkeley, where he researched and experimented on cowpox and smallpox. In 1796, a milkmaid visited Dr. Jenner for treatment of cowpox. He tested a process he called vaccination (from the Latin word for cow, *vacca*) wherein he inoculated his gardener's son with cowpox taken from the young milkmaid. The boy suffered a mild case of cowpox but when subsequently inoculated with smallpox did not get the disease. Jenner repeated the process on twenty-three other patients, including his own son. He proved that vaccination with cowpox prevented infection by smallpox. Based on his work, a smallpox serum, a vaccine, was developed. Compulsory vaccination was used in Bavaria, Denmark, and Prussia, and the practice soon became widespread throughout Europe, but outbreaks of the disease continued to spread when unvaccinated travelers brought the disease after visiting places where smallpox was endemic. Jenner's work on vaccination of smallpox and other diseases paved the way for modern immunology. He died in 1823. Ultimately, a campaign by the World Health Organization eradicated the disease by 1980 (see LeMay 2013, v.2: 55–56 for Jenner's importance to immunization).

Similarly, Lord Joseph Lister, a British surgeon, made the important contribution of developing effective antiseptic surgery. He was influenced by the work of Louis Pasteur. He, like all the surgeons of his time, struggled with surgical sepsis. Lister developed carbolic acid sprays and compresses to combat infection during and immediately after surgery. He said of his insight: "Just as we may destroy lice on the head of a child who has pedicule, by poisonous applications which will not injure the scalp, so I believe we can use poisons on wounds to destroy bacteria without injury to the soft tissue of the patient" (cited in Nuland: 345).

Yet another pioneer was George Miller Sternberg, a hygienist and epidemiologist and surgeon-general of the United States. He was born in 1838 in New York state. He was first educated in a seminary and began teaching school in New Germantown, New Jersey. But at age 19, he began the study of medicine, first with a doctor in Cooperstown, New York, and then at the College of Physicians and Surgeons at New York City, from which he graduated in 1860. With the outbreak of the civil war, he was appointed assistant surgeon in the U.S. Army. He contracted typhoid fever in 1862 but recovered and continued his military medical service. At Fort Harker, Kansas, where he was posted, his wife died from yellow fever during an epidemic that broke out among the troops there. He went on to become post surgeon at Barrancas, Florida, during which epidemics of yellow fever flared in 1873 and 1875. He contracted the diseases there in 1875. In 1879, he was a member of the Havana yellow fever commission. In 1893, he was consulting bacteriologist to New York City, at which time he was appointed surgeon-general of the U.S. Army. He held the position until his retirement at the age limit in 1902 (Kaufman, Golishoff, and Savitts: 716–717).

Sternberg's work on the etiology of yellow fever disproved two commonly believed etiologies. He organized and appointed Major Walter Reed to head the U.S. Army Yellow Fever Commission. This commission proved that the *Stegomyia* mosquito was the true carrier of the dreaded disease. Dr. Sternberg's preliminary work and techniques overthrowing the claims of other bacteriologists led to the discovery of the specific organism causing the disease. His organization of the commission and its effective campaign were critically important to that discovery.

In 1878 he was stationed in Walla Walla, Washington, and conducted valuable experiments on the practical value of various disinfectants, using putrefactive bacteria to test germicidal activity. He later continued those experiments in Washington, D.C., and at the Johns Hopkins University Hospital under the auspices of the American Public Health Association. He received the coveted Lomb Prize in 1886. Along with Robert Koch, Dr. Sternberg was a pioneer of scientific disinfection. As surgeon-general, he established the Army Medical School. He died in 1915 (Garraty and Carnes: 1158–1159).

Dr. Walter Reed first came to medical fame as chairman of the U.S. Army Yellow Fever Commission and discoverer of the mode of propagation of the disease. He was born in 1851 in Virginia. He was educated at different private schools and then entered the University of Virginia to study medicine. He became the youngest-ever graduate of this school in 1869. He served at the Bellevue Medical College and received his M.D. there at the end of the year. In 1874, he entered the U.S. Army as an assistant surgeon. In 1889, he began pursuing medical research, attending the courses just opened at the Johns Hopkins Hospital, where the science of pathology and bacteriology, then new fields, attracted him. He published a number of research papers that brought him some attention.

In 1898, when the Spanish–American War broke out, he was appointed chairman of the commission to investigate the cause and mode of propagation of the epidemic of typhoid fever, and his report brought him further attention as a groundbreaking researcher.

In 1899, Surgeon-General Sternberg appointed him chair of the yellow fever commission. Their investigation proved that the two bacilli then thought to be the cause of the disease were not the true bacilli of the human disease (one was of the hog-cholera). In June 1900, he observed an epidemic of yellow fever at Pinar del Rio and conducted experiments that proved that the disease was not transmitted by contact or by contaminated clothing, bedding, or such like. In 1882, Dr. Carlos Finlay conjectured that the mosquito *Stegomyia fasciata* transmitted the disease from one person to another. Dr. Reed set up experiments at Camp Lazear that proved the mosquito the carrier. This established that disinfection of articles supposedly contaminated with yellow fever was unnecessary. His work demonstrated the life cycle and twelve-day incubation period of the disease. The commission report showed that the mosquito was capable of infection for at least fifty-seven days after its contamination, possibly longer

The Reed Yellow Fever Commission built on the pioneering work of Sir Ronald Ross, 1902 Nobel Laureate, who proved that the mosquito was the carrier of malaria (and yellow fever). After he proved it the vector spreading the disease, "what he now realized was that the way was clear to prevent malaria, since the anopheles mosquito bred chiefly in stagnant water. Malaria could be controlled by destroying the pools and puddles. Here was an opportunity to become a leader in a campaign to eradicate malaria" (Magill: 46).

After the commission work, Dr. Reed returned to Washington, D.C., as professor of bacteriology and clinical microscopy at the Army Medical School. He was a natural teacher, delving into little-known subjects and developing his own methods of instruction, making him a particularly attractive instructor. In 1902, Harvard University conferred an honorary degree on him, and the University of Michigan made him an LL.D. Dr. Reed investigated typhoid fever. His influence as a teacher was deep and far-reaching. He died, much revered, in 1902 (Garraty and Carnes: 1018–1020).

William Crawford Gorgas is famous as the pioneer who halted the epidemics of yellow fever and malaria and as the conqueror of the mosquito that transmitted the diseases. Born in 1854, in Mobile, Alabama, he joined the army and was appointed to the commission studying yellow fever. He was stationed in Cuba at the time and learned of the research of Cuban doctor Juan Carlos Finley, who had made the connection between mosquitoes and disease transmission. In 1898, Sir Ronald Ross, an English scientist knighted in 1911, showed that certain mosquitoes could transmit malaria to birds. His pioneering work on malaria won him the Nobel Prize in 1902 (Fox et al: 474–477). After the Reed Commission's study proved the connection between the mosquito and the transmission of yellow fever to man, Dr. Gorgas was transferred to Panama, where he implemented a far-reaching sanitation program based on Finley's and the commission's work. He realized that the best way to stop the diseases was to exterminate the mosquito that carried them. It was a Herculean task inspecting and controlling every possible breeding place in the city. Gorgas's work stopped the spread of the diseases (yellow fever and malaria) in the Isthmus of Panama and was instrumental in the construction of the Panama Canal.

Dr. Gorgas was later appointed surgeon general of the U.S. Army, and was heavily involved in the army's attempt to cope with the 1918–1919 influenza pandemic. He died in 1920.

CONCLUSION

These pioneering efforts paved the way for modern medicine, for bacteriology, and for immunology. They greatly limited the number, duration, and mortality rates of numerous pandemic diseases, particularly bacterial ones. Their work demonstrated that findings in bacteriology grew out of the research conducted in laboratories and such research was an effective investment in the war on disease. They contributed greatly to the prestige of certain research institutes and hospitals, paying great dividends on the money invested in them and on the hospitals that supported them (Rosenberg, 1987: 163; Winslow, 1971).

No less important, they demonstrated the value of investing in public health. Public health was and is where the largest numbers of lives are saved, usually by understanding the epidemiology of a disease—its patterns, where and how it emerges and spreads—and attacking it at its weakest points. This usually means prevention. Science first contained smallpox, then cholera, then typhoid, then plague, then yellow fever through large-scale measures—everything from killing rats to vaccinations. Public health measures lack the drama of pulling someone back from the edge of death, but they save lives by the millions.

Chapter 3

THE ANGEL ISLAND QUARANTINE/IMMIGRATION STATION, 1891–1946

The quarantine station in San Francisco bay was established as a result of epidemics. Angel Island faced several epidemic outbreaks. The major battles at Angel Island concerned coping with bubonic plague and influenza, although smallpox was a feared disease in the early years of operation. Medical examinations also screened for trachoma, hookworm, liver flukes, and filariasis as nondeadly but "loathsome" conditions for which an immigrant could be excluded. They were directed especially at Chinese immigrants. Fortunately for the residents of San Francisco, and especially those in its Chinatown, the onslaught of the plague arrived at the turn of the century, when doctors leading the campaign against bubonic plague benefited from the medical developments of the 1880s and 1890s. This resulted in the deaths of a few hundred rather than thousands.

The saga of Angel Island focuses on the impact of two doctors in particular. One doctor, Dr. Joseph James Kinyoun, remained relatively unknown and unheralded despite playing an important role at a critical time. A true and trained medical microbiologist, Kinyoun developed important innovations in the apparatus useful to fight several epidemic diseases. He became embroiled in political conflict and fell out of favor with his superiors, in his case the surgeon general of the United States, Walter Wyman. He retired into relative obscurity. The other, Dr. Rupert Blue, was not a medical scientist, but he was politically more astute and diplomatic than Kinyoun. Like doctors Reed and Gorgas, Rupert Blue did not make a scientific breakthrough such as discovering the cause of the disease. His significant contribution came in administrative innovation. He applied insights from scientific breakthroughs of others to the battle against a pandemic. Like them, he did not attack the disease directly. Instead, he fought to eradicate the transmitters—the vector. In Rupert Blue's case, the vector was rats and their fleas. Unlike Dr. Kinyoun, Rupert Blue went on to higher office, being appointed, in 1912, surgeon general of the United States. But like Dr. Kinyoun, Dr. Blue's career ended with his falling out of favor with his political superiors, in part at least due to the failure of the Public Health Service to cope well with the great influenza pandemic of 1918–1919 (Barry, 2005).

The story of Angel Island illustrates that public health policy saves more lives by prevention and mitigation of the ravages of pandemics than doctors do in saving individual lives, bringing the sick back from the brink of death. At Angel Island, their very successes against epidemic disease brought about the closing of the station when its role as a major barrier against the invasion of epidemic disease became obsolete.

A BRIEF HISTORY OF THE ANGEL ISLAND QUARANTINE/IMMIGRATION STATION

Angel Island is the largest of several in San Francisco Bay. Until Europeans arrived on the west coast, it was uninhabited, used by small and temporary hunting-party settlements of the Miwok Indians, who came out in balsa boats to hunt deer on the island. Angel Island received its name in 1775 when Spanish explorer Don Juan Manuel Ayala, aboard the ship *San Carlos*, stopped there while exploring the bay and mapping the region. Ayala named it "Isla de Los Angeles"—Island of the Angels—as its position seemed to protect the bay (Soennichsen: 8–92; this section draws on his history and on Flanagan: 10).

The Spanish put the first settlement on the island in 1839, when it was granted to Don Antonio Maria Osio, a native of Baja California and customs collector at Monterey. He was granted the island to prevent its settlement by the Russians or Americans. Don Antonio Osio raised cattle on the island in 1846. He visited the island for some months at a time and put a portion of land under cultivation. When the Bear Flag revolt erupted in northern California, Don Osio fled south. With onset of the war between Mexico and the United States, the U.S. Navy took possession of Angel Island. They killed Osio's cattle for a meat supply for the troops. In 1849, his claim to the island was challenged by Henry W. Halleck, a military officer who had found a flaw in Osio's legal title in how the initial grant was processed (Soennichsen: 10).

In November 1850, President Millard Fillmore, by executive order, reserved for public purposes land around the bay and several of the islands in the bay, including Angel Island. Osio disputed the seizing of the island, and in 1854, the Board of Land Commissioners confirmed his title. That decision was in turn disputed by the U.S. government, and Osio lost the island in the land-grabs that prevailed in the 1850s, when the U.S. Supreme Court ruled against him. He returned to Mexico in 1852. After the Court rejected Osio's claim, the secretary of the interior and E. M. Stanton, the attorney for the government, wrote President Buchanan, noting its strategic value and pressing the federal government to take possession of it.

For about a decade, the island remained in the U.S. federal government domain, home to a number of squatters. The U.S. government finally exercised its option on the land and occupied it, establishing Camp Reynolds (1863–1865) to provide fortifications for the defense of San Francisco Bay. In 1861, the Civil War precipitated the building of two forts at the entrance to the bay, one on Alcatraz Island and an inner line of defense on Angel Island. Then General in Chief of the Army Henry W. Halleck, who had detected the flaw in Osio's title, called for batteries to guard the bay, and a fort with ten to twenty guns was ordered for Angel Island. In September 1861, troops began construction of a battery, christening it "Camp Reynolds" in honor of Major General John Reynolds, commander of the First Corps, Army of the Potomac, who had been killed at Gettysburg two months earlier.

The first hospital on the island was finished in 1864, at Ayala Cove, some distance from the army post, as was the custom of the time. Germ theory had not yet been proven, but medical officers at the time did know that distance lessened contagion. The hospital included separate quarters for a surgeon and steward, and the cove became known as Hospital Cove (Chase, 2004).

After the Civil War, the batteries were removed, Camp Reynolds abandoned, and management of the property assigned to the commanding officer at Alcatraz Island. The camp was reopened—not as an artillery post, but as a depot for recruits, particularly infantry, on their way to posts in the west. The recruit depot remained in active status until 1896.

In 1867, the first steamboat, the *General McPherson*, went into service between San Francisco, Alcatraz, and Angel Islands. It was named after an army engineer who had been in charge of fortifying Alcatraz before being killed in the Civil War. A small, tuglike boat, it served for twenty years. The ship was replaced by the *General McDowell* in 1886, and the last quartermaster steamer, the *General Frank Coxe*, took over in 1922 (Flanagan, 2006; Lucoccine, 1996).

As immigration increased in the late 1870s, concern rose about establishing a quarantine station in the area to protect against disease being introduced by ship from Asia. Fear was heightened with the outbreak of a smallpox epidemic in Hong Kong in 1888. The city of San Francisco had no isolated place suitable for a detention center. Fear of smallpox led to establishment of a quarantine station away from the city, which had been using inadequate facilities on the waterfront (RG 90, File 2796, Box 240; Shah: 58–60). Angel Island was viewed as a possible site. The U.S. Marine Hospital Service, which became the Public Health Service in 1912, concluded that "a more desirable place for a station could scarcely have been found on the entire seaboard of this coast" (cited in Soennichsen: 84).

The army fought the decision to locate a quarantine station on the island to no avail. When the army realized that it would not win, it sought to change the location of the station from Hospital Cove to Quarry Point. The Treasury Department, then in charge of U.S. immigration policy, refused to change the site, noting the lack of suitable anchorage and fresh water supply at Quarry Point.

The Treasury Department acquired ten acres of land at Hospital Cove to construct the quarantine station in 1888. Construction began in March 1890. The government took possession of the buildings on January 28, 1891, though construction continued until 1893. The cost to construct the quarantine station was $98,000. The station initially consisted of a wharf and boathouse, a warehouse, a disinfection building with three steam chambers, two detention barracks, a barrack and kitchen building for staff, a pump house, a surgeon's house, officers' quarters, a lazaretto (leper house, or isolation hospital), and a convalescent building. The initial staff was comprised on nine attendants, one hospital steward, and one medical officer, plus a medical officer engaged as needed during quarantines. It opened officially on April 29, 1891, under overall command of Surgeon Robert H. Bailhache of the Marine Hospital Service (Soennichsen: 86).

The steamship *China* arrived on April 27, 1891, the first ship placed in quarantine when two cases of smallpox were found aboard. Two hundred fifty-seven passengers and the ship's crew were quarantined for fourteen days, and the ship was fumigated using pots of sulfur and manganese. In May, the steamer *Oceanic* arrived with a case of smallpox detected, and 340 immigrants were placed in quarantine while the ship was fumigated. Whenever inspection detected disease on board a ship, a yellow flag was raised, and the vessel anchored at the station. With construction of the station not yet complete, these two incidents of quarantine exceeded the station's ability to accommodate the passengers, who remained in quarantine for fourteen days. Dr. Bailhache requested more barrack space. His urgent appeals over several months were not acted on. The year 1892 continued the serious overcrowding when more than 600 persons were in quarantine, far beyond the capacity of the barracks. In May 1892, the Occidental and Oriental Steamship Company was granted permission to construct temporary barracks to hold up to 500 passengers. Before such construction could begin, more steamships arrived, and hundreds of passengers were forced to sleep on the floor (Flanagan, 2006).

Between December 1891 and May 1892, the station detained nearly 2,500 persons. It lacked adequate barrack space and water supply, and Bailhache urgently requested that a pump be installed to bring in salt water for purposes other than cooking and drinking. The army post surgeon complained that patients under quarantine were not being sufficiently guarded and isolated and recommended that a fence be built around the station to isolate it from the rest of the island. In June, Dr. Bailhache promised him that the fence would be built, though a year later no action had been taken; the controversy over the fence continued for months. The fence was not begun until the end of May 1893, two years after the initial request (RG 90, File 2392, Letter of 10/23/1897).

Construction of various buildings and facilities continued until 1902, by which time the station included twenty-nine buildings. These included the quarters for the commanding officer, a double set of officers' quarters, a large building for cabin passengers, two other large buildings for ship's officers, custom officers and such, and a hospital for noncontagious diseases and two compounds for contagious ones. In the latter, one compound comprised two buildings for smallpox cases and one for plague and cholera cases. These three buildings were placed in an isolated cove. There were three large barracks for steerage passengers, two for Chinese and one for Japanese. The station had a 271-foot wharf with a boat house and a ninety- by fifty-two-foot building known as the disinfecting shed. It housed probably the largest disinfecting apparatus ever built. Three steam disinfecting chambers, each forty by seven feet, were fitted for disinfection with steam and a chemical solution of 20 percent formaldehyde followed by ammonia. These were supplied by a bank of three large boilers and weighed thirty-three tons each. Carts with luggage, clothing and bundles of other such items to be disinfected were pulled into the tubes on rails. The station also had two long bathhouses with dressing rooms, one for cabin and one for steerage passengers. The capacity of the station was 1,104 persons, not counting the personnel of the station (www.angelisland.org).

The quarantine and immigration station was served by a fleet of vessels. The quarantine station's flagship was the U.S.S. *Omaha*, built in 1867 at the Philadelphia Navy yard as the *Astoria*. It was 250 feet long and launched on June 10, 1869. In August 1869, she was renamed the *Omaha*, then was commissioned as a U.S. Navy frigate on September 12, 1872. The

Omaha served in the South Atlantic Squadron, then the North Atlantic Station, from 1873 to 1879. She was refitted in Philadelphia in 1880 to 1884 and served around Cape Horn from 1885 to 1891, at which time she was decommissioned and turned over to the Marine Hospital Service, anchored at San Francisco, and used as the quarantine ship.[1] She continued in service until struck from the U.S. Naval Register on July 10, 1914. In April 1915, she was sold to Smith and Bond.

The *George M. Sternberg* served as the fumigating steamer, a disinfecting barge. It was equipped similar to the *Protector*. Built in 1901, the barge was 118 feet long and had two 9′6″ Kinyoun-Francis disinfecting chambers with a formaldehyde attachment, one forty-horsepower vertical boiler, one sulfur furnace, a bichloride force pump, and four shower baths. The quarantine station was also served by a steam launch, the *Bacillus*, the disinfecting barge.

The station's flagship was the *Angel Island*, 144 feet long and able to carry 16,000 passengers a month. There was a cutter, the *Inspector*, and a boarding launch, the *Jeff D. Milton*, and three tugs, the *Woodward*, *Bailhache*, and *Argonaut*. Rounding out the fleet were three launches, the *Marion*, *Albatross*, and *Q17*.

The station processed between 1 percent and 16 percent of immigrants arriving in the United States, the most in 1918 (16 percent). Typically, 30–48 percent of its total immigrants were Chinese; 28–38 percent were Japanese. The remainder was other Asian or other races (Barde, 2003: 186). The total volume of immigration through Angel Island was small in comparison to Ellis Island and several of the East Coast stations, generally running about 1 percent of total U.S. immigration. During its thirty years of operation, it was the principal gateway for Asian immigration, and roughly two-thirds of immigrants entering through Angel Island were Chinese, Japanese, or other Asian—for example, southeast Asian Indians. A number of other nationalities also entered via the Pacific station, including Australians, New Zealanders, Russians, and a number of Latin Americans (Barde, 2008).

The increase in volume of Chinese and Japanese steerage passengers that had to be transported to the station for bathing and disinfection led to further improvements. A powerhouse was built and the station wired for electricity. The disinfecting shed was enlarged and covered walkways constructed so that work could be done more efficiently during the rainy season. The lack of water supply was remedied by the weekly delivery of 36,000 gallons of water by the Army steamer *General McDowell* (Soennichsen: 117; Shah: 179).

By 1899, the quarantine station was dealing with nearly 7,000 detainees, about 10 percent of immigrants inspected. That year it began a three-year battle against the smallpox outbreak that spread across much of the United States. A regiment of troops, the 26th, New England militiamen, were headed for the Philippine war. While encamped at the Presidio, smallpox broke out, and they were quarantined on Angel Island and given a fresh round of vaccinations (Willrich: 117).

Even more serious, in March 1900, bubonic plague broke out in San Francisco. City officials and business leaders conflicted with quarantine officers over whether the epidemic was the plague and over the nature of the quarantine imposed. Local health officials resented the Marine Hospital Service and disputed its procedures. Months of investigation by a special commission confirmed the plague cases, and local opposition to the Marine Hospital Service work declined. Tragically, 112 deaths resulted from this first outbreak of the plague, despite a rat eradication program (Barde, 2008: 110).

By 1907, the quarantine station comprised forty-five buildings, the size of the station until it closed. Proposals to enlarge the quarantine station were considered when the Panama Canal opened in 1912, but lack of funds and local community support delayed a decision. With the advent of World War I, the decline in immigration ended any further consideration of major expansion.

The need for the quarantine station declined with the reduction of threat of infectious diseases due in part to developments in medicine to vaccinate against diseases, and improved conditions at ports of embarkation to disinfect ships and passengers before departure. In 1914, for example, the station inspected more than 85,000 persons aboard about 500 steamships, but that year, of 491 ships fumigated, only one was placed in quarantine. In 1919, the station inspected about 72,000 persons, fumigated over 525 ships, and killed nearly 3,000 rats. In 1920, it inspected and fumigated 679 ships and killed 5,000 rats. In the early 1900s, the quarantine station dealt with cases of smallpox, diphtheria, leprosy, typhus, yellow fever, cholera, typhoid fever, and—most notable—bubonic plague. The last suspected case of smallpox infection among arriving passengers was in 1935. By 1936, the station's officers were inspecting and disinfecting the China Clippers, flying boats used by Boeing to transport passengers from Asia to the United States. Later, they disinfected military aircraft at Hamilton Field. In 1946, it was declared surplus and all its functions moved to San Francisco. In 1954, the cove became a state park, and in 1957 most of the buildings of the station were torn down, the huge disinfection chambers removed, and the station grounds bulldozed. The station's attendants' quarters and mess hall, built in 1935, now serve as the park's visitor's center. Only the surgeon, assistant surgeon, and pharmacist's quarters remain of the original 1891 buildings. They now house park rangers and their families. Only the faintest vestiges of the old Hospital Cove remain, now replaced by the green lawns and picnic tables of Ayala Cove (Sakovich, 2002: 11).

THE IMMIGRATION STATION

Angel Island operated for several decades separated from the immigration process then handled directly at the port of San Francisco to which immigrants were transported after their inspection stop at Angel Island. San Francisco was the main port of entry on the west coast for Japanese and Chinese immigrants but had no immigrant building per se. Immigrants were handled either aboard ship before disembarking at the wharf or, if nonquarantine detention was necessary, in quarters furnished by the shipping lines—principally the Pacific Mail Steamship Company, whose ships transported roughly 50 percent of all passengers arriving at the port of San Francisco. The other steamship lines bringing traffic to the port were the Japanese-owned Toyo Kisen Kaisha (TKK) and the Chinese American–owned China Mail Steamship Company (Barde, 2003: 40; Shah: 180–183). Steamship-line facilities were disgraceful, cramped, and lacking facilities for cleanliness and decency. Nor were they secure. In the early 1900s, numerous detainees escaped from the quarters, and only a few were recaptured. A 1902 investigation called for the construction of an immigration detention facility to be administered by the government. A second congressional investigation was conducted in 1904. It confirmed the inadequacy of the port accommodations and recommended that a new station be constructed on government land in the harbor—along the lines of Ellis Island in New York City—where both the immigration and the quarantine functions could be administered. The 1904 report specifically recommended Angel Island (www.angelisland.org).

The secretary of commerce and labor, whose department then housed the Bureau of Immigration and administered immigration policy, wrote Secretary of War William Howard Taft. The army gave permission to locate a station on the island and allotted ten acres of land to Commerce and Labor. The site selected for the immigration station was China Cove, on the east side of the island.

The project began in 1905, when surveying took place, but the devastating earthquake in 1906 delayed actual construction work. In July 1906, work began on constructing a wharf. The terrain of the China Cove site required that an additional four-and-a-half acres be allotted to the station so that employee housing could be located on relatively level ground. Another problem was inadequate water supply. Inadequate funding and construction problems and delays postponed the department's planned opening of the facility in 1909. After pressure from California's senators and representatives, and San Francisco city government officials, President Taft urged the secretary of commerce and labor to open the station. It was officially opened on January 22, 1910 (Flanagan: 9–11; see also LeMay, 1987: 53–55; and "Angel Island: Guardian of the Western Gates," 1998). During its years of operation as the immigration station on the west coast, Angel Island processed an estimated 300,000 persons, about 70 percent of the estimated 340,000 alien arrivals to San Francisco who were detained at the station. Over its thirty years of operation, the station inspected an estimated 579,000 aliens.[2]

The cutter *Inspector* transported immigrants from the station to San Francisco, making several trips daily. In 1911, the steamer *Angel Island* was added, and she and the army ship *General Frank Coxe* served as the primary means of transportation for the immigration station until it closed in 1946. After the *Angel Island* began service, the *Inspector* was used as a boarding launch, meeting steamers in the bay.

During its first year of operation, Luther Steward, acting commissioner of immigration, inspected the station and wrote a lengthy, scathing report on the inadequacies of the facilities. He severely criticized the layout of the station, the arrangement of the buildings, the use of canvas flooring, inadequate toilet facilities, filthy conditions, and poorly designed heating. His report was the first of several to list the station's faults and recurring problems that plagued the station throughout its years of operation. In 1911, improvements were made to the general hospital, the detention barracks, the administration building, and the sanitation facilities, but they did not eliminate all the problems of faulty design. In 1919, the San Francisco Commissioner of Immigration made complaints similar to those of Commissioner Steward's. The station's facilities remained disliked by its administrators and the medical staff stationed there and resented by detainees (Lucoccine 1996: 92; and Lee, 2002).

Angel Island was the port of entry for Asian immigrants—mainly Chinese, Japanese, and Koreans, but including Filipinos and East Indians. From 1910 until 1915, the largest Asian immigrant group was the Chinese. They made up from 70 percent to as much as 90 percent of the immigrants detained at Angel Island (Flanagan: 12; Lai, Lim, and Young: 10; LeMay, 2006: 77). The Japanese became the most numerous after 1915. Whereas at Ellis Island the immigrants were from Europe and the station intended mostly to facilitate entry, at Angel Island, racial prejudice and more restrictive laws aimed at Asian immigrants meant that the station was used more as a barrier to restrict their flow than as a station to facilitate their entry. That role is suggested by the name some used to refer to the station: "Guardian of the Western Gate" (LeMay, 1987: 56–59; LeMay and Barkan, 1999: 55–69; Flanagan: 22–23; and www.angelisland.org/immigr02.html).

The few European immigrants coming through the west coast, and many of the Japanese, were processed quickly, their paperwork completed, and sent on to San Francisco soon after their ships docked at Angel Island. Immigration officials detained more often and for longer periods of time Chinese immigrants, whom they wanted to keep out. As at Ellis Island, steerage passengers were more often detained, and were detained for longer periods, than were first-class (or cabin) passengers. Chinese immigrants, and Asian immigrants generally, were more likely to be steerage passengers than were European immigrants. Europeans entering through Angel Island (and of course, far more often through Ellis Island) were processed in hours or a few days unless detained for medical reasons. At Angel Island, Asian immigrants were detained, on average, four to six days (Barde, 2006: table 6).

The Chinese came to the United States mostly after the 1848 Gold Rush. They were pushed to emigrate by wars and extreme poverty and were pulled by stories of the streets of America being "paved with gold." The Chinese called California "Gam Saan"—the Land of the Golden Mountains. They were sojourners, young men intending to stay a short while, get rich, and return to China to take a place of honor in their families. Few achieved that goal. Most never reached the gold fields, for discriminatory laws kept them out, and taxes took money away from those who did. Despite its name, the Foreign Miner's Tax, collected by the state of California between 1850 and 1870, was in fact imposed only on Chinese miners. San Francisco passed laws such as the 1870 Cubic Air Ordinance, aimed at the Chinese renters having fewer than 500 cubic feet or air per person; the Sidewalk Ordinance, which prohibited Chinese from using poles to carry laundry loads on the sidewalks; and the Queue Ordinance of 1873, which required Chinese prisoners to cut their hair short, a disgrace to Chinese nationals at the time (Shah: 187–189; Markel: 535).

Being among the early arrivals, many Chinese came by sailing ship where conditions were grim. Food and water were in short supply, particularly for those in steerage—the vast majority. Steerage was overcrowded, and many of the Chinese had to take turns sleeping in the same bed because of the crowded conditions. As a result, illness spread quickly, and many died during the voyage.

A second wave of Chinese immigrants was drawn in the 1860s by the railroads, then building the transcontinental railroad from the west eastward. This wave continued until 1864. When the railroad construction project was completed, in 1869, they took various jobs on farms and ranches, in the fishing and canning industry along the west coast and in San Francisco, where they opened up grocery stores, restaurants, and laundry shops in a distinct ethnic enclave that became known as "Chinatown." Between 1849 and 1882, when the Chinese Exclusion Act was passed to drastically restrict their entrance, more than 300,000 Chinese laborers came to the Unites States. Initially welcomed as cheap labor taking jobs no one else wanted and working long hours for low pay, resentment against them soon grew. The Know-Nothing Party, the Workingmen's Party, and the Ku Klux Klan, among others, led campaigns against the Chinese. Discriminatory laws and violence forced many to flee further east or return home. Laws restricted their travel and ownership of land and made them carry papers to prove their right to live in the United States. They were arrested and returned to China if found without papers (Lai, Lim, and Young: 15; Soennichsen: 121–123; Lee, 2002).

The culmination of laws to restrict Asian immigrants was the Immigration Act of 1924. Section 13a specifically excluded all aliens ineligible for citizenship—essentially barring all Asians (LeMay and Barkan: 150). Policy at the Angel Island was designed more for exclusion than for admission. Chinese immigrants were subjected to intensive cross-examinations to screen out paper sons. Japanese immigrants underwent less intensive examination, and Japanese picture brides were typically cleared in a few days if there were no health issues (Lai, Lim, and Yung: 29; and "Interrogation of Chinese Immigrants at Angel Island," 1).

Delays in examining Chinese immigrants meant that they consistently remained the largest ethnic group held in detention. This difficult situation was compounded by the often chaotic conditions of life in China. It was wracked with political turmoil, politically disintegrating. Extreme poverty was endemic. Such conditions pushed many to immigrate despite the risk of rejection.

When immigrant ships arrived at San Francisco, those seeking admission were transported to the station on Angel Island. Once there, whites were separated from all other races, and the Chinese were separated from all other Asians. Men and women, including husbands and wives, were separated and not allowed to communicate with one another until they were admitted. Small children remained with their mothers. Immigrants were given a physical examination, described in greater detail hereafter. Immigrants were especially inspected for trachoma, a process used to bar the entrance of many (LeMay, 1987: 62–68; NARA, RG 90, File 219, Box 036).

After the physical exam, they were assigned to quarters until questioned by immigration inspectors. The process for Chinese immigrants was long, difficult, and designed to trick them. A 1910 committee of San Francisco merchants, all white, found young children being asked questions about the names of grandparents and of neighbors living blocks away. These exams, the committee concluded, "were unreasonable, and to answer the questions correctly was an impossibility" (RG 90, File 219, Box 036). Critics maintained that the policy used for the Chinese was inhumane, inequitable, and cruel in its treatment of hapless humans.

> Aware of their strategic role as gatekeepers, a number of these officials took advantage of the situation in which so much was at stake for the Chinese, particularly the merchants. They extorted bribes and engaged in other corrupt practices. Compounding these problems . . . was the fact that many of these officials were drawn from California with its pathological dislike of the Chinese. As a result, they resorted to technicalities to reject the credentials of Chinese, detained many others unnecessarily while their credentials were being checked, and demanded payoffs from still others. (Ringer: 670, cited in LeMay, 1987: 66)

In the early years, men and women were housed in separate areas on the first floor of the detention barracks. In 1926, women were moved to the second floor of the Administration Building (Lucoccine, 1996: 94).

The detention and examination process became something of a game. Immigration officials suspected that the documents of many, maybe even most, were fraudulent. And many Chinese immigrants held documents of questionable validity. They felt, however, that the immigration laws were patently discriminatory and unfair—that the only way they could enter was to circumvent them. A method of claiming citizenship was having a citizen father. Children whose father was a citizen could enter the country as a citizen. A man who was a citizen could maintain a family in China, visiting them at intervals, report the birth of the child, and in due time bring the child in as a citizen. Such citizens could essentially report the birth of non-existent children and thereby create slots for others to use to enter the country. These slots were paid for by those using them, entering as paper sons, with a new name and identity. Documentation rarely existed, especially after the 1906 San Francisco earthquake, which caused fires that destroyed many records that would have verified citizenship. Immigration inspectors used rigorous questioning to determine the claims of citizen paper sons. Even legitimate immigrants could fail the tests, and they, as well as the paper sons, resorted to coaching to commit necessary details to memory.

The interrogations of the Chinese applicants were intricate and extensive to a degree unheard of in United States immigration history. They can only be described as traumatic experiences, their nature alluded to in many of the thousands of poems carved into the wooden walls of the detention barracks. Life on the island for the detainees undergoing the interrogation process was strange, stressful, demoralizing, and humiliating. Separated from family members, they were housed in crowded communal living quarters where one hundred persons would sleep in bunk beds, stacked three high in columns, in a room about 1,000 square feet (Lee, 2002).

Despite interrogations, most immigrants were ultimately admitted, though for some the wait was days to perhaps a week and, on a few occasions, even months. In 1923, for example, of 5,009 applicants, 4,806 passed. Between 1910 and 1940, 175,000 Chinese immigrants were processed through the Angel Island station. The deportation rate at Angel Island, however, was much higher than at Ellis Island (Barde, 2008).

Japanese immigrants, though experiencing less rigorous examinations than those faced by Chinese immigrants, were treated differently from European immigrants. Japanese immigration rose in the 1890s, when the supply of Chinese laborers dwindled, and their rate of entry increased tenfold. Their peak year was 1907–1908. In 1870, there were only fifty-six Japanese immigrants on the mainland. By 1890, their numbers exceeded 24,000. By the 1910 census, they numbered 72,000. In 1920, they exceeded 111,000, at which level they essentially stabilized by being barred by the 1924 Immigration Act, known as the Johnson–Reed Act (Act of May 26, 1924, 43 Stat. 153: 8 U.S.C. 201; summarized in LeMay and Barkan, 1999: 148–151).

Increased Japanese immigration aroused a growing anti-Japanese movement, and the west coast echoed with fears of the "Yellow Peril," particularly after Japan defeated Russia in the Russo–Japanese War of 1905. In 1905, the Japanese/Korean Exclusion League was formed, with a claimed membership of over 100,000 in California alone. Renamed the Asiatic Exclusion League in 1907, it was a coalition of 231 affiliated groups, eighty-four of which were labor organizations that considered the Chinese and Japanese as undesirable races. They agitated for restrictions against Japanese immigration. In 1907, the Immigration Act (Act of February 20, 1907, 34 Stat. 898; U.S.C.) raised the head tax on immigrants from 50 cents to $4. It also banned persons who had tuberculosis (endemic in much of Asia, particularly China and Japan), imbeciles, and persons of moral turpitude, and added stringent enforcement machinery. That year, the United States government reached a diplomatic agreement with Japan, the so-called "Gentlemen's Agreement," in which Japan reluctantly agreed to restrict emigration of skilled and unskilled laborers (Executive Order 589, March 14, 1907). Immigration declined dramatically. The total number of Japanese immigrants dropped from 30,824 in 1907 to 16,418 in 1908 to 3,275 in 1909. By 1910 it was fewer than 3,000. Picture brides were allowed, and from 1911 to 1920, 87,000 Japanese were admitted, but 70,000 returned to Japan, for a net gain of a mere 17,000 for the decade. Among them, an estimated 6,000 to 19,000 picture brides were processed through Angel Island (Barde, 2008; Lee and Young, 2010).

The picture bride aspect was almost unique to Japanese immigration. Marriage outside their ethnic group was unacceptable to most Japanese, and many states had laws banning whites from marrying across racial lines. Moreover, a 1907 federal law terminated the citizenship of any American woman who married a foreigner (Act of March 2, 1907, 34 Stat. 1228; 8 U.S.C. 17). There were few Japanese women living in the United States in 1907, so Japanese men arranged marriages with women in Japan. Japanese law did not require both parties to be physically present at the ceremony, and Japanese culture fostered arranged marriages through families and intermediaries. As a result, pictures were exchanged. A simple registration sealed the marriage, and the new bride was eligible to join her husband in the United States under an exemption in the Gentlemen's Agreement that allowed the spouse of a resident alien to enter. Picture brides began arriving in numbers. They were given physical exams and their papers checked, but the procedure was routine in nature, as their status was predetermined. Their reception in the United States was mixed. They presented a romantic image, having traveled thousands of miles to meet a husband they had never seen. They were dressed in traditional garb while on Angel Island, offering the newspapers a steady stream of photographs of demure women awaiting arrival of their mates. Others felt that the brides were merely a means for the Japanese to evade restrictions on Asian immigration, and they resented the legal loophole allowing their entrance. Many of the brides were shocked when they saw their husbands for the first time, as the photographs were often taken when the men were ten to fifteen years younger, or touched up to conceal their real age. The men often exaggerated their social and economic standing. Some disillusioned brides refused to join their husbands and returned to Japan. The era of the picture brides ended in 1920, when Japan stopped issuing passports to proxy brides. By then, thousands of Japanese picture brides had passed through Angel Island (Soennichsen, 2001: 133–134).

Restrictionists kept pushing to ban or discourage Japanese immigration. In 1913, the state of California passed the Webb–Henry Bill, also known as the California Alien Land Act. It restricted Japanese aliens from owning land, limited them to leasing land for three years, and forbade land already owned from being bequeathed. When the Supreme Court ruled the law constitutional, similar laws were passed by neighboring states. California Attorney General Webb frankly described the racist nature of the law he co-authored:

> The fundamental basis of all legislation . . . has been and is, race undesirability. It seeks to limit their presence by curtailing the privileges which they may enjoy here, for they will not come in large numbers and long abide with us if they may not acquire land. And it seeks to limit the numbers who will come by limiting the opportunities for their activities here when they arrive. (cited in Kitano: 17)

Despite their dramatic decline, political pressure continued until enactment of the Immigration Act of 1924, which barred Asian immigration altogether. Sentiment on the west coast resulted in the immigration bureaucracy's becoming increasingly important in the process of admission or denial. Boards of special inquiry, established by the act of 1893, heard, on an annual basis, tens of thousands of cases nationally. In 1910 alone, for example, they heard 70,829 cases (RG 90, File 219, Box 036).

In 1916, charges of corruption were made against officers at the Angel Island Immigration Station. They were accused of a widespread conspiracy to smuggle illegal aliens into the country. A special investigation by the Department of Labor found pervasive fraud allowing large numbers of Chinese to be illegally landed. The conspiracy included three attorneys, an interpreter, an inspector, record room clerks, watchmen, and others. Widespread corruption was induced by the paper son industry (RG 90, File 219, Box 036).

The immigration station not only dealt with immigrants seeking admission, but it also processed persons in transit and persons awaiting deportation. A majority of the latter group were Europeans. The vast majority of the former were Asians, though there were applicants from east India, Russia, Armenia, Mexico, Central and South America, Korea, India, and Europe. During the period of highest activity, the station could handle up to 2,500 immigrants per day and had sleeping accommodations for 1,000. A 1929 report found that 15,000 people from thirty-nine "races" had passed through the station. In some years, the emigrants exceeded immigrants, resulting in a net loss of population. In most years, emigrants made up roughly half the traffic through the station. In 1917, for instance, 11,629 immigrants entered through the station and 9,234 emigrants departed. In 1923, there were 13,710 immigrants and 14,474 emigrants, and in each of the years between 1931 and 1936, more aliens emigrated than immigrants arrived. In 1935, Chinese emigrants exceeded immigrants by 1,605 (RG 90, Arrival Files, Box 1211).

In 1917, thousands of stranded Germans and other enemy aliens were arrested and detained. The immigration bureau took charge of all seamen from all interned German ships. Those arrested in Pacific ports were brought to Angel Island, and the station held several hundred enemy aliens. In 1918, 740 enemy aliens were held at the station (Soennichsen: 135–140).

The federal government used Angel Island briefly as a maximum security prison in the 1920s, but the practice ceased after several escape attempts and vigorous protest by the Immigration Bureau. In October 1920, a three-month meningitis epidemic broke out, largely the result of overcrowding, poor sanitation, and limited water, hospital and medical services.

The station received national attention when it became the site for the deportation hearings of a notorious labor leader, Harry Bridges. He led a strike at twelve major ports in 1934, culminating in a general strike in San Francisco, in which two men were killed and sixty-seven injured. Some members of his union were communists, and the party supported the strike. He was a powerful leader of a powerful union. Efforts to deport him failed, but the hearings went on for months.

The station's conditions engendered continuous complaints and, in 1915, suggestions for moving station from Angel Island to Alcatraz Island. The War Department refused to make the change. In the early 1920s, complaints surfaced again, including a 1922 report by the commissioner general of immigration, who called the station the worst he had ever visited. In another report, the assistant secretary of labor called it a "fire trap." In 1924, 1937, and 1938, proposals were made to move the station to another location, but it remained on Angel Island. In 1940, an event occurred that had long been predicted—a major fire started in the Administration Building, caused by faulty wiring, and it burned down. The immigration authorities were moved to San Francisco, and in November, detained immigrants were relocated there as well. With those departures, the station on Angel Island was closed after thirty years of operation (Soennichsen, 2001; Sakovich, 2002).

In 1941 the property reverted to the army and became the North Garrison of Fort McDowell. The hospital was converted into barracks, and the attendants' buildings became noncommissioned officers' quarters. After Japan's attack on Pearl Harbor, the site was improved and expanded with the addition of a 1,600-man mess hall, an infirmary, a guard house, a recreation building, and a post exchange. The North Garrison used the old immigrant detention barracks to house German and Japanese prisoners of war during World War II, and a few enemy aliens were processed at the center but not detained; nor was the site used as an internment camp. In 1946, the North Garrison was closed. The former Immigration Station is now Angel Island State Park, in recognition of the historic importance of the Immigration and the Quarantine Stations, and the site has been designated a national historic landmark (www.angelisland.org).

COPING WITH EPIDEMICS AND PANDEMICS

The Marine Hospital Service was first established by an Act of Congress in 1798 to provide for the health needs of merchant seamen. In 1870, the service underwent reorganization; the first supervising surgeon was appointed in 1871. He appointed a corps of uniformed physicians, and his title was changed to surgeon general in 1873. The role of the service in quarantine work was embroiled in controversy between federal responsibility and states' rights advocates. Surgeon General Dr. John Woodworth believed that states' regulations were inconsistent from locality to locality and that only a federal enforcement effort could halt the spread of infectious diseases. In 1877 a yellow fever epidemic that started in New Orleans spread throughout the Mississippi Valley, and Woodworth pressed for an effective system of quarantine to be established at the federal level. In 1878, Congress passed the Quarantine Act, which assigned responsibility to the Marine Hospital Service, although with strings attached in that its regulations could not conflict with or impair those of state and municipal authority. As Mullan notes, it took fifty years before the service assumed complete responsibility for quarantine in all states (22–25). In 1891, as immigration increased dramatically, the Marine Hospital Service was assigned responsibility for the medical inspection of all arriving immigrants (Willrich: 78; law summarized in LeMay and Barkan, Document 41: 66–70).

When the quarantine station at San Francisco opened in 1891, it faced possible epidemics of bubonic plague, cholera, scarlet fever, yellow fever, smallpox, and typhus fever. Many epidemics were occurring in outbreaks in Asian countries and spreading to Europe and North America. A decade after the quarantine station opened, it had to cope with the most severe epidemics of bubonic plague ever experienced in the United States.[3] After fewer than two decades, it had to cope with the Spanish flu, the most deadly pandemic in American, and world, history. Fortunately, the doctors at Angel Island benefited from breakthroughs in medical science that occurred in the 1880s. As a result, they were better prepared to cope with epidemic diseases, more able to manage against a pandemic event. Research by the founders of bacteriology and microbiology, along with the work of medical pioneers, had proven the effectiveness of public health hygiene approaches. The early exponents of germ theory and their discoveries about how bacillus-caused disease was transmitted and spread demonstrated the effectiveness of combating disease by vector analysis and control, by eradicating the carriers of the disease.

Sanitary reformers demonstrated that the greatest numbers of lives are saved by an understanding of epidemiology and by attacking the disease at its weakest points. Prevention was the best weapon in the war on disease. Medical science eventually showed how to contain smallpox, cholera, typhoid, bubonic plague, and yellow fever. Large-scale public health measures involving filtering water, testing and killing the vermin carriers, and vaccination saved countless thousands, if not millions. These lessons had been learned and spread among the medical profession by the late 1890s. An epidemic of smallpox in Hong Kong in 1888 spurred Congress to authorize the quarantine station. Doctors of the U.S. M.H.S. became leading advocates of scientific medicine and innovators in the movement from simple quarantine methods to scientific maritime sanitation. In the words of historian Michael Willrich, doctors of the U.S. M.H.S. "were the vanguards of a modern, national public health system" (76).

The station had barely been opened when the 1893 immigration act (28 Stat. 7) empowered the surgeon general to send assistants abroad to infected ports to examine immigrant passengers before embarkation. The 1894 act established a Bureau of Immigration (LeMay and Barkan: 76, 28 Stat. 390; 8 U.S.C. 174). Ports of embarkation had to comply with regulations promulgated by the Secretary of the Treasury that required detention of immigrants for four to five days before departure and the disinfection of baggage and personal effects by steam and disinfecting chemicals. By 1894, twenty-three major ports in the United States were equipped with steam-disinfecting chambers, including San Francisco's Angel Island (RG 90, File 544 and Box 505).

Discoveries by Pasteur, Koch, Chamberland, Gaffky, Loeffler, and others proved that sterilizing materials by heat was effective in preventing the spread of contagious disease. Dry heat killed bacteria but required long exposure and high temperatures for effectiveness, particularly for bacteria in the spore state. Moist heat was even more effective. But moist heat worked better in combination with steam of low degree and slight pressure passing over articles in a slow current, and it worked best when in combination with chemical disinfectants. The New Orleans station tested, over three years, virtually every chemical on the then-known table of chemicals for effectiveness as germicides, experimenting with different chemicals and different temperatures. The steam chambers at Angel Island were fitted for steam at 230 °F with 20 percent formaldehyde followed by ammonia. Some of the earlier versions of these chambers had problems with the fittings and leaked some of the chemical-laden steam when formaldehyde was added. Dr. Joseph James Kinyoun, the bacteriologist with the U.S. M.H.S., perfected the steam apparatus and, together with the manufacturer of the apparatus, developed the Kinyoun–Francis chambers and designed plans for the apparatus suitable for use on disinfection ships, at quarantine stations, in marine hospitals, and even portable devices for use in municipal hospital service (these latter devices used sulfur fumigation—RG 90, File 4605, "Sterilizing Machines," Box 505).

Dr. Joseph Kinyoun joined the U.S. M.H.S. in 1886.[4] He established the first bacteriological laboratory at the Quarantine Station in New York, an unimposing one-room facility in the attic of the Marine Hospital on Staten Island. In examining slides taken from a passenger, he saw a swarm of short, rod-shaped bacteria with hair-like fringes, called flagellae. It was *Vibrio cholerae*, the bacteria that causes cholera. His was the first diagnosis of cholera anywhere in the Western Hemisphere. He was only 27 years old at the time, and his work marked him as a force with which to be reckoned. In 1891, he moved to Washington, D.C. to work as the first director of the National Hygienic Laboratory, which decades later would be world renowned as the National Institutes of Health.

Dr. Kinyoun was born in 1860 in North Carolina, the son of a physician, with whom he first studied medicine as an apprentice. In 1880, he studied at the St. Louis Medical College, then at Bellevue Hospital Medical College of New York University, where he took his M.D. degree in 1882. Kinyoun was captivated by Pasteur's pioneering work in microbiology and studied it along with microscopic examination of diseased tissue. He studied bacteriology with Herman Biggs at the Carnegie Laboratory at New York's Bellevue Hospital. While he was posted as director at the National Hygienic Laboratory, Kinyoun examined yellow fever, whose viral etiology was then unknown. There he also designed the Kinyoun–Francis sterilizer, a disinfecting apparatus for ships, and demonstrated the superiority of sulfur dioxide as a fumigating gas. The chambers were developed and produced at the Kensington Engine Works, Ltd. Company in Philadelphia. The "Francis" portion of the name of these chambers is from the owners and executives of the company, H. C. and W. H. Francis (Kelly and Burrage, 1971: 737).

In 1894, the laboratory began to manufacture diphtheria antitoxin after Dr. Kinyoun had traveled to Europe to study the process with Emile Roux of the Pasteur Institute. He learned and refined the procedure for developing antitoxins for diphtheria in horses. State and local public health officials soon came to the laboratory for instructions in the new technique under Kinyoun. Dr. Kinyoun worried about the consistency and quality of the manufacture of antitoxins and for some years advocated that the federal government regulate the marketing of such products to ensure their quality. These efforts resulted in the enactment of the Biologics Control Act of 1902, giving the Hygienic Laboratory regulatory authority in the production and sale of vaccines and antitoxins. As Mullan argues, the law exemplified the achievement of the public health reformers of the Progressive era, and its regulatory function remained an important part of the work of the Hygienic Laboratory for the next thirty years (Mullan: 39).

Dr. Milton J. Rosenau, who had earlier served with Kinyoun at Angel Island, succeeded him as Director of the Hygienic Laboratory in 1901 and served there until 1909 (Garraty and Carnes, vol. 4: 875–876). It is through his work there that he had his greatest effect on the development of public health. The public health pioneer was born in Philadelphia in 1869. He took his M.D. from the University of Pennsylvania in 1889, and joined the U.S. M.H.S., serving two years at the Hygienic Laboratory under Kinyoun and studying a year at the Hygienic Institute in Berlin. He served as an assistant surgeon at Angel Island from 1895 to 1897 and as a quarantine officer at the Philippine Islands in 1898. Upon his appointment as director of the Hygienic Laboratory, Rosenau began secretly buying up samples of eight different vaccine makers on the open market to test them for their purity and potency. His 1902 report to the New York Academy of Medicine showed great unevenness in the quality of the vaccines being produced. Doctor Rosenau did pioneering research on diphtheria, typhoid fever, yellow fever, malaria, botulism, bubonic plague, and tuberculosis. After the Biologics Control Act of 1902 gave enforcement of regulatory power to the U.S. M.H.S., Rosenau administered the act and established at the separate laboratory divisions of bacteriology, chemistry, pathology, pharmacology, and zoology—paving the way to its development as the National Institutes of Health. He studied the germicidal effects of glycerin for vaccination points and wrote the highly influential service-published *Disinfection and Disinfectants: A Practical Guide for Sanitarians, Health, and Quarantine Officers* in 1902. In 1912 he published the influential book regarding milk sanitation *The Milk Question* (Kaufman, Galishoff, and Savitts: 649).

After directing the National Hygienic Laboratory in Washington, D.C., with great distinction, he served as the quarantine officer in Santiago at the close of the Spanish–American War. His studies of the vaccines being produced, and their often poor quality, demonstrated that the regulation of vaccine production "was a national problem requiring a national solution" (Willrich: 194–195). Rosenau taught bacteriology at the Army and Navy Medical School, 1904–1909, and tropical diseases at Georgetown University, 1905–1909. In 1909, he became the first professor of preventive medicine and hygiene in the United States when he left public service to teach at Harvard University in a teaching career that lasted twenty-six years. His 1913 published textbook, *Preventive Medicine and Hygiene*, became the standard textbook on the subject. While at Harvard, he organized the Harvard and Massachusetts Institute of Technology School for Health Officers and from 1914–1921 was affiliated with the Massachusetts State Board of Health as chief of the Division of Biologic Laboratories and director of the antitoxin and vaccine laboratory for the state. Dr. Rosenau served as president of the Society of American Bacteriologists in 1934 and of the American Public Health Association in 1944. He died in 1946, and the University of North Carolina named a building after him at Chapel Hill, where his papers are housed at the UNC Southern Historical Collection.

On July 1, 1902, then President Theodore Roosevelt signed the Biologics Control Act. By January 1, 1903, the law established a system of licensing and inspection of all biologics (vaccines, sera, etc.) sold in interstate commerce or imported from abroad. In the 1902 act, Congress enlarged the authority of the M.H.S. and gave it a new name: the U.S. Public Health and Marine Hospital Service. Rosenau's Hygienic Laboratory (since 1930 called the National Institute of Health) administered the licensing and inspection provisions of the act and by 1904 had inspected thirteen manufacturing concerns, most for the sale of diphtheria antitoxin and smallpox vaccine. By 1921, the lab was inspecting forty-nine companies marketing a hundred different products, and its staff grew to thirteen in 1904 (Willrich: 206–207).

While Dr. Kinyoun was the first director of the Hygienic Laboratory, he began courses of instruction in bacteriological techniques for junior service officers. He continued his own studies in bacteriology at Johns Hopkins University and Georgetown University schools of medicine, receiving a Ph.D. from Georgetown. He served, from 1890 to 1899, as professor of hygiene, bacteriology, and pathology at Georgetown, and he traveled to Europe several times to study laboratory techniques with such pioneers of bacteriology as Dr. Robert Koch and Elie Metchnikoff. In 1899, Surgeon General Walter Wyman removed him as director of the Hygienic Laboratory and sent him to assume command of the Marine Service's quarantine station at Angel Island. Kinyoun essentially traded places with Dr. Milton

J. Rosenau, who had been the medical chief at the Angel Island quarantine station (Willrich: 206).

At Angel Island, passengers were ordered into quarantine after being checked by a doctor when they arrived and were separated by type of ticket (cabin or steerage), then sent through a disinfection process. They stripped, washed with carbolic soap, and donned coveralls provided by attendants. While they were being disinfected, their clothing and luggage was loaded into wire cages that were placed on a track system that carried the cages through the Kinyoun–Francis disinfecting tubes, where dry steam under very high pressure was used as a disinfectant. The process often slightly affected the color of the clothing. Money and small items were dipped in carbolic acid.

All passengers and crew members exposed to smallpox were vaccinated. If cases were detected aboard ship, the steerage passengers and crew underwent quarantine. Cabin passengers (almost always whites) were allowed to leave. Twice daily (morning and evening), those in quarantine were lined up and inspected by a medical officer to ensure that there were no new outbreaks of disease and to check for escapes. The barracks were fumigated with sulfur dioxide and flushed out with salt water every morning. At the end of the quarantine period, clothing and personal effects were again disinfected before they were allowed to leave. The lazaretto, where those who had contagious diseases were kept, was thoroughly fumigated, and the bedding and clothing of patients burned, in preparation for the next quarantine. When the passengers had disembarked, their ship would be disinfected using the station's fumigating steamer, the *George M. Sternberg*, and later by the "disinfecting hulk," the U.S.S. *Omaha*. Dry steam was pumped into the infected vessel, and pots of sulfur dioxide were burned in tubs of water in the vessel's hold. Over the years, the station used a number of disinfectants in the station and the fumigation ships: sulfur, manganese, hydrochloric acid, sodium cyanide, formaldehyde, ammonia, and sodium chlorate (Soennichsen: 89–90).

The fumigation of ships was a dangerous business. The chemicals used were deadly, and ships varied in the problems they presented for the fumigation crews. The fumigating devices often leaked gas from their fittings. Three stevedores were killed in 1919, a steerage passenger died in 1921, and two crew members died in 1922. That year, three crew members of a Japanese ship were overcome but did not die. In 1922 also, the most tragic accident at the station occurred. Six men, including four employees of the quarantine station, were killed by hydrocyanic gas during fumigation. No cause for the accident was ever determined. Hydrocyanic gas was not detectable by ordinary means, and fumigation by cyanide could never be made totally safe by any rules or regulations, though Dr. Kinyoun worked to improve the design and fix faulty fittings. In October 1899, he wrote the M.H.S. a report on the status of the steam chambers at Angel Island, noting that they were of an obsolete design and urging adoption of the "Kinyoun–Francis" design with metal hood and better fittings. He also ordered new autoclaves.[5]

In 1896, news of an outbreak of the plague in China resulted in all Chinese passengers' entering San Francisco bay being taken to the quarantine station from any vessel, even if sickness was not found on board. This increased demands on the station. Plague probably arrived in San Francisco aboard the ship *Australia* on January 2, 1900—on some four-legged stowaways that somehow escaped detection and fumigation. The first case of the bubonic plague was diagnosed on March 6, 1900, when one Wong Chut King died. The city bacteriologist, Dr. Winfred Kellogg, suspected plague and asked Dr. Kinyoun to confirm that the long-feared disease had come to Chinatown.[6]

> Plague traveled in stealth. No one yet knew how it spread. Nineteenth century theories of its transmission focused on dirt, tainted food, and a "miasma," or cloud of infectious vapors. In the boomtown of San Francisco, the business and political elite believed plague to be an alien scourge that would tarnish their trade and tourism. So from City Hall to the dome of the state capitol, officials dismissed the threat. The little people would die of it while the powerful debated its existence. (Chase: 10)

Business interests and city government officials at first denied that plague existed, and the press and public opinion sided with them against the doctors of the Marine Hospital Service. Previously, local health officials had performed quarantine procedures, and they resented the federal quarantine station's taking over the process. Dr. Kinyoun, in particular, was attacked in the press and by a coalition of public officials who resented his quarantine and his authoritarian manner of dealing with Chinatown residents.

The issue and the diagnosis were sufficiently sensitive that Kinyoun and Wyman sent telegrams to one another in code. One such coded message, dated July 1, 1899, from Kinyoun to Wyman, for example, concerned the arrival of plague to Honolulu. Translated it read: "Carmichael reports plague on a Japan-America liner arriving in Honolulu June 18, 1899. Autopsy confirms diagnosis. Detained in quarantine, expected to arrive [in S.F.] ten days. Lazaretto inadequate for plague and smallpox. Recommend

250 dollars for epidemic related purchase for necessary lumber for tent floors, barbed wire, piping. Absolutely necessary for emergency."[7] In a letter of March 6, 1900, Kinyoun wrote to Wyman requesting full information from Surgeon Perry at the Manila station regarding a plague outbreak there. Kinyoun expressed deep concern that U.S. soldiers would bring it to San Francisco. He stated that informal reports indicated that the Manila outbreak was more severe than in Honolulu, as in Manila "discharged soldiers are subject to little or no discipline during the time they are awaiting transportation to the U.S." (RG 90, File 5608, Box 627, Letters from Surgeon Kinyoun, 1899–1902).

In an October 8, 1900, letter to Wyman, Kinyoun noted the arrival of a British steamer, the *Coptic*, which had arrived at San Francisco from Kobe, Japan. It had three dead rats found aboard, and Kinyoun ordered her placed alongside the *Omaha* and disinfected with sulfur dioxide gas for the ship's hold, steerage decks, store rooms and forecastle areas. He placed the steerage passengers and oriental crew in quarantine and ordered them bathed and all their effects disinfected. Kinyoun reported that he had ordered the *Coptic* held for twenty-four hours after fumigation gas had been sufficiently strong to kill vermin. He allowed the vessel to dock on October 2, 1900 (RG 90, folder for June, 1900).

Despite his awareness that dead rats indicated a threat from the plague and his taking appropriate precautions, Kinyoun failed to make the connection when plague erupted in San Francisco that the eradication of rats may be a key measure to take in combating the epidemic.

As Chase, in his chronicle of the epidemic, notes,

Two doctors in federal uniform—Joseph Kinyoun and Rupert Blue—would each try in his own way to quell the pestilence. One doctor would try to subdue the outbreak from his laboratory at the quarantine station on Angel Island. The other doctor would work at the street level, purging the infection from boardwalk and basement. The public health efforts of the day were handicapped by limited scientific knowledge and bedeviled by the twin demons of denial and discrimination. One man would fail, the other would succeed to become the top physician in the land. Today, few people know their names. But their mission would foreshadow the challenges posed by epidemics for centuries to come (4).

Dr. Kinyoun's diagnosis was confirmed. Between 1900 and 1905, 119 cases of plague were confirmed in San Francisco, resulting in 113 deaths. The third Asiatic plague began in Hong Kong and spread quickly along trade routes, no longer slowed by wind- driven sails. Cholera migrated with the speed of coal-fired steamships (Chase: 6).

Plague symptoms were violent. Rampant fever, crushing headache, overwhelming nausea, and debilitating weakness downed a person who had been strong only hours before. As inflamed lymph glands swelled with the invading bacteria, a painful red bubo erupted and inky hemorrhages burst from small vessels, giving the skin a blue-black tattooed appearance—the characteristic look of the Black Death. Delirium and pain drove people to near madness and stirred the limbs in an agitated dance of death. In their final agonies, victims tore at their bedclothes, unable to bear the slightest touch on their swellings. It was usually a speedy death. When bubonic, plague killed in five days. Pneumonic plague, in which the buboes invaded the lungs and victims spat black blood, was the deadliest form, known to be contagious from person to person by saliva as the coughing victims helplessly infected caretakers and family members. Pneumonic plague killed in two to three days. Both forms, however, were caused by the bacteria known as the *Yersinia pestis*.

The co-discoverers of the bacterium were Alexandre Yersin of Paris and Shibasaburo Kiasato of Tokyo, who went to Hong Kong in 1894 when the plague first broke out. Yersin's discovery prevailed and prompted a name change from *Bacillus pestis* to *Yersina pestis*. Their landmark discovery enabled scientists at long last a way to identify the deadly germ. It gave Joseph Kinyoun's culprit a face and a quick tool with which to identify it. On culture plates (petri dishes), colonies of plague looked like ground glass. Kinyoun applied Koch's postulates to prove that the plague germ was in fact what killed Wong Chut King. He isolated the bacteria, injected the germs into lab animals, and when those animals died, isolated the germ again—proving that it was bubonic plague (Chase: 46).

When he diagnosed it as the plague, he instituted quarantine on all Chinatown. He became embroiled in controversy as local officials first doubted his findings (fearing, no doubt, the economic effect of the quarantine on city business and tourism). Even when an outside commission appointed to investigate the case confirmed his diagnosis and his recommendations for prevention of its spread as standard service policy, Kinyoun became the symbol of unwelcome federal intervention in state health matters. Kinyoun was a scientist who knew he was right and who expected others simply to comply with the wisdom of his prognosis. He dealt imperiously with Chinatown residents and local health officials. They resented him and his attitude. They complained to the service. Local residents began to hide bodies and, when family members were interviewed, seemed to respond in ways that suggested to him that they had been coached to conceal the plague.

Surgeon General Wyman tried to respond with diplomatic maneuvers. He urged China's envoy to Washington to use his influence on Chinese residents in San Francisco to comply with the necessary measures of health officials and to confer with Surgeon Kinyoun at Angel Island. Wyman telegrammed Kinyoun to cordon off suspected areas of infection, to guard ferries and railroad stations, to conduct house-to-house inspections with Haffkine inoculation, to quarantine Chinatown, to move suspected victims—if deemed necessary—to Angel Island, and to assemble a disinfecting corps to destroy rats in the city. His last point, the destruction of rats, received little attention in the spring of 1900. Surgeon General Wyman recognized mounting evidence that rats were the chief agent in the spread of plague from port to port, though their connection to the infection of people had not yet been confirmed. A report from Sydney, Australia, noted that doctors there had discovered plague bacteria in the stomachs of fleas, but the report received scant attention. Only later did medical science recognize the significance of the role of the rat and the flea (Chase: 58; Shah: 128). As Shah puts it: "Throughout the crisis, municipal and federal officials believed they could divide the contaminated from the uncontaminated along racial lines" (121).

Complying with Wyman's suggestions, Kinyoun met with an official and a lawyer of the Chinese Six Companies. Tough negotiators, they would not have public health forced on them and their people. Kinyoun believed that this meeting was the main source of opposition to the service and to himself in particular. In Chinatown and in the press, Kinyoun was dubbed the "wolf doctor," a reference to his snappy and officious manner. They knew of some of the risks of the Haffkine vaccine—fever, weakness, and, in some percentage of cases of inoculation, death. The Chinese Consolidated Benevolent Association (CCBA) led a campaign against Kinyoun and his quarantine and objected to the compulsory vaccine order of Chinatown residents issued by Kinyoun. They vigorously sought his removal (Chase: 59; Shah: 123, 129–146).

In a long letter (eighty typed pages) to Doctor Bailhache, at the Presidio, Kinyoun complained of the politics involved: the newspaper coverups, the friction between the city board of health officials and the state board of health, the intense opposition of the Merchant's Association, and the governor of California's selection of a Dr. Winslow Anderson, whom Kinyoun saw as a leader of the coverup. Kinyoun was sued in court in a case that was not resolved for some months, during which time he faced the threat of a six-month jail term. The court issued an injunction against his quarantine. He complained to Bailhache:

If you have read over the decisions and the injunction, as well as the habeas corpus proceeding and my writ of discharge, you will see that the U.S. Court assumes a position in the first case whereby the Board of Health or myself cannot interfere whatsoever. According to this decision, a Chinaman could be suffering from bubonic plague, with smallpox, with leprosy, with diphtheria, with cholera, and go anyplace within San Francisco, and pass and repass to places within the state of California without fear or hinderance. (Letter of JK to Doctor Bailhache, Files of J. Kinyoun, National Library of Medicine, Folder 5)

Dr. Kinyoun filed a detailed report on the plague in San Francisco to the M.H.S. that was twenty-three pages long. In it he noted at that time that there were thirty-one confirmed deaths to the plague, as well as that he suspected many other bodies of being hidden from his inspectors, or local doctors of having made other diagnoses of the cause of death (Ibid., File 6, Report of January 23, 1901). When the independent commission appointed to investigate the issue confirmed the plague, Kinyoun felt vindicated and expected the support of Surgeon General Wyman and the M.H.S. He continued to recommend drastic measures, for he considered the outbreak "a smoldering fire" (Letter to Bailhache: 64).

Instead of the support he expected, Surgeon General Wyman transferred Kinyoun out of San Francisco. Before he could leave, however, Dr. Kinyoun was delayed by legal action filed against him. He reported this in another coded telegram to Wyman on May 6, 1901, in which he wrote:

Just as ready to depart for Detroit, warrant issued for my arrest on trumped up charges of attempt to murder, by shooting at a fisherman, near Island in November last. Facts are these: military authorities mistook a deaf mute fisherman for an escaped convict and fired three shots, two striking the boat. Seeing incident, I took launch and went out to him. On finding out not convict, explained matters. By interference, I saved the man's life, as soldiers would have killed him. No shots fired by me. Whole matter a part of a plan of certain parties here who will go to any extreme to place me in false light. This incident may result in a slight delay, in compliance with instructions [i.e. from Wyman to Kinyoun to transfer]. Wire instructions. Kinyoun. (RG 90, File 5608, Box 627, Folder 1901)

The charges against Kinyoun were dropped, and he was allowed to leave. The incident illustrates, however, the degree to which he was opposed by the San Francisco business and political elites. They were delighted to see him depart San Francisco for good.

Kinyoun was worn out by his experience in San Francisco and bitter in professional exile. He wrote long, rambling letters blaming the press, the politicians, and Surgeon General Wyman, whom Kinyoun felt sought to "simply relegate [him] to oblivion" (cited in Chase: 90). He was sent to represent the service on a brief trip to Japan, where he conducted research on tropical diseases. He was then stationed briefly in Hong Kong and in British Columbia. In April 1902, he resigned from the service, bitter about the lack of support for his actions in San Francisco. In 1903, Kinyoun was named director of the H. K. Mulford Company in Pennsylvania, a commercial manufacturer of biologicals such as diphtheria antitoxin and smallpox vaccine. He held that post until 1907, when he returned to Washington, D.C., as professor of pathology and bacteriology at George Washington School of Medicine, and from 1909 to 1919, he directed the bacteriological laboratory for the District of Columbia. He developed a technique for detecting tubercle bacilli in sputum samples that is still used, known as the "Kinyoun method." During World War I he served as an expert epidemiologist in the army in North and South Carolina. He also served a term as president of the Society of Bacteriologists and was a member of many medical associations. In December 1918, he was appointed pathologist at the Armed Forces Medical Museum, where he served until his death in 1919 (Kelly and Burrage: 737).

Surgeon General Wyman selected Dr. Rupert Blue to replace Kinyoun and lead the campaign against the bubonic plague outbreak in San Francisco. Blue was born in North Carolina in 1868. He attended the University of Virginia and earned his M.D. from the University of Maryland in 1892. He joined the Marine Hospital Service for a nine-month internship in 1892–1893, after which he applied for entrance and was commissioned an assistant surgeon in March 1893. He spent his first years in the service as a medical inspector of immigrants. Blue was 33 at the time and stationed in Milwaukee, Wisconsin, caring for sick boatmen on Lake Michigan. Wyman dispatched him to oversee the campaign against the plague outbreak in San Francisco in 1902–1904 and again in 1907–1908 after the earthquake and fire there in 1906 (www.surgeongeneral.gov/library/history/bioblue.htm).

Probably one reason why Surgeon General Wyman sent Dr. Blue was that he correctly assessed that Blue would be diplomatic in dealing with city and state officials, the Chinese community, and the Anglo business community in the city.[8] The assistant surgeon at Angel Island, Dr. Joseph White, was given temporary authority over the station after Kinyoun's transfer and until Blue assumed control. Dr. White felt helpless to cure the plague in Chinatown, puzzled by how to deal with the community and their hiding of dead bodies. He pleaded for reinforcements, remarking: "The difficulties here are so great that never before in our history has there been a greater need for tactful and forceful officers, and mediocrity is I think clean out of place" (cited in Chase: 91). Dr. White had been most impressed with Kinyoun and his brilliance as a bacteriologist and was, frankly, very skeptical that Rupert Blue would do the job. His first impression of Blue increased his doubts. Yet soon after Blue's arrival, Dr. White wrote to Wyman in a letter dated April 30, 1901.

> Finally, regarding Blue, I wish to say that his work up to date has been excellent, and that the impression, which has for some reason or other, gained currency to the effect that he was not a man of pronounced personality and executive ability, although a very nice gentleman, is utterly erroneous. He has untangled a good many rather difficult snarls, has an immense amount of self- possession and good temper, and is altogether fully capable of acting as executive officer, and it may be, of ultimately taking my place should you conclude to return me to Washington. (RG 90, File 5608, Letters from Surgeon White to Surgeon Glover (1901–1904), Folder 2, Letter of April 30, 1901)

In his letter Dr. White refers to Mrs. Kinyoun having sent him a telegram to the effect that doctors Kinyoun and Wyman had reached a "satisfactory understanding," and that he, White, was glad of that fact. In subsequent reports, Dr. White informed Drs. Glover and Wyman that deaths had continued to mount in the epidemic, fifteen deaths between April 20 and July 6 and another eight deaths in October/November. By January 6, 1902, Wyman authorized White to report to both City of San Francisco and the California State Boards of Health on both the provisional and positive diagnoses of plague and authorized payment for one Wong Chung to be chief interpreter in the campaign to cope with the outbreak (Letter of January 6, 1902, Folder 1).

Blue had arrived in the city just as it launched a frenzied beautification project for a visit by President William McKinley. He arrived during a political tug-of-war over the corpse of a Chinese resident who had been suffering from tuberculosis, but whom Dr. White suspected had actually died of bubonic plague. The state board of health officials appointed by Governor Cage ridiculed Dr. White and his diagnosis. Although the state had earmarked $25,000 of its $100,000 plague fund for cleaning up Chinatown, the state board's main job seemed to be to dispute the plague diagnosis. Rupert Blue handled the wrangling diplomatically. Rather than engage the state board and the Chinese community head on, he met all with a genial smile and gave all sides the impression that he saw things from their respective viewpoint. While White wrangled and tried to find hidden bodies, Blue inspected the area for sanitary problems. He found cellars afloat with sewage and vermin, garbage heaps in backs of stores and on vacant lots, squalor galore, and rotten meat dumped in hundred-pound mounds.

President McKinley and his wife arrived in mid-May for a brief visit. In early June, Wyman granted Dr. White's request to be returned to Washington, D.C. Blue and two assistants were left to oversee the floundering campaign against the plague—which the state board declared, predictably, non-existent. Rupert Blue saw that the money earmarked for cleanup could be used to begin a massive sanitary effort. He set up headquarters for a "rat crusade" and leased a morgue and laboratory on Merchant Street (Chase: 93–94).

Outbreaks of plague cases returned in July 1901, spreading from Chinese residents to Japanese women, several of whom died. Blue wrote Wyman in code about the renewed outbreak. Like Kinyoun and White, he at first faced a wall of denial and deceit, but rather than collide head-on with them, he circumvented them, allowing their doctors to handle the deaths and only using his lab to assess the cause of death. A few more deaths, suspected victims of the plague, occurred among Chinese residents. Blue used a Chinese interpreter who proved to be a font of medical and political intelligence, tipping off Blue and his doctors to cases of suspected plague deaths before the bodies could be hidden. Then a white sailor, not a resident of Chinatown, came down with the plague. He survived the illness, but Blue's interview of him led Blue to suspect waterfront rats as the source of his infection. That hinted at a far wider plague infestation. Then a 53-year-old white matron, a laundress, was struck and died of the illness on September 27 (Shah: 153–157; Chase: 96–97). Blue filed weekly reports on the number of deaths and mapped the location of their spread. Blue noted that the Italian family lived within a few blocks of Chinatown, a distance easily covered by rats in their migration. Dead rats had been a signal of plague outbreaks for years, although doctors had not yet accepted their direct link to transmission of the disease. "Diseased rats bred and spread, heedless of skin color or scientific fashion."[9]

As more deaths—and, important, more white deaths occurred—opposition to the plague campaign declined. A new governor replaced Cage in November 1902, and state opposition ceased. The city began to lay traps for rats in earnest. City labs found that they had been infected—sixteen infected rats were found in two weeks from traps in city streets and sewers. Blue led the massive campaign to clean up the city and eradicate the rats. He ordered debris from condemned buildings dredged with powdered lime—making it unusable for firewood—then burned. In summer 1903, Blue headed a systematic cleanup. Thousands of rats were killed and dissected and tested for plague. Wooden cellars were replaced with concrete. A bounty was placed on dead rats. Blue proposed a wholesale eradication of the rats of San Francisco. Thousands of rooms were inspected, and nearly 1,000 sites were limed and disinfected. Sidewalk sanitation was promoted as medicine. Poured concrete became rat barriers. Blue courted city officials and aroused public support and awareness. In the fifth year of the smoldering plague, cases of pneumonic plague occurred among a white Italian American family. Blue met with state and local health officials and the city merchants over how best to fund the plague campaign (Chase, 2003: 90).

The Public Health Commission of California was formed, with Rupert Blue as president. Blue's drive began to get impressive results. Instead of focusing on quarantine only of Chinese residents, he got the entire community to see "rats" and appallingly unsanitary conditions as the common enemy. The cleanup campaign seemed to slash the rates of sickness generally—the overall death rate dropped to 388 compared to 466 the preceding year. As Chase documents, by early 1905, the city's plague seemed to be over, with 121 cases of plague and 113 deaths (138). In April 1905, Blue was transferred to Norfolk, Virginia. Unlike Kinyoun, who departed being vilified in the press, Blue left something of a hero for having ended the deadly epidemic. But the hiatus was to be short-lived.

On April 18, 1906 the devastating San Francisco earthquake struck, with huge fires erupting in its aftermath. Refugees were housed in crowded tent compounds. Sanitation was disrupted. The city quickly erected thousands of two- and three-room wooden cottages. Occupants cooked in communal kitchens and used earthen trenches for latrines. The earthquake shook tens of thousands of rats from their hiding places. From fractured walls and ruptured sewer pipes, rats and their fleas poured forth, joining the river of refugees as resourceful camp followers. They feasted on the garbage and bred in abundance. Wyman sent Blue back to the city to report on its sanitary conditions. He did so, dreading another plague outbreak. After his inspection trip, Blue returned to his post in the east. His premonition was right. On May 29, 1907, the first death from bubonic plague occurred. The second wave of epidemic struck. By August 22, additional cases were confirmed.

This time, there was no denial, no reluctance, no opposition to federal efforts. The city officials called by name for Rupert Blue to be reassigned to head the effort to combat the disease. Blue returned with no illusions. He formed a "rat crusade" of inspectors, assistants, and rat catchers in a massive effort to exterminate them, centering his headquarters and lab on Fillmore Street. It became the "rattery," the center of his war on rats.

Blue's campaign soaked the 750 Red Cross cottages in carbolic acid. By May 1908, they had inspected 20,907 houses, placed 190,104 poisoned baits, trapped 4,063 rats, collected another 2,518 rats from bounty hunters, and found 691 dead rats. They tested 2,952 rats for bubonic plague bacteria (Chase: 181). The unprecedented efforts to eradicate rats and the massive sanitary hygienic measures launched by Blue and his team proved successful in stopping the epidemic. The last reported case of the plague was September 26, 1908.[10] Blue was hailed by the *San Francisco Call* as the hero and conqueror of the San Francisco plague. By the end of the campaign, the total sick from the second outbreak (1907–1908) were put at 281, with 190 confirmed plague deaths. The statistics of the campaign were staggering. The team had inspected and disinfected 11,000 houses. More than 250,000 square feet of Victorian boardwalks had been replaced with concrete sidewalks. More than 6 million square feet of homes, shops, and stables were girded with rat-proof cement floors. More than 10 million pieces of rat bait were placed. More than 350,000 rats had been trapped, killed, and collected from bounty hunters. Bacteriological tests were conducted on 154,000 rats in the rattery. The total estimated kill of rats was 2 million—five times the city's human population (Chase: 194–195).

By 1910, the role of the station changed. A U.S. naval ship anchored off-shore was found to have smallpox aboard. The ship and crew were disinfected. By 1912, the station provided medical inspections for the Immigration Station, identifying diseases in its lab tests to prevent them from entering the country. In 1914, the station provided disinfection and bathing facilities for the 452 enemy aliens incarcerated on Angel Island. During World War I, it fumigated Army transport ships arriving from overseas and disinfected clothing and bedding from the Fort McDowell hospital. Some 6,500 blankets and 1,000 mattresses were treated with steam (RG 90, File 5608, Box 616).

In 1919, army transport ships returning with troops from Siberia were brought to Angel Island to be disinfected. The soldiers bathed in an emulsion of gasoline and soap, and their clothing and gear were disinfected with hydrocyanic gas. The station received complaints that it was inadequately supplied with towels, bathrobes, and dungaree suits.

When the 1918–1919 influenza pandemic swept the country, San Francisco was one of a few cities that publicly acknowledged the epidemic, dispensing 100,000 gauze masks and thousands of doses of vaccine (which were ineffective, being for a different strain). The quarantine station was used to cope with its outbreak among returning servicemen. As in other cities, the efforts were largely futile. The number of cases of the disease seemed no less than in other western cities suffering from the killer flu, and its final death rates were the worst on the west coast (Barry: 375).

In 1920, another case of smallpox was discovered on the U.S. Army transport *Mount Vernon* while moored at the Mare Island naval yard. The

510-man crew was brought to Angel Island and quarantined, overtaxing the capacity of the station. The inadequate barracks there forced about 100 men to sleep on the floor.

In 1924, a rat infected with bubonic plague was found in a garbage dump in near-by Oakland, California. Officers from the quarantine station instituted a rat eradication program that lasted several years. Thousands of rat traps were set, and some 80,000 rats were killed in 1926 alone. Two were found to be infected with the plague. The surgeon in charge at the station was sent to Imperial County, California, in 1924, to oversee an outbreak of trachoma among migrant workers' children.

SPREADING INNOVATIONS

The Angel Island station was the source of several important innovations for better coping with contagious disease epidemics that were spread throughout the Public Health Service network and to public health doctors and hospitals beyond those of the service. Of significance to the early 1900s were improvements in sterilizing equipment. Kinyoun's design improvements for the steam chambers, for example, involved adding a metal hood and redesigning fittings that greatly improved the chambers' operations. Early designs of the chambers developed leaks from the fittings, particularly when changing from sulfur dioxide to formaldehyde gas.[11] A circular sent to the U.S. M.H.S. from the surgeon general's office in 1899 requested reports on the status of the steam chambers (most stations had gotten their chambers in 1893). In October, 1899, Kinyuon ordered new chambers and autoclaves, and a new steam injector boiler for the Angel Island Quarantine station from the Pacific Coast Boiler works. Soon the Kinyoun–Francis apparatus was being used in numerous places: Delaware, Reedy Island, Cape Charles, Southport, South Atlantic Station, Brunswick, Fernandia, Dry Tortuga, Key West, San Diego, Port Townsend, Pittsburgh, Brooklyn, New York, Santiago, Cuba, and Washington, D.C. The design of the steam chamber and related equipment was being used in a number of disinfecting vessels in the service: the *Zamora*, *Jamestown*, *Koch*, and *Protector* (RG 90, File 4605, Box 505; Letters of July 6, 14, September 30, October 7 and 9). Numerous shipping orders were made and reports on their safe arrival filed after August 1898, when the shift to formaldehyde gas apparatus was made. In June and August, large steam chambers were shipped to the Marine Hospital in Baltimore, along with boilers and sulfur furnaces. On February 1, 1899, Surgeon G. W. Stoner ordered eight steam disinfecting chambers and steam boilers and sulfur furnaces for the Port of New York. In December 1899, the U.S. M.H.S. began purchasing that design of steam chamber as the standard chamber for foreign quarantine stations (e.g. in Manila, Havana, and so on) (Ibid.: folder 16).

The Kensington Engine Works Ltd. produced a booklet on the steam chamber and related apparatus for equipping disinfecting vessels, quarantine stations, hospitals, and even portable devices for municipal public health agencies. This was widely distributed (Pamphlet, Kinyoun Papers, National Library of Medicine, Box 1, Folder 16, "The Kinyoun–Francis Disinfecting Machinery"). When the plague epidemic broke out in San Francisco in April 1902, Dr. Hugh Cumming, surgeon in charge, moved one chamber, owned by the San Francisco Board of Health, from the Port of San Francisco to the Angel Island station for its use on board a floating disinfection plant, it having those design innovations.

In 1910–1911, the assistant surgeon in command at Angel Island worried that the *Omaha*, outfitted to fumigate vessels and in service since the late 1890s, had outgrown her usefulness and that if a transpacific liner arrived with plague on board, it would be impossible to place the *Omaha* alongside the infected vessel. He urged the service to build a new wharf at the station, equipped with the better-designed chambers, saying that this must be done before the Panama Canal was finished in order to do thorough and efficient fumigation (RG 90, File 2392).

Kinyoun influenced a new generation of bacteriologists through his work at the hygienic laboratory in Washington, D.C., and in his teaching after leaving the service. He imbued them with lessons learned during his years in the service battling various infectious diseases.

Perhaps even more extensive an effect came from Rupert Blue as a result of his San Francisco plague outbreak experiences. In a report dated February 23, 1909, entitled "Rat Fleas and Their Relation to the Transmission of Plague," Carol Fox and Rupert Blue shared insights from their experience that were published as a P.H.S. bulletin.

On April 13, 1909, Rupert Blue wrote "Rodents in Relation to the Transmission of Bubonic Plague," introducing standards by which the service operated. In late 1909, the U.S. M.H.S. (not yet the P.H.S.) received reports of plague in Honolulu and in Kentucky. Wyman ordered reports from all stations on their processes and efforts for the destruction of rats. Reports on the extermination of rats poured in from around the world: Alaska, Africa, Argentina, Australia, Austria, Burma, Chile, China, Colombia, the Congo, Denmark, the Dominican Republic, Great Britain, Hawaii, India, Hong Kong, New Zealand, Russia, Siberia, South Africa, Syria, Uruguay (RG 90, File 2392; File 114, Box 16, Folders 1 and 2). In 1911, all quarantine stations were ordered to conduct a rat quarantine during the first week of December and to report numbers of ships fumigated and numbers of rats exterminated. American consulates from key ports around the world sent in reports to the service on their efforts and the number of rats exterminated using the Blue pamphlet guidelines: Bordeaux, France; London, England; Odessa, Russia; Antwerp, Belgium; Genoa, Italy; Edinburgh, Scotland; Liverpool, England; Hamburg, Germany, Vancouver, B.C.; Panama City, Panama; Montreal, Canada; Kingston, Jamaica; Havana, Cuba; Christiania, Norway; Puerto Cortes, Honduras; Colon, Panama; and Havre, France (File 2392, Folder 544).

Blue's influence was spread at meetings of the Association of Military Surgeons, which many Public Health and Marine Hospital Service doctors regularly attended—for example, at Atlanta in 1908; Richmond in 1910 and 1911; and Norfolk, Virginia, in 1910. Blue's right-hand man in the San Francisco campaign became secretary of the Association of Military Surgeons in 1913. Another of his close colleagues, Surgeon J. W. Kerr, then at Ellis Island, presented at St. Louis a report on their efforts to contain infectious diseases among U.S. troops in 1919. When bubonic plague broke out in New Orleans in 1914, the lab established there by the National Health Service conducted research on rats and used the extermination approach developed by Blue in San Francisco in 1908–1909.

Blue extended his "extermination of the carriers of disease" approach in his other work. He directed mosquito eradication efforts against yellow fever in New Orleans (1905), at the Jamestown Exposition (1907), and in Honolulu (1911). He represented the United States at a number of sanitation projects in South America and attended the London School of Tropical Medicine in 1910. Blue's success in the field enhanced his growing reputation, and he was promoted to position of surgeon in May 1909. When Walter Wyman died unexpectedly, President William Howard Taft promoted him to surgeon general, in which role he served from January 1912 to March 1920, having been reappointed by President Woodrow Wilson for another four-year term in 1916. Under Blue's leadership, physician researchers at the P.H.S. used bacteriology and refined versions of age-old sanitation practices and public education and turned them into effective campaigns to battle infectious diseases, especially those linked to poverty in both rural areas and urban slums. He oversaw a dramatic, if short, expansion of the P.H.S. during World War I. The service battled venereal disease with control programs among troops. Funded by the Red Cross, it provided industrial hygiene and health services for thousands of workers laboring in the war plants and, in communities surrounding them, emptied swamps and sprayed for mosquitoes to prevent malaria. The service built sanitary privies. The Hygienic Laboratory in Washington, D.C., produced vaccines against tetanus, diphtheria, typhoid, and smallpox. Blue created a new public health infrastructure that was up and running when Congress supported it with earmarked dollars in a statute covering the control and prevention of venereal disease (the Chamberlain Act of 1918) (www.surgeongeneral.gov/library/history/bioblue.htm).

Recruiting and training physicians during wartime challenged Blue and the P.H.S., especially when the influenza pandemic hit in 1918. The P.H.S. struggled, inadequately, to battle the outbreak, all the time underfunded and understaffed. Blue advocated enacting a national health insurance program as part of an overall federal public health strategy (an idea decades ahead of political opinion and a climate to support it). When the leadership changed in the Department of the Treasury, then the Public Health Service's home, Blue fell out of favor. He stepped down as surgeon general in March 1920. He was sent to Paris, France, to oversee P.H.S. operations in Europe and served as the U.S. delegate to the Office of International d' Hygiene Public (1920–1923) and, subsequently, to the League of Nations. He retired from the P.H.S. in December 1932. He died in April 1948 (www.surgeongeneral.gov/library/history/bioblue.htm).

CONCLUSION

The Angel Island story illuminates the service's battles against the ravages of pandemic diseases and critical epidemics of smallpox, bubonic plague, and influenza.

Doctors serving there waged valiant battles against these diseases while helping process millions of immigrants entering the United States through the west coast. Numerous nondeadly contagious diseases, most notably trachoma, hookworm, and liver fluke, exemplified the "loathsome and contagious" disease category used to bar many from entrance, especially those hailing from China and those from Asian countries more generally.

Doctors at the station exhibited the racial attitudes prevalent at the time, and racial assumptions as well as local politics influenced their campaigns to battle the deadly epidemics they faced, particularly the bubonic plague outbreaks between 1900 and 1908.

Important innovations they developed or refined there, both in sterilizing devices and in administrative processes to conduct massive public health and sanitation reform, became the standard for a scientific medicine approach to public health. They influenced another generation of medical scientists and public health officers and shaped the infrastructure of the federal public health service. Their effects were felt at the largest quarantine facility and program in the world—Ellis Island in New York City harbor. And it is to that station's story that we next turn our attention.

Chapter 4

THE ELLIS ISLAND STATION

Ellis Island is unquestionably the most famous and—in terms of volume of immigrants processed through it—most important station in the United States. It had a special role in American immigration history and saw more than 16.5 million immigrants pass through its portals. The Ellis Island station typically handled 70–80 percent of all the immigrants coming into the United States. It averaged nearly 69 percent for its entire period of operation. It experienced a decline in total number of immigrants coming to the United States, and a dramatic decline in the percentages it processed, during the World War I years (1915–1918), the Great Depression Years (1931–1938), and the World War II years (1942–1945). Those data indicate the importance of push factors in immigration to the United States over official policy—which is focused on pull factors. Forces such as worldwide depressions and wars influenced the decision of millions about whether to emigrate to a much greater degree than did any law enacted by the United States.

Today as well, violence in Central American countries is pushing illegal immigration of children and some adults that comes unabated by laws or efforts to tighten control at the borders. This is not to say, of course, that "pull" policy has no effect. A dramatic effect on the total legal permanent migration resulted from the quota acts of 1921, 1924, and 1929, when immigration to the United States and through Ellis Island declined from many hundreds of thousands to tens of thousands annually. During World War II, however, the numbers declined to mere thousands.

The medical staff at Ellis Island struggled with enormous waves of immigrants. In each of its zenith years of operations, from 1903 to 1914, Ellis Island processed from more than 700,000 to more than 1 million immigrants (Willrich: 224–225, LeMay, 2006: 30–31). During its all-time peak year of 1907, when 1,004,756 persons arrived, the station averaged 2,750 persons inspected per day, and the typical day that year exceeded 5,000! Ellis Island inspected ten times the numbers of persons who entered through Angel Island and even more than that of those who came through New Orleans. To handle so many while effectively screening for highly infectious disease was a remarkable accomplishment. The doctors at Ellis Island faced numerous epidemic diseases: cholera, smallpox, diphtheria, yellow fever, measles, trachoma, and influenza. They used microbiology techniques in their medical laboratory to test for contagious disease. They developed procedures to screen the thousands of persons who daily attempted to enter the United States through the station and to safely and scientifically disinfect many thousands of ships and their cargo, and the personal belongings of immigrants, to prevent the vermin carriers of disease, the silent travelers, from infecting the population of New York City and cities beyond. Like those at Angel Island, Ellis Island doctors were, in Parascandola's words, unsung heroes in the fight against the spread of pandemics (7).

Service physicians never sat on the boards of special inquiry that made the final decisions to admit or exclude despite numerous attempts by the Immigration Service to pressure them to find more of the arrivals to be physically or mentally unfit. Service doctors at Ellis Island, Angel Island, and New Orleans did not suffer from the graft and favoritism that so often notoriously plagued the Immigration Service. As historian of the service Mullan notes:

> The white, male, predominantly southern physicians of the Public Health and Marine Hospital Service were certainly liable to a variety of cultural biases, but given the press of newcomers, and the paucity of their own numbers, they served as evenhanded—even benevolent—keepers of the gate. In all, almost twenty million immigrants passed under their examining eyes from 1891 to 1924, making them midwives, of a sort, to the American nation. (46–48)

Finally, as it has been at Angel Island, the epic story of Ellis Island has been memorialized by a national historic park at the site (Benton, 1998: 144–145).

A BRIEF HISTORY OF ELLIS ISLAND
QUARANTINE STATION

Castle Garden—the Predecessor

For decades before Ellis Island was opened, in 1892, New York City was already established as the port of entry for millions of immigrants. It was preferred by the shipping lines for discharging immigrant passengers, and it, as well as New York City, grew rapidly as the immigrant flow rose from a trickle, to a stream, and then to a flood of arrivals. In the 1820s, 1830s, and 1840s, immigrants were generally met on the wharf and asked a few rudimentary questions (their names, relationships to fellow passengers if traveling as a family group, their ages, country or place of origin, and destination in the United States). Manifests were checked against that information, and the ship's logs were examined with regard to the presence of any incidents of illness or death during the voyage. During those decades, immigration processing was under the policymaking, implementation, and control of *state* governments. Federal government policy focused merely on the "census" aspect of the millions of arrivals (LeMay, ed., 2013, vol. 2: 197–208).

One vexing problem that developed as the wave of immigrants increased in size and complexity was that the newcomers were being swindled by dishonest boardinghouse operators and railroad ticket agents who met the immigrants as they disembarked. Germans established immigrant-aid societies in 1784. The Irish followed suite in 1841. They quickly developed into ethnic organizations that lobbied New York state legislators on the issue. They called for New York to establish a board of commissioners of emigration. The legislature did so in May 1847. The board first created the Emigrant Hospital and Refuge on Wards Island, which treated noncontagious illness among immigrants. The Marine Hospital was placed under the board's control.

As immigration swelled to hundreds of thousands annually, the flow became too great for local inspectors and the immigrant aid societies. In 1850, for example, more than 2,000 ships delivered over 200,000 immigrants. The need for a central receiving station became apparent.

In New York City, implementation of immigration policy was through the Castle Garden station, the first center specifically established for receiving immigrants. By the early 1850s, 1,000 immigrants a day were arriving at the New York City port. Castle Garden opened on May 5, 1855. The creation of Castle Garden was motivated by a desire to better deal with the corruption and exploitation that occurred on the wharfs and at nearby inns that accommodated the newly disembarked immigrants, but soon the volume was such that Castle Garden itself was noted for lesser but still significant levels of corruption, cronyism, inefficiency, and exploitation. The danger posed by epidemic disease outbreaks remained ever present, and outbreaks were a prime motivation to establish the Castle Garden reception station. New York City suffered cholera epidemics in 1832 and cholera and smallpox epidemics in 1834, which collectively resulted in several thousands of deaths. In 1849, a severe cholera epidemic occurred. The massive numbers of immigrants arriving in 1847–1848 (typhus epidemic years referred to as "ship fever" at the time) led policymakers to conclude that the epidemic came with the immigrants. In 1851 another smallpox outbreak occurred, and in 1854 more than 2,500 people died in a cholera outbreak (LeMay, 2006: 41, and 2013, vol. 2: 51–52).

During the era of the sailing vessels, epidemic diseases took many lives during the voyage itself. We now recognize that typhus was spread by lice. It resulted in some horrific losses. Some 7,000 persons succumbed to ship fever in voyage during 1847, with some 10,000 more dying at or near Quebec City and Canada's Grosse Isle station. Nearly as deadly was Asiatic cholera, caused by an intestinal microbe and spread in contaminated water. In 1853, an estimated 15 percent of passengers on some ships died from cholera.[1]

The transatlantic journey during the era of the sailing vessel was a terrifying experience. Many ships were lost in storms or shipwrecked near arrival. During the winter of 1853–1854, for example, 200 German immigrants died in a ship wreck off the New Jersey shore, and 480 passengers, the crew, and two ships sailing out of Glasgow disappeared altogether.

In 1847 over 200,000 Irish fled the poverty and disease of their homeland for North America. They boarded sailing vessels hungry, weakened, and often already ill. Most of them set off with scarcely enough money for their passage and with inadequate amounts of food for the long voyage of a month or two. At that time, passengers were required to provide their own food for the voyage rather than the ship captain's doing so. An estimated 9 percent of those who embarked in England, Ireland, and Germany, destined for the United States (the vast majority of whom were headed for the port of New York City) died during the voyage. The news of that staggering death toll shocked immigration authorities and moved policymakers to enact legislation requiring ship owners or their agents to provide food for the journey, increased ventilation for passengers during the voyage, and to be inspected on arrival, with increased fines imposed for those breaking the laws. Such penalties, however, were set too low to effectively deter greedy sailing ship owners or masters, and the death rates on board remained quite high until steamship lines developed to manage the transatlantic migration. They became the prominent, although not the exclusive, mode of travel by the 1880s. As Guillet notes about the New York City port's immigration processing:

> The course of events in the ship-fever year, 1847, indicates careful management on the part of the Commissioners of Emigration which contrasts

very favorably with the congestion at Grosse Isle. In the first place stringent sanitary regulations and other restrictions were enforced at American ports, so that when the plague broke out, many overcrowded vessels bound for New York altered their destination to the St. Lawrence, where two or three times as many might be landed as in the United States. Such protective measures saved American ports from the calamity which descended upon Montreal, though the disease was widespread enough to require extensive hospital accommodation. In New York all the quarantine hospitals were first filled with the ill and destitute; then all spare rooms connected with the City Almshouse were rented at $1 per week for those who were destitute and $1.50 per week for the sick. But the risk attendant upon placing fever patients in the Almshouse led to the construction of special buildings on Staten Island. As these were still inadequate, the buildings on the Long Island Farms were leased, but the fear of contagion so alarmed the neighborhood that they were burned by incendiaries. The United States Government then permitted the use of warehouses at the Quarantine Station; and when they were almost immediately filled, all the chief hospitals, public and private, were called into requisition. Finally, at the height of the plague, a large stone building on Ward's Island was leased, which, with structures subsequently added to it, afforded ample accommodation for all. (183)

From 1820 until 1860, roughly 70 percent of the nearly 5.5 million immigrants who came to the United States arrived through New York City. Immigrants arrived at a rate of about 5,000 per year. They were processed casually at whichever port of call they arrived. In those years, many immigrants entered at the ports of Boston, Philadelphia, Portland, Maine, New Orleans, and Galveston. Typically, the shipping company merely presented a list of passengers (a manifest) to the collector of customs. The immigrants made their customs declaration for items being brought in that were subject to customs law and then went on their way. By the 1850s, the numbers arriving increased to the tens, even the hundreds, of thousands annually. As numbers soared, political pressure to better screen and process them led to the establishing of reception centers specifically organized to do so. As said, the very first such immigrant reception station established in the country was the Castle Garden station, then still a state-run operation.

New York established the receiving station at Castle Garden in 1855 to protect its residents from the spread of epidemic diseases and to protect the immigrants from a host of swindlers who met them as they disembarked. Agents met them on the piers, enticing them with offers to find housing, food, and railway tickets to destinations beyond New York City. City political connections and cronyism often victimized immigrants by a network of crooked shippers, innkeepers, railroad ticket agents, porters, and moneychangers operating out of Castle Garden. Even some compatriots who had arrived earlier participated in their exploitation (Reeves: 16–17).

Thanks to a lack of knowledge about how epidemic diseases were spread, visual medical inspection followed by detention was the established procedure for epidemic outbreaks associated with the ever-increasing numbers of arrivals. Because many disease carriers arrived in a nonsymptomatic stage, or while their conditions were not sufficiently noticeable to be detected by what was still fairly casual inspection, illness was spread to the broader population. The 1860s and 1870s saw smallpox and cholera outbreaks that took thousands of lives. By then the association of smallpox and cholera with "the filthy poor" was long-standing, based more in class and racial bias than on medical reality (Willrich: 27; see also Williams, 1951).

An 1866 newspaper article illustrates the plight of immigrants at Castle Garden:

Many are the weeping eyes and widowed hearts, that now under the great exodus going on are leaving their native shores. . . . There was one among the group of women who was the object of great commiseration. She had lost her little one on the voyage, from fever, and the poor child had to be thrown overboard, she, poor mother, being left, like Rachel, weeping for her child and would not be comforted because it was no more. It is indeed a sad thing to have to hide one's offspring in the grave on land, but there is something about death and burial in the cold canvas winding sheet at sea, in a fathomless grave, yet harder and more galling. (www.members.tripod .com/~L-Alfano/castle.htm)

Only after the medical breakthroughs of the 1880s did epidemic outbreaks take the lives of only a few hundred rather than a few thousand. Changes in medical knowledge and procedures came at an opportune time, since during the decade of the 1880s more than 5 million immigrants came to the United States, about 3.8 million through the port of New York, the busiest seaport during the peak decades of Euro–American transatlantic shipping. Most immigrants and goods bound for most American destinations passed through New York's port, then the primary hub of commerce and trade.

The advent of steamships eased the journey and made it merely uncomfortable rather than potentially deadly. Though typhus and smallpox still occasionally cropped up, by the 1880s new laws enacted in sending countries required ship owners to employ doctors on board during the journey, and improved conditions even in steerage, enabled sufficient control to cut considerably outbreaks of typhus and smallpox. The better ship lines provided cooked meals three times a day, though ventilation continued to be a problem in steerage.

The main steamship transportation line serving the port of New York was the famous Cunard Line. It began as the Royal Mail Steam Packet Company to deliver mail from Liverpool to Halifax, Canada, and the line started service with four steam paddle ships. Its very first one, the *Britannia*, made the crossing from Liverpool to Halifax in fourteen days, with founder Samuel Cunard and sixty-three passengers aboard. His company stressed safety over speed, and during his lifetime the company lost no ship. As Fox notes, the first and only liner the company lost was the sinking of the *Lusitania*, torpedoed by a German submarine on May 7, 1915, fifty years after Cunard's death (405–407). The line moved its headquarters to London in 1848 and eventually developed a fleet of forty ships, mostly steel-hull steamships. In contrast to the grim voyage described by the Irish immigrant in Guillet, cited in chapter 1, a Swiss journalist described the era of the steamship transport even in "steerage class" as follows:

> There are 280 berths in all, disposed in two single ranges along the sides, and one double range in the centre of the ship. Air and light are abundant and there is no lack of space to promenade when the deck would be a doubtful source for bodily exercise. About a ninth of the whole number of berths are boxed off from the rest for the use of unmarried females. There are also two hospitals for the use of steerage passengers, one for males and the other for females. . . . [and describing the transatlantic crossing by steamship] She opened up a new era in which sustained speed and reliable passages were complemented by superior standards of accommodation. With choices ranging from luxurious cabins in terms of the day, by those who could afford them, to relatively spacious communal mess-decks for travelers of more modest means, all passengers had steward service of some kind and cooked meals. In general the coming of the *Canadian* marked an efficient and humane approach to emigration at a time when many sailing ships . . . were still carrying unfortunate people as they had done for the previous century. (cited in Sevigny, 1995a: 213–214)

During 1855–1890, about 8 million immigrants passed through Castle Garden, accounting for 75 percent of all immigrants to the United States. Castle Garden was located at the tip of lower Manhattan in Battery Park. It was originally part of a chain of forts constructed to defend against naval attack and known first as West Battery, then renamed Castle Clinton, in 1815, after the first governor of the state of New York. In 1855, New York State's Board of Emigration Commissioners decided to convert it to an immigration landing depot. It opened on August 3, 1855 (LeMay, ed., 2013, vol. 2: 205).

In 1847, the emigration board established a 350-bed hospital and other buildings on Ward's Island. A refuge building was erected for destitute women and children. A New Barracks building temporarily housed destitute alien males. Though the Ward's Island facilities provided needed detention facilities, Castle Garden enabled authorities to process, better protect, and medically screen arriving immigrants. It was operated under contract with the federal government which relieved New Yorkers of caring for the destitute or sick foreigner. The emigration board also operated a smallpox hospital on Blackwell Island.

Castle Garden quickly grew to a staff of about one hundred, managed by a superintendent. It sent boarding officers to inspect ships for cleanliness. They either passed a ship for landing or ordered it to quarantine. When allowed to dock, the ship was met by Castle Garden duty officers and agents from the Labor Department to transport immigrants to the depot's pier via tugboats and barges. Arriving immigrants were marched into the Castle Garden building for medical examinations. Those assessed as sick were put on a steamboat bound for either Ward's or Blackwell's Island. Anyone determined likely to be a public charge was admitted only under a bond. Immigrants were then sent on to the rotunda of the station, where registration clerks processed as many as 3,000 immigrants daily. They were divided and sent to English-language and foreign-language desks to be interviewed and their names, nation of origin, and destinations in the United States recorded. Those traveling on were directed to railroad agents to purchase tickets to their destinations in the United States or Canada. Those intending to settle in the New York area were sent to the City Baggage Delivery, which sent their luggage to a local address. The Information Department handled family reunions. It had qualified interpreters for German, French, Italian, Spanish, Dutch, Czech, Swedish, Norwegian, Danish, Polish, Portuguese, Swiss–German, Russian, and Latin. The Forwarding Department, located in the main reception area of the rotunda, forwarded letters, remittances, and held any telegrams waiting for arriving immigrants. A letter-writing department composed letters in most European languages for the many illiterate immigrants. An exchange broker changed foreign currency into United States currency. An Employment Department, latter called the Labor Exchange, helped immigrants find work. Men and boys typically worked in cabinet-making, shoemaking, baking, weaving, and gardening. Women were often hired as domestic laborers. A posting of approved boarding-house keepers listed room prices in English, German, French, Italian, and the Nordic languages (Moreno, 2004: 3).

The Ward's Island department for the sick and the destitute handled admissions for immigrants sent there. It operated the main hospital, the Verplanck State Emigrant Hospital, supervised by a surgeon-in-chief. The hospital provided basic care for noncontagious diseases. There was also an insane asylum on the island for those suffering from dementia, melancholia, epilepsy, chronic alcoholism, and mental retardation.

In July 1876, a fire destroyed the building within the walls of the old stone fortress, destroying most of the station's records. Only the buildings outside the Castle Garden walls survived—the Labor Exchange, a small hospital, and the intelligence office. The depot was quickly reconstructed and reopened in late November 1876 (Foreign Language Information Service, New York, Index No. 4939, February 24, 1941).

When immigration swelled in the 1880s, the pressure at Castle Garden grew. In 1875, the United States Supreme Court ruled that only Congress should control immigration. Congress did not act on the matter until the August 3, 1882, with the passage of the Regulation of Immigration Act (22 Stat. 214; 8 U.S.C.), which authorized the secretary of the Treasury to contract with states for enforcement of that law. The 1882 laws were aimed at denying entrance to "undesirable aliens," then defined in the law to include Chinese laborers (often called "coolies"), prostitutes, and "any convict, lunatic, idiot, or any person unable to take care of himself or herself without becoming a public charge."[2]

From 1882 until 1890, the station was administered as a joint state/ federal system. For some years, complaints increased about abusive behavior by employees toward immigrants, political patronage, and excessive profits from the sale of railroad tickets. Congress responded with an official inquiry into all phases of immigration in 1890. On April 1, 1890, the secretary of the Treasury, then responsible for immigration policy, terminated the contract. On April 18, 1890, the Treasury Department assumed control of all immigration at New York. Castle Garden was closed when the federal government opted to build a new station on Ellis Island.

Secretary of the Treasury William Windom revoked all contracts with local officials (though they remained in effect for an additional year at Portland, Maine, Boston, Philadelphia, Baltimore, Key West, New Orleans, Galveston, and San Francisco). He announced his decision to build a new facility on one of the federally owned islands in the harbor. An island site was viewed as best in that it would better enable quarantine of the contagiously ill and better protect the immigrants from exploitation. They could be transferred directly from the island to the railroad terminals in New Jersey. The secretary initially intended to use Bedsloe's Island, site of the Statue of Liberty, erected in 1886, which had almost immediately become the national symbol of immigration. The statue's sculptor, Auguste Bartholdi, was horrified at the idea, calling the plan "monstrous," and a "desecration." The hue and cry over its likely effect on the Statue of Liberty site prompted federal authorities to consider Governor's Island, but the military rejected that possibility, and the decision was made to use Ellis Island, named after one of its previous private owners, a butcher named Samuel Ellis. Of the three islands in federal possession, it was the least attractive, but the only one not facing substantial political opposition.

Angered by the new federal policy, the state of New York refused to let the federal government use Castle Garden under lease while Ellis Island was under construction, so the Treasury Department, then the supervisory department for immigration policy, set up a temporary center at the Old Barge Office near the Battery at the tip of Manhattan. Federal officials conducted immigration services there until Ellis Island was opened two years later, on January 1, 1892. In its two years of operation, the Barge Office processed more than 500,000 immigrants, about 80 percent of all who entered the country then. A staff of about 100 persons worked there, many of whom had been at Castle Garden and who went on to service on Ellis Island.

The Office of Superintendent of Immigration in the Treasury Department was created by an act of Congress of March 3, 1891 (26 Stat. 1084: U.S.C. 101), and was designated as a bureau in 1895, charged to administer the alien contract labor laws. The bureau eventually became the Immigration and Naturalization Service, under the auspices of the Department of Justice. It administered immigration policy until March 1, 2003, when it was dissolved after its functions were moved to the Department of Homeland Security.

The Ellis Island Station

Ellis Island was about 2.5 acres. The main reception center was located there. Using fill from the rubble obtained from the construction of the city's subway system and ballast from ships, engineers eventually expanded the size of the island to fourteen acres in three islets linked by ferry dock. The unnamed second and third islets (created by fill) held the hospitals, quarantine buildings, and detention centers (Highsmith and Landphair: 1). The island, previously known as Oyster Island, was purchased by the state of New York in 1808 to be used for storage of naval materials and as a powder magazine. In 1880 the island, along with two others in the port of New York, were granted by the state of New York to the U.S. government. The first station constructed on Ellis Island (opened on January 1, 1892) had twelve wood-constructed buildings. There was a large main processing center, a two-story pine timber, and galvanized iron building designed to deal with up to 10,000 immigrants per day. There were four separate buildings used as hospitals, a surgeon's quarters, record storage building, disinfection house, boiler house, and tank and coal house. Water was supplied by artesian wells and stored in cisterns. Construction of the first station cost more than $500,000, about double the original estimate. The first immigrant processed through the new station was Annie Moore, a 15-year-old Irish girl. Ultimately, its volume was such that Highsmith and Landphair estimate that a third of all Americans had at least one ancestor immigrate to the United States through the Ellis Island station (Foreword).

In the 1880s, immigration increased nearly exponentially, especially through Ellis Island, because steamship lines could transport millions from around the world, cutting the journey from months to days. Emigrants poured out of Europe. Approximately 9 percent of the entire population of Norway came to the United States. Whole families migrated, drawn by the offer of cheap land. About a quarter of the population of Ireland emigrated during the peak period of the transatlantic flow.

On June 13, 1897, a fire broke out that burned to the ground most of the structures, including the main processing center and its record storage space in the basement. All the administrative records for the first five-year period were lost, as well as records transferred there from Castle Garden and the Barge Office sites (www.members.tripod.com/LAlfano/immig.htm.1).

In 1898–1903, the five-year epidemic of smallpox previously mentioned struck the United States. In 1900, it broke out in New York City, starting in what was called the "All Nations Block" of tenement slums, which had high populations of Italian, Irish, Jewish, German, Swedish, and Austrian immigrants, as well as African Americans. The city opened a smallpox hospital, "the pesthouse," on North Brother Island, located between Riker's Island and the Bronx mainland (Willrich: 2–4). A "vaccination corps" worked, in 1901–1903, enforcing compulsory vaccination in New York City, concentrating especially in the "Little Italy" section, where the density of population spread smallpox (Ibid.: 211–245). This corps, however, met considerable resistance from the "anti-vaccinationist" movement, led by the Anti-Vaccination League of America (Ibid.: 246–284). In addition to those who feared the vaccination process on health grounds, the movement had religious group opposition as well—especially the Christian Scientists, who opposed all vaccination, not just that against smallpox (260). By 1901 the city recorded 2,000 cases of smallpox, resulting in 410 deaths, the worst smallpox epidemic to strike the city since 1881, and twice as many as the previous year, In 1902 there were 309 deaths among 1,516 cases, which tapered off to only sixty-seven cases and four deaths by 1903 (Willrich: 236–237).

On Ellis Island, after the fire of 1897, a new, brick, stone, and steel structure in a French Renaissance style was constructed. While it was under construction, immigrants were once again processed through the old Battery Barge Office site. The new brick and stone station opened in December 1901.

Initial construction cost more than $1.2 million. Though impressive in style, it was soon inadequate to meet the demands placed on it, and over the next sixteen years numerous new constructions and remodeling took place, including repairs and enlargements. The central processing building dealt with steerage passengers and in its first year of operation processed nearly 389,000 immigrants. In 1907, its peak year of operation, it dealt with more than 1 million immigrants, with a record of 11,747 immigrants in a single day, on April 7, 1907 (Highsmith and Landphair, 2000: 1).

In 1904, administration of the station was transferred from the Treasury Department to the Department of Commerce and Labor. A new dining facility was completed that accommodated about 200 immigrants. In 1908, it was expanded to seat 1,000. That same year, the Baggage and Dormitory building, located behind the main building, was completed. A new surgeon's house and a psychopathic ward were added. In the decade before World War I, a third story was added to the main building and to the Baggage and Dormitory buildings, and a new ferry house, an incinerator, a greenhouse, a bakery, and a carpentry building were constructed. A new concrete and granite seawall was completed. Island 3 was filled in on which a Contagious Hospital was built.

Steerage passengers were processed through the central reception building, climbing stairs up to the first floor under careful observation of doctors who watched for any mobility problems, breathing difficulties, or similar signs symptomatic of the need for a more thorough medical screening. They filed past doctors who gave them a cursory examination and asked them rudimentary questions. Most were passed through—on average only about 2 percent were refused entry and sent back to their country of origin. But considering the huge numbers seeking entry, 2 percent still meant that annually several thousand suffered that fate. Immigrants who passed the medical exams were then sent on to answer to immigration officers a detailed questionnaire about their origin, destination, level of education, job skill level and occupation if any, relatives who might meet them or aide them in finding housing and work, and so on. About a third of those passing through in its early decade settled in the New York City area. Those who arrived with the means to do so arranged for railroad passage to the Midwest, where land was still available and comparatively inexpensive (Parascandola: 2–3; Benton: 56).

The Boarding Division comprised a chief inspector and twelve assistants, plus four or five surgeons from the Medical Division and five attendants from the Matrons' Division. They worked in crews boarding incoming vessels. They inspected the first and second-class passengers, mostly giving perfunctory examination of their paperwork. The Boarding Division sent all questionable cabin aliens, as they were called, to Ellis Island, separating American citizens from the steerage so that they could land with admissible cabin passengers at the piers. The boarding officers collected the manifests and accompanied all immigrants (mostly from steerage) going to Ellis Island for close examination. Steerage passengers were sorted into groups of 250. Anyone older than 2 was required to walk, unaided, up the stairs to the mammoth Registry Room on the second floor. They were observed while ascending, a rather simple screening device. In the Registry Room, physicians looked for contagious diseases and mental or emotional impairments and administered a "thirty-second medical" exam. Immigrants were "chalked" with a code and separated into more lines for questioning, in some cases for hours, about their paperwork, criminal records, and work status. The immigrants were then funneled down the "Stairs of Separation," where they were divided into three streams—those on the right proceeded to a New Jersey train station, those on the left to a ferry to Manhattan's tenement district, those in the center, detainees, to legal hearings, hospitalization, or deportation. Approximately 97 percent were eventually allowed to enter the United States.

The Medical Division was staffed by U.S. Marine Hospital Service personnel (after 1912 called U.S. Public Health Service). A few were attached to the Boarding Division. Their primary responsibility was to detect possible contagious diseases, especially cholera, smallpox, and yellow fever. If detected or suspected (sometimes accurate diagnosis required confirmation by the lab), the sick immigrants were sent on to Public Health hospitals in New York. Eventually a contagious diseases hospital was constructed on the island's expanded area where cases of "loathsome or contagious" diseases were sent. Medical Division personnel were stationed at the top of the stairs of the Registry Hall where doctors gave the general exam, working in pairs to determine whether the alien met the physical and mental requirements to enter. The screening process was done in stages.

One doctor observed them at the beginning of each line, the other about thirty feet down at a right angle turn in the piping that separated immigrants passing through at a steady but slow enough pace to keep about ten to fifteen feet apart. The physicians divided aspects of the examination between them, depending on their specialties and experience. They watched for various defects, physical and mental, observing each immigrant straight on and in profile. They observed the immigrant's general manner and demeanor, conversation, style of dress, or any unusual appearance. They noted posture and gait, the condition of the face, hands, skin, and scalp. Clothing that might conceal a part of the body needing observation was removed. A hat or a wig might obscure a scalp condition such as favus (a highly contagious fungus resulting in baldness and discoloration). A high collar might hide a goiter. A shawl over the arms might conceal a deformity or paralysis. All children had their scalps inspected. A third doctor, positioned at the end of the line, stood with his back to a window and faced the approaching immigrant. He spoke to the immigrant briefly to check for his or her mental awareness. He then examined the eyes for signs of trachoma or other optical problems or disease. Typically, they used their finger or a special instrument, something like a button hook, to invert the lids. This was a dreaded part of the exam, but generally was quick and painless for persons with healthy eyes. A diagnosis of trachoma could exclude the immigrant without hope of appeal (Willrich: 224–225). One service doctor, Dr. John McMullan went on to become the P.H.S. specialist on trachoma, traveling extensively to consult and assist local public health agencies, especially in the Appalachia region, in diagnosis and treatment of trachoma.

Doctors had but two or three minutes to search for signs of contagious or loathsome disease or for any condition for which the immigrant might become a public charge. If the doctor had any doubt, the immigrant was marked with a chalk to indicate the suspected condition: B for hunchback, C for conjunctivitis, Ct for trachoma, E for eyes generally, Ft for foot problems, G for goiter, H for heart, K for hernia, L for lameness, P for physical and lungs, Pg for pregnancy, S for senility, X for mental retardation, and a circled X for insanity. Some people had several chalk marks, and all persons with marks were channeled into examining rooms or compartments for extensive exams. There were separate examining rooms used for males and females, the latter having a matron to accompany and assist the physician. Eventually the service added several female physicians to the staff.[3] Some examinations resulted in immediate clearance, and the immigrant proceeded to join his or her family. If the illness or suspected condition were confirmed, the immigrant was sent to the hospital. Depending on the condition, some were sent on to deportation hearings. The medical personnel did not make the determination to admit or deport but only reported on the conditions, making out certificates of health abnormality and sending immigrants on to the next phase of inspection. The actual decision for admission or rejection (deportation) was made by immigration officers and the Boards of Special Inquiry. The immigrants could be detained based on any number of diseases that put them into the classes debarred by law. The most common such were trachoma, tuberculosis, favus, ringworm, and other parasitic illnesses. Another set of classes of illness that could bar admission were ones that affected the ability to work, such as hernia, arthritis, heart disease, malnutrition, deformity, varicosity, severe arthritis, and poor vision. Victims of any one of these diseases were sent to special medical boards, or a board of special inquiry. If not cleared for admission, they were deported within a day or two.

During the early1900s, the Medical Division typically comprised twelve doctors responsible for all medical inspections as well as the care of all hospitalized aliens. At its peak, the medical staff was comprised of thirty doctors. The challenges facing the staff are illustrated in a letter, dated March 31, 1913, from the Office of Commissioner of Immigration (then Robert Watchorn) to the Commissioner General of Immigration in Washington, D.C.:

Broadly speaking then, the medical officers at Ellis Island are expected to detect each person with a serious mental or physical defect, and they must do this as to some eight or nine hundred thousand aliens a year. It is difficult to exaggerate the magnitude and importance of such a task. It would be difficult enough of performance if it were to be carried out with an adequate staff of medical officers, at convenient times and places, and in reference to peoples of intelligence, speaking the English language. But only few, if any, of those favorable conditions surround the medical work at Ellis Island. Some of the unfavorable conditions under which it is performed are indicated in what follows:

– The total number of medical officers attached to Ellis Island is only twenty-five, which number includes hospital "interns" [whose duties include]
– The care of the sick at the Ellis Island hospital;
– The medical examination of first and second cabin passengers on ship between the quarantine station and the docks;
– The medical examination of immigrants at Ellis Island. (Letter 18524/100, RC 90, Box 37, File 219)

A 1912 report indicates the volume of work at the station during 1911, when 637,003 immigrants were processed, among whom 1, 361 where certified with a loathsome or dangerously contagious disease, of whom 85 percent had trachoma. More than 6,000 were treated at the general hospital on the island and another 725 at the State Quarantine Hospital, at which 100 deaths occurred, mainly from complications associated with measles, scarlet fever, and meningitis. Approximately 200 deaths in total occurred on the island.

The largest division was Registry, a portion of whose inspectors were assigned, on a rotating basis, to the Special Inquiry Division, who determined whether a detained alien would be allowed to land or had to be deported. Each board was made up of three members appointed by the commissioner. They also had assigned interpreters, stenographers, and messengers. They typically heard fifty to 100 cases daily. The clerk of the board oversaw the massive clerical work involved in processing aliens to and from the boards and keeping track of the outcome of all cases.

An Information Division kept records and supplied interested parties with information on the immigrants' status and whereabouts—that is, whether landed, detained, sent to hospital, or deported. It adjoined the Discharging Division, responsible for all detained aliens until friends or relatives called for them. If after five days no relatives appeared, detained aliens were turned over to the Special Inquiry Division.

In 1893, the station received disinfecting chambers from the U.S. Marine Hospital Service. These were used in the disinfecting of luggage and other personal belongings. The service also had disinfecting barges to fumigate the holds of vessels ordered into quarantine (sometimes for up to ten days). After a fire, when the station was being rebuilt, on February 1, 1899, the surgeon in charge, G. W. Stoner, ordered eight new steam disinfecting chambers, of the Kinyoun–Francis design, steam boilers, and sulfur furnaces for the port of New York operations. These new apparata used formaldehyde (RG 90, File 4605, Sterilizing Machines, Box 505, Folder 16).

The sheer volume of immigration through Ellis Island contributed to administrative problems, many of which plagued operations for years— charges of corruption, swindling, brutality, exploitation; ineptitude in medical screening, attacks from both restrictionist and anti-restrictionist forces, and misunderstandings with distant superiors in Washington, D.C. Periods of economic depression and rapid industrialization challenged the station and threatened to overwhelm it (Pitkin: 65).

President Theodore Roosevelt ordered reform and appointed a new commissioner, William Williams, in 1902, who struggled valiantly to bring better management. Williams served for three years, annually reporting on the need for increased staff. He stressed the need for additional interpreters, each of whom could speak at least two languages, to work in the hospitals, listing the languages for which the need of interpreters was desperate: Italian, Polish, Yiddish, German, Greek, Russian, Croatian, Slovenian, Lithuanian, Ruthenian, and Hungarian (RG 90, File 2855, Box 258, Report to the Surgeon General).

Williams pressed for expanding both the physical plant of the station and the staff to operate it. The newly rebuilt station was up and running before the hospital had been completed, and both Williams and Surgeon George W. Stoner, chief of the Medical Division, argued that the hospital was insufficient in size. When the general hospital opened, in March 1902, it was determined to have inadequate ward space. Contagious disease cases had to be sent to the New York City Health Department, as they had been during the years of operation out of the Barge Office. Dr. Stoner pressed for added ward space and construction of a special contagious disease hospital. Special appropriations in 1903 were allocated to enlarge Ellis Island for construction of more hospital quarters, and the contagious disease hospital was built on a new connecting islet, where its location was sufficiently distant from the main facilities to eliminate the danger of infection. A battle over the title to Ellis Island delayed construction of the hospital until after the appointment of a new commissioner general, Robert Watchorn, in 1905 (Pitkin: 105–106; 65–111).

Robert Watchorn, himself an immigrant, was a veteran service officer. He had labored in the English coal mines. He migrated to America, entering through Castle Garden. He worked in the coal mines of Pennsylvania, bringing over his parents and siblings in less than two years. In the evenings he went to technical school. He joined the Knights of Labor and soon became president of the local lodge, then took over the district office in Pittsburgh. Watchorn helped found the United Mine Workers of America, which became one of the largest and most powerful unions, and served as its national secretary. The governor of Pennsylvania appointed him chief factory inspector for the state. When the governor's term ended, Watchorn was also out of office. He was offered a position of inspector at Ellis Island. His reports on sweat shops in New York City attracted the attention of Washington, D.C. His reform efforts created opposition there, and they attempted to shelve him by assigning him to the port of Victoria, in Canada, on the Pacific Coast—about as far away as they could send him. He discovered that many immigrants were coming to the United States uninspected by going underground, traveling with immigrants through small places, like Winnipeg and other centers in western Canada. He pressured railroad and steamship companies by threatening to stop all trains at the border until every train was inspected. The companies gave in, and Watchorn set up stations across Canada from Quebec to Victoria. President Theodore Roosevelt, familiar with the problems at Castle Garden and then Ellis Island, decided that reforms at Ellis Island were in order, and he appointed Watchorn to do the job ("Robert Watchorn—The Man Who Climbed Out," www.freepages.genealogy.rootsweb.com/quarantine/watchorn.1.htm).

Watchorn had few illusions about the enormity of the task. Soon after his appointment as commissioner general, he stated: "To receive, examine, and dispose of 821,169 aliens in one fiscal year is a work so stupendous that none but painstaking students of the immigration service could possibly have any intelligent conception of what arduous duties and unusual considerations are involved" (cited in Pitkin: 65).

Watchorn sought to protect arriving immigrants with great fervor. He pressed for an additional $250,000 to complete the contagious disease hospital on an adequate scale. Like Commissioner Williams, Commissioner Watchorn bickered with steamship lines concerning their manifests, over who would bear the costs of detentions, and over matters of detention policy. Like Williams, he annually called for increased personnel. And like Williams, he oversaw the expansion and remodeling of the physical plant of the station.

The station experienced a lull during World War I. When war broke out in Europe in 1914, emigration was markedly reduced as the hostilities led the British to blockade major sending ports in Germany and as individuals who might otherwise have joined the flow decided, or were compelled, to remain, some no doubt fearful of the dangers of transatlantic migration as submarine warfare developed and increasingly threatened shipping. Immigration dropped dramatically. In 1914, more than 1,200,000 immigrants had come to the United States, nearly 900,000 of them through Ellis Island. In 1915, those totals fell by 75 percent to only 326,700, among whom 178,000 came through Ellis Island. Not only was the total volume reduced, but by 1916, more than half of those who did come entered from places other than New York City. In 1918, at the height of the war, the number of immigrants passing through Ellis Island shrank to 28,867. By 1919, as the war was ending, it fell to under 27,000, fewer than 20 percent of those entering the United States. In 1919, Ellis Island suffered an epidemic of influenza (then called the Spanish flu). Ellis Island was used as the port of embarkation for a group of Russian immigrants being deported in response to the Red Scare hysteria that year, and the influenza outbreak arrived with them.

A consequence of the reduced traffic was a reduction in staffing that affected the ability of the station to perform its functions. The prewar efficiency of operations at the station was never again achieved. The reduction in traffic, however, enabled much-needed reforms. At the beginning of the war, President Woodrow Wilson appointed a new commissioner of immigration at Ellis Island—Dr. Frederic Howe, a well-known municipal reformer (Frederic Howe: 113–126, 252–258). Reduced volume allowed for more thorough medical exams of those who did arrive. The old line inspections were replaced by a system of more intensive examinations.

Two female physicians were added to the staff. Howe used the wartime interlude to conduct a systematic check on the missionary operations conducted by some forty organizations represented on Ellis Island. Many sent arriving immigrants to "migrant-aid homes" that the various societies and organizations operated. The commissioner's office conducted periodic inspections of their operations, and some were closed down when they were found to be acting as ticket agents of railroad and steamship lines (Parascandola: 2; Frederic Howe: 260–261).

Commissioner Howe resolved to humanize the process. He had an advantage neither of his two immediate predecessors enjoyed. The reduction in volume from 700,000 to 1 million a year down to fewer than 30,000 allowed an increase in the human warmth with which immigrants were met. Howe brought out benches from storage to provide seating on the lawns, and he let people out of detention quarters to sit on them. He installed a playground for children and hired a teacher to supervise it. He opened a wall that had separated the detention quarters for husbands and wives, creating a common social hall where family members could see each other at times other than meals. Sewing materials were provided for women and toys for children. On Sunday afternoons, band concerts entertained detainees to which the public was invited.

Howe was at the forefront of the movement to Americanize the immigrants, advocating that the government set up an internal bureau to prepare them for citizenship. During 1914–1915, when New York City suffered serious unemployment, he opened up two buildings on the island for the local unemployed, most of whom were immigrants, daily rounding up some 750 men from the waterfront area and giving them shelter during the winter months. The island's ferry took them to Battery daily to look for work, and charitable organizations set up a soup kitchen for them there, so the expense to the government was minimal (Pitkin: 113–115).

Howe's reforms created enemies for him and his administration. He requested that cabin passengers be required to be landed and their inspections conducted on Ellis Island. When shipping lines protested, the order was rescinded and an investigation into the matter conducted (Frederic Howe: 260–262). Headed by the Solicitor of the Department of Labor, the commission held hearings at Ellis Island. Congressmen from New Jersey, and assorted representatives from cities in New York and New Jersey, who stood to lose business, merchant's associations and hotel associations, steamship line and railroad line agents—all protested the order requiring that second cabin passengers be landed and examined on Ellis Island rather than aboard ship. When the steamship lines promised to improve lighting and other facilities for shipboard examinations, the order was revoked.

Howe tangled with the shipping lines over the rates charged to them for aliens detained in the hospital. He found the rate to be a nominal one based on a loose calculation of costs made years before. He recalculated the actual costs worked out by an accountant and obtained an order fixing the rate based on the actual cost. Although this generated thousands of dollars in revenue, it precipitated organized hostility. His efforts to reform the railroads' procedures for transporting immigrants inland, a process open to all sorts of graft, raised the ire and opposition of various railroad companies.

Deportations became nearly impossible during the war, and Ellis Island began to fill up with alien men and women rounded up from all over the country, often pursuant to the "White Slave Act," which aimed at cracking down on prostitution and immoral trafficking (Act of June 25, 1910, 36 Stat. 825; U.S.C. 397–404; see LeMay and Barkan: 101–103; and Frederic Howe: 266–268). During the crackdown, many women were detained on Ellis Island awaiting deportation with little due process. Howe invited a group of prominent New York women to the island to listen to evidence of some of the arrested women, and on the basis of this committee's report, he proposed to the secretary of labor and commerce that casual offenders in the group be paroled. Many were released. This, too, made him enemies.

When the food contract at Ellis Island expired in 1916, Howe advocated operating the restaurant rather than contracting. His proposal was approved but raised the ire of a congressman from New York who had been an attorney for the food contractors. Howe was denounced as a "half-baked radical with free-love ideas." An investigation was demanded. Though Howe was able to defend himself at hearings before the House Immigration Committee, some of the "mud" hurled at him clung.

At the height of the controversy, an explosion occurred at Black Tom's Wharf, just behind Bedloe's Island, on the wharf and on a number of barges moored there that were piled with explosives bound for Russia. It was suspected to be the work of German saboteurs. Ellis Island's seawall caught fire. Ferry boats evacuated the detention quarters to the Barge Office, and hospital patients were taken outdoors on the sheltered side of the island. No lives were lost among the 600 occupants of the island, but shrapnel and fire debris rained down on the buildings, and considerable damage ensued. Estimates for repairs were set at $400,000. Congress appropriated $150,000 to begin restoration, later supplemented by another $247,000. Pitkin notes that while these repairs were being made, funding for other improvements already ordered was delayed (116–119).

When the United States entered the war, in April 1917, Ellis Island was used for internment of crews of German ships, ultimately totaling 1,150 internees. This required the complete reassignment of quarters and the shifting of other detained aliens to other rooms, as well as considerable reorganization of the administration. A detachment of soldiers from the War Department provided military guard, and the ground floor of a dormitory building was used as their barracks. Ellis Island became the site of internment of prisoners of war as enemy aliens were rounded up by the Department of Justice throughout the country and brought to the island for custody. The Immigration Service made arrests of people suspected as being German spies and saboteurs, and these were kept under guard on Ellis Island. Complicating matters, the staff of the station was reduced as interpreters and inspectors were transferred to other stations and other government agencies.

The Immigration Act of February 5, 1917 (39 Stat. 874; 8 U.S.C.), passed despite President Wilson's veto, added a literacy test and required more stringent examinations just as the staff was being reduced. The classes of excluded aliens increased to thirty-three, and full medical examination of all arriving alien ships' crews was ordered. All foreign-flag merchant ships had to be boarded and their crews inspected, even if the vessel carried no passengers. This greatly strained the Boarding and the Medical Division's medical staff (Pitkin: 119–120; see also LeMay and Barkan, Document 63: 109–112).

Commissioner Howe complained bitterly about the roles Ellis Island and he were forced to play due to the wartime hysteria:

> The administration of Ellis Island was confused by by-products of the war. The three islands, isolated in New York harbor and capable of accommodating several thousand people, were demanded by the War Department and Navy Department for emergency purposes. They were admirably situated as a place of detention for war suspects. The Department of Justice and hastily organized espionage agencies made them a dumping- ground of aliens under suspicion, while the Bureau of Immigration launched a crusade against one type of immigrant after another, and brought them to Ellis Island for deportation. No one was concerned over our facilities for caring for the warring groups deposited upon us. The buildings were unsuited for permanent residence; the floors were of cement, the corridors were chill, the island became submerged in war activities. Eighteen hundred Germans were dumped on us at three o'clock one morning, following the sequestration of the German ships lying in New York harbor. The sailors had been promised certain privileges, including their beer, which was forbidden by law on the island. Several hundred nurses were detained for their training prior to embarkation; each day brought a contingent of German, Hungarian, Austrian suspects, while incoming trains from the West added quotas of

immoral men and women, prostitutes, procurers, and alleged white-slavers arrested under the Mann White Slave Act and the hysterical propaganda that was carried on by moralistic agencies all over the country. I was custodian of all these groups. Each group had to be isolated. I became a jailer instead of a commissioner of immigration; a jailer not of convicted offenders but of suspected persons who had been arrested and railroaded to Ellis Island as the most available dumping-ground under the successive waves of hysteria which swept the country . . . . I found that we were lawless, emotional, given to mob action. We cared little for freedom of conscience, for the rights of men to their opinions. Government was a convenience of business. Discussion of war profiteers was not to be permitted. The Department of Justice lent itself to the suppression of those who felt the war should not involve equal sacrifice. Civil liberties were under the ban. Their subversion was not, however, an isolated thing, it was an incident in the ascendancy of business privileges and profits acquired during the war—an ascendancy that could not bear scrutiny or brook free discussion, which is the only safe basis of orderly popular government. (266–267)

The War Department took over the Ellis Island hospital on March 2, 1918. Its patients were transferred to hospitals in Georgia and North Carolina. The U.S. Army operated the hospital for the remainder of the war (Letter from R. H. Creel to Surgeon General, RG 90, File 2832, Box 258). It was not returned to the immigration and quarantine service administration until August 15, 1919 (RG 90, File 2855, "Hospital, Ellis Island," Box 258). The U.S. Navy took over baggage and dormitory buildings and some considerable space in the main building to quarter several thousand Navy personnel pending assignment to ships. This required the service to conduct all inspection of arriving aliens on board ship or at steamship piers, adding to the difficulty of the work. The chief medical officer, J. Perry, asked for additional medical officers and inspectors in his 1918 and 1919 reports, even though the head count of arrivals was the lowest in the station's history, noting the war-time duties required, in 1917, inspection of on average 500 vessels per month, for which they had only sixteen inspectors and eight boarding officers to examine all passengers and crewmembers (Pitkin: 120–121).

On May 9, 1918, Congress passed a law on the Naturalization of Persons with Military Service, Citizenship Education, the Naturalization of Other Special Classes of Persons; and Alien Enemies.[4] This law, with the backing of the Department of Justice and the Bureau of Immigration, eased the deportation of any alien considered an anarchist or radical. It enacted into law the principle of guilt by association, authorizing the deportation of any alien simply for belonging to any organization deemed by the attorney general to have advocated revolt or sabotage. Ellis Island became the point of concentration of this "class of undesirable aliens," suspected as wartime enemies.[5]

The summer of 1919 saw Attorney General A. Mitchell Palmer conduct raids. The Red Scare summer culminated a two-year period of fear of Red revolutionaries, anarchists, and alien enemies "in our midst." Alleged "reds" were rounded up and shipped to Ellis Island. Members of the Industrial Workers of the World, known as the "Wobblies," were summarily sent to Ellis Island aboard a special train out of Seattle, Washington, dubbed the "Red Special." They were held at Ellis Island in anticipation of swift deportation. Howe insisted on strictly following procedures for deportation and was soon himself labeled a "Red." Some members of Congress (New York's LaGuardia and Siegel) suggested his impeachment. In the Senate, Utah's Senator William King called for his immediate removal as a Bolshevist sympathizer. Howe soon found himself in constant and increasing conflict with the commissioner-general, who was insisting on the swift deportation suggested by the Department of Justice. Howe was summoned to Washington. The House Committee on Immigration and Naturalization investigated his administration, critically noting that although some 600 aliens were arrested and sent to Ellis Island, only sixty had been deported, and that Ellis Island was filled with enemy aliens.

During their enforced detention, an influenza epidemic broke out, undoubtedly brought to the island by some of the enemy aliens rounded up from around the country while the pandemic raged. On December 21, the army transport *Buford* popularly dubbed "the Soviet Ark," sailed from New York carrying 249 deportees, anarchists and others, bound for Russia by way of Finland, Russia still being under British naval blockade. The deportees left many wives and children behind. Further raids in January 1920 filled the island as more than 4,000 people were arrested, many not pursuant to warrants. Many were sent to Ellis Island. The hospital facilities were not up to the task, and when the flu epidemic broke out and several deaths occurred, the commissioner-general ordered an investigation. Three of the deaths that occurred at the hospital were found to have been radical aliens who had arrived with symptoms of pneumonia.

The general public clamored for the wholesale deportation of all the radicals on Ellis Island. The Department of Justice reopened cases against ninety alleged "reds" even though by law such deportation proceedings were under the Department of Labor, making the Department of Justice proceedings illegal. Assistant Secretary of Labor Louis Post began a meticulous examination of all the radical cases, deciding against the Department of Justice determination in many cases. Eventually he ordered the deportation of some 700 but canceled the warrants against 2,700 others. Resisting the public hue and cry for immediate and mass deportations, Secretary Post put a stop to Commissioner-General of Immigration Caminetti's freewheeling methods. He ordered Caminetti to keep his "hands off" the appeals, stipulating that only the secretary of labor had "primary and final authority" over such appeals (Pitkin: 128).

After World War I, immigration increased from 26,731 in 1919 to more than 225,000 in 1920, more than doubling to over 560,000 in 1921. The literacy test imposed by the 1917 law failed to achieve its goal of drastically reducing immigration, but it complicated and slowed the processing of immigrants. The rate dropped from an average of 5,000 per day before the war to about 2,000 per day in the early 1920s. Ships awaiting inspection were backlogged in the harbor because there was no room for their passengers on the island. Complaints about the pace of processing immigrants led to the appointment of a new commissioner, Frederick Wallis, but the job soon overwhelmed him. Great publicity arose over the problem of vermin and the postwar rise in the incidence of typhus. The station was seen as a danger to public health. As Pitkin notes:

> One byproduct of the war was an outbreak of typhus and other epidemics in Europe. Some of these were still raging or endemic in parts of the continent. Body lice, carriers of typhus, common enough among some classes of prewar immigrants, were now regarded as a national health hazard. Sometimes the discovery of lice among them held up whole barge loads of immigrants for hours at Ellis Island. The U.S. Public Health Service, the New York City Health Department, and New York State medical officers at quarantine agreed to cooperate to prevent any landing of an immigrant until he and his baggage had been put through a delousing plant. Superintendent Baker of Ellis Island notified shipping companies that 'the immigration authorities would receive no more aliens not in presentable condition.' Shipping companies and health agencies scoured the neighborhood for delousing facilities. (133)

The New York City commissioner of health, Dr. Royal Copeland, visited Ellis Island and declared conditions there "a menace to the country," citing the inadequate number of medical inspectors (forty to examine 4,000 immigrants per day). He saw filthy blankets on the floors and was dismayed to learn that immigrants had been sleeping on the floor the night before. When 15,000 immigrants were backlogged on ships waiting in the harbor, he pressured Washington, D.C., to send more medical personnel to clear the congestion. The British ambassador to the United States inspected Ellis Island (at the invitation of Commissioner Tod) late in 1922. He stated that he would prefer "imprisonment in Sing Sing to incarceration on Ellis Island awaiting deportation" (cited in Pitkin: 146–147).

The obvious failure of the literacy test and other measures in the 1917 law to drastically reduce immigration increased the fervor and political effectiveness of the restrictionist forces, and Congress responded by passing the quota acts. The 1921 act, known as the Emergency Quota Act (42 Stat. 5; U.S.C. 229), established the quota principle. It affected the station's operations. Arrivals dropped from more than 800,000 in 1921 to just more than 200,000 in 1922. That spurred restrictionist forces to greater efforts, and in 1924 the Johnson–Reed Act was passed, implementing even greater restrictions (LeMay and Barkan, Document 73: 133–135).

By the time its provisions were operating, the rate of arrivals processed through Ellis Island fell to about 150,000 annually, roughly half of those entering the nation. As more immigrants were turned away, rioting ensued as entire boatloads of hysterical immigrants, having disposed of their homes and other possessions to begin life anew in America, protested their treatment. Commissioner Wallis urged using a screening process at the ports of embarkation to avoid the tragedy. When his superiors failed to institute the policy, Wallis resigned in disillusionment.

Wallis was succeeded by Robert Tod, an able administrator who improved operations at Ellis Island, but he, too, was soon inundated by continuing political pressure. He complained especially about the detention policy and the delays that process caused. After 1924, the steamship lines altered their operations, essentially replacing the old steerage class with more comfortable (and, in terms of controlling illness, more effective) third-class cabins.

After July 1924, most immigrants were processed aboard ship. Ellis Island was limited to those being held for hearings, essentially changing its role to an administrative and detention facility until it was closed in 1954.

COPING WITH EPIDEMICS

Island medical staff grappled with many of the same epidemic disease outbreaks as found at Angel Island and New Orleans. Compared to those stations, however, the outbreaks were relatively small, brief, and less deadly. In 1891, New York City and Ellis Island experienced a smallpox epidemic that took 132 lives. In 1892, there was the typhus outbreak previously referred to that took 200 individuals, and a small cholera outbreak in which nine died. Smallpox flared up again in 1893, taking 302 persons, and in 1901 and 1902 some 2,100 smallpox cases took 410 and 310 lives, respectively. These latter outbreaks were effectively the last epidemics of smallpox to strike New York City, as by 1907 the city had achieved efficient control of the typhus carrier (human lice) by a combination of delousing at ports of embarkation, quicker and cleaner transatlantic passage aboard much improved steamship liners, and effective fumigation and more thorough delousing upon arrival. This reflected the experience with how better to cope with epidemics that developed and spread with the breakthroughs in medical knowledge about epidemic diseases, how they were carried and spread, and better methods of vector control. Whereas New York City had suffered epidemics of cholera and smallpox in the 1870s that took the lives of between 1,000 and 2,000 persons when immigrants were processed through Castle Garden, by the time Ellis Island was effectively under way after 1900, deaths dropped off to the dozens or, at most, a few hundred.

By 1900, inspectors at Ellis Island were inspecting all immigrants arriving at the port. The size of that task is well illustrated in a 1906 fiscal year-end report by Assistant Surgeon L. L. Williams, in which he stated that the station had inspected 935,860 persons (immigrants and crews), certified illness for 7,573 persons, and deported (for all classes) 2,920. By 1905–1906, cholera and smallpox were no longer significantly the basis for certification and deportation. The biggest categories for exclusion that year, as detailed in the Williams' report, were trachoma, with 802 certified; tuberculosis, with 41 certified; and mental illness, used to exclude 176 persons (RG 90, File 219, Box 038).

Incidents of trachoma were first noted in a July 7, 1897, report from Ellis Island in which the medical staff asked whether trachoma was to be considered a dangerous contagious disease and thus grounds for barring entry. That was answered in the affirmative from surgeon general's office (then Surgeon General Walter Wyman) on October 21, 1897. On December 28, 1901, in a letter from the surgeon general, tuberculosis was included as a basis for certification and rejection of entry under the law, but the diagnosis was to be certified by a panel of three medical officers on the basis of bacteriological examination.

Ellis Island staff became particularly proficient in trachoma inspection and established a reputation of expertise in its diagnosis. A report by the station in 1907 (by Chief Medical Officer and Surgeon-in-Charge George W. Stoner) details how the examiners process immigrants for trachoma inspection and follow-up medical exams (Ibid.: Box 036). Dr. Stoner filed a similar report (seven pages long) on the treatment for the mentally defective subsequent to criticism of their operation at Ellis Island (Ibid.: Report of January 2, 1907).

Bacteriological lab work was increasingly used after 1900 to confirm diagnoses to certify illness for exclusion/deportation purposes. Physicians serving at Ellis Island, by necessity given the volume during the decade 1900–1910, became notably adept in their diagnostic abilities despite the speed with which the line inspections were made. John Thill, a P.H.S. physician who served on the island, noted the following, in admiration of the skill of the chief medical officer: "I can recall what a clever diagnostician and acute observer our chief medical officer was, Dr. Billings. A German lady was in the line and he took one look at her and he said, [in German] 'take off the wig', which we had not noticed, and we were astounded to see a totally bald lady who had had favus" (cited in Parascandola: 2).

From 1902 through 1911, the rate of inspections was typically between 600,000 and 900,000 annually, with over 1 million in the peak year of 1907. Refusals to entry based on medical certification of contagious or loathsome diseases ranged from 670 per year in 1902 to a high of 1,735 in 1910 (RG 90, File 219, Box 038).

In 1903, amid controversy over the inspections and how thoroughly they were being conducted, the chief medical officer asked the surgeon general's office whether it was necessary to strip-search all aliens for vermin carriers. In September 1903, they received the response that a strip search was not necessary, but thorough fumigation and delousing was ordered (Ibid.: Folder 4).

That year the physical plant was expanded and the three-story contagious disease hospital opened. The general and contagious disease hospitals typically treated about 10,000 patients per year. Deaths at all hospital facilities on Ellis Island for all causes averaged between 100 and 200 per year. The diseases requiring hospitalization included: tuberculosis, measles (then still an often-deadly disease, especially for young children), pneumonia, and pleurisy. The latter two conditions resulted as complications of other illness and were the proximate cause for the largest number of deaths. In addition to noncontagious illnesses, the general hospital treated patients who were injured in mishaps aboard ship (RG 90, File 219; Box 037, Letter of March 31, 1913 to the Office of Commissioner of Immigration from Dr. D. L. Williams, Chief Medical Officer at Ellis Island).

The contagious disease hospital contained a new bacteriological lab. A 1911 report by Surgeon R. H. Creel, then a surgeon in charge, details changes in procedures used at the lab, "Methods Employed at N.Y. Quarantine Station for the Detection of Cholera Carriers." It specifies how specimens were obtained, cultures and subcultures done, how smears were collected, and the identification of vibrios for the bacteriological determination of cholera. To document the thoroughness of the lab work, the report noted that from mid-July to mid-November 1911, the total number of immigrants examined was 26,930, with lab work completed on

3,900 patients, among whom twenty-seven cholera carriers were detected, including one ship on which two carriers were discovered even though the cases were not recognized nor even suspected by the physician aboard the ship en route (RG 90, File 219, Box 039).

Commissioner L. L. Williams requested, in 1913, approval to purchase medical equipment for the lab to detect uncinariasis (hookworm). He also pleaded for increased medical staff, noting that each day they typically treated 100 cases of measles and overall 200, and at times up to 400, patients per day. He complained that the online inspection was usually done by five medical officers when he was recommending that twelve to fourteen be used. He noted that at the time they were inspecting 4,000 to 5,000 immigrants daily and that the lack of interpreters and medical officers on the line was a particular problem. He recommended assessing the steamship line companies a $25 fine for transporting an alien who had obvious illness that would prevent the earning of a living, advising that the income from such fines could be used to employ more interpreters and medical staff. He observed that because the registry lines were fed by the medical lines, the inadequate number of medical inspectors resulted in the disarrangement and interruption of the work being done by the immigration officers on the registry floor (RG 90, File 219, Box 037, Letter of March 31, 1913).

The effectiveness of the work at Ellis Island was greatly facilitated by a policy implemented in 1901–1903 as a pandemic of typhus spread from Asia to Europe, whereby the Department of State established medical facilities at the major foreign ports of embarkation. Service medical officers posted abroad supervised sanitary conditions in those ports, operated fumigation chambers from land stations or aboard specially equipped vessels, and monitored outbreaks of diseases in the countries and ports, alerting the State Department, the surgeon general's office, and usually the station at the port of destination of ships bound for the United States. This policy of foreign-port operations continued throughout the decade.[6]

In early September 1909, such reports helped the station medical staff avoid a cholera outbreak. They were warned about cholera on board a Japanese vessel, the *Daian Maru*, which had left port in China, where a cholera epidemic of great virulence was raging. The ship had an outbreak of ten cases on board, including one death. That same month, an outbreak struck Rotterdam, with nineteen cases and ten deaths. In Wollenberg, inspectors determined bacteriologically that unfiltered river and canal water was cholera-infested, though the filtered city water was negative. Stringent precautions and rigorous inspection of vessels from those ports prevented any incidence at Ellis Island (Assorted reports, RG 90, File 219, Box 037).

In 1913, responding to restrictionist and anti-restrictionist criticisms, Surgeon L. L. Williams, chief medical officer at Ellis Island, reported on the Immigrant Hospital for Contagious Diseases:

> Infectious cases developing among aliens on ship-board or at Ellis Island are admitted. The majority are children suffering from measles, scarlet fever, and diphtheria. The death rate is materially influenced by the reception of a considerable number of moribund patients and those suffering from more than one infectious disease. On account of the increasing number of patients handled and the congestion in the wards, at certain seasons a larger staff, especially a larger nursing staff, is needed. The sick are brought to Ellis Island from the ships on barges, along with steerage passengers, and it has been the practice [of the shipping lines] to place all patients, irrespective of the nature of their disease, in a single room on these vessels. This abuse, which accounts for at least some of the multiple infections treated in the hospital, has been brought to the attention of the Commissioner of Immigration who has made vigorous representations to the steamship companies and a betterment of these conditions is in sight. (in RG 90, File 219, Box 37)

Restrictionist forces pressured for more vigorously enforcement of the mental deficiency grounds for exclusion. The medical staff increased the number of deportations based on that class. In a letter to William McAdoo dated December 9, 1913, Mr. Holmer Folkes, Secretary of the State Charities Aid Association, noted that the number of "insane and mentally defective" immigrants certified at Ellis Island during fiscal year 1912 was 212. In 1913, that number rose to 500, and at the time of the report, 100 such certificates were being issued per month, resulting in an anticipated 1,000 such exclusions in 1913–1914. The medical staff at Ellis Island was busy and certainly zealous in that category of examination. In their 1913 end of fiscal year report, they noted that of 1,211,035 arrivals, 10,381 persons were treated at the hospitals (9,011 in the general hospital, with ninety-seven deaths and 1,316 in the contagious hospital, with 180 deaths), and 22,733 aliens were certified for either physical or mental defects, including 1,176 who had "contagious and loathsome" diseases (Ibid.: Reports for years 1914–1917).

The station reported dramatic increases in the number of exclusions based on mental defects, which resulted in counterpressures from the Hebrew Sheltering and Immigration Aid Society. They issued a report, on November 20, 1913, alleging serious errors in certifying the condition of aliens by the then U.S. P.H.S. surgeon stationed at Ellis Island. The medical chief, L.L. Williams began, in 1915, a two-year study on the procedures used. These were detailed in a "Manual for Mental Examination of Immigrants," published by the P.H.S. in 1917, and became a standard for Ellis Island and most other stations (1915 F.Y. Report, RG 90, File 219, Box 037).

The trend set in 1880–1910 continued in the pre–World War I years. In FY 1914, Ellis Island saw 1,009,864 aliens arrive along with 167,105 citizens, resulting in 1,176,959 inspections. Of those, 19,616 medical certificates were issued, with 1,547 certified for loathsome and contagious diseases, resulting in 1,496 deportations. Likewise, the hospitals were busy: 8,933 were admitted to the general hospital and 1,246 to the contagious disease hospital, of whom ninety-eight died.

In 1915 the lab was improved and equipped well for the times. The lab examined 43,069 aliens, resulting in 637 certifications for loathsome and contagious diseases, 509 of whom were among the year's total of 1,738 deported. Twenty-eight died in the General Hospital and seventeen in the Contagious Diseases hospital.

In 1916, a total of 176,461 aliens and 48,735 citizens were processed, with 6,303 admitted to the hospitals, and 496 certified, leading to 384 being deported. Sixty-eight immigrants died in the hospitals of all causes.

In 1917, before the official U.S. entry into World War I, but after hostilities were raging in Europe, the total number of arriving alien passengers dropped to 160,105, plus 39,439 citizens processed and 16,028 crewmembers, for a grand total of 215,572 being handled by the station. Among them, 4,291 were hospitalized, and of those, 1,214 went to the contagious disease hospital. The total number certified was 488, with 333 deported. That year, forty-one deaths occurred among those hospitalized. The lab processed 3,101 cases.

In the fiscal year ending July 1918, then Surgeon-in-Charge J. W. Kerr reported that the station received 222,024 aliens, and processed 257,707 when including crew and returning citizens to be inspected. Kerr reported 1,354 certified, with 593 certified with contagious diseases, of whom 233 were deported. The general hospital admitted 1,617 patients, of whom twenty died. The contagious disease hospital received 257 patients, with eight deaths that year (RG 90, File 219, Box 038).

Medical diagnosis made by the P.H.S. doctors figured heavily in the fate of an immigrant. Noted medical historian Alan Kraut observed: "They did not decide to admit or deport. Rather, they reported findings to immigration officers to rule on admissibility. Physicians refused to sit on the Boards of Special Inquiry, which made the final decisions on exclusions" (Parascandola: 3, citing Kraut's book, *Silent Travelers: Germs, Genes, and the "Immigrant Menace,"* 1994).

Of particular concern at the time was the fear of mental health among the flood of immigrants during the prequota period. The "Manual of the Mental Examination of Immigrants" provides a good picture of the procedures for detecting mental deficiencies. During the online inspections, doctors relied on the appearance, attitude, and conduct of the immigrants filing by them trying to endeavor aliens with mental defects. Appearance alone was not a very dependable guide, but the manual noted the "idiots and many imbeciles generally presented some physical signs that attracted the physicians attention to their mental condition." The manual advised physicians to look for people who seemed unusually dull or apathetic, or those unusually agitated. They asked these immigrants a few key questions, like "What is the name of the month of the year?" or "Count from 1 to 20." Anyone suspected of having mental defects was held over. The manual recommended that before such follow-up examination the immigrant have a bath, a good meal, and adequate sleep. The manual advised the examiner and the interpreter to be calm, patient, and sympathetic. Considering the importance of the diagnosis for the alien's admissibility or exclusion, the manual cautioned that the decision should not be made hastily. The follow-up tests were designed to ascertain both the amount of acquired knowledge and the person's general cognitive abilities. It was assumed that the mentally competent person had knowledge of the ordinary affairs of his or her life. Thus a person from a farm family should know the seasons for sowing and reaping of crops, perhaps things like the quantity of milk the cow gives, and so on, regardless of his or her level of formal education. Persons were expected to know the days of the week and months of the year. Examiners were cautioned about making judgments based on acquired knowledge. It noted, for example, "it is almost impossible for Americans to realize the narrowness of experience of some of the poorer classes of the countries of Europe." It gave an example:

> The farmer of southern Italy, tilling a few acres of land and living in a hut, the bare walls of which contain only one ornament, an unframed picture of the Madonna, and the only articles of furniture of which are a bed, a chair or two, a few kitchen utensils, and a little bedding, can hardly be expected to define the word "charity." He has never been 50 miles from his place of birth. He could not go into a room in an ordinary American home and give the name in his own language for even a small part of the things he would see there, because he has never seen or heard of them before. His possessions, his ideas, his vocabulary, and his experiences are all extremely limited, and he must be judged and measured accordingly. (cited in Parascandola: 5)

The manual evinced ethnocentrism when talking about those from southern and eastern Europe, but at least it recognized the limits of the testing methods and cautioned examiners not to mistake lack of experience for lack of intelligence. An array of methods was used to assess the ability to reason abstractly, to form correct judgments, and to draw logical conclusions. For instance, an examiner might describe an imaginary situation calling for a conclusion on the part of the subject. An example given was to tell the immigrant that a young woman's body was found cut into eighteen pieces and then to ask him or her whether or not it was likely that she had committed suicide. The hospital's psychiatric ward was at once a maternity ward and an insane asylum. More than 350 babies were born on Ellis Island.

The fact that the P.H.S. officers wore uniforms and were the immigrants' first contact with Americans caused intimidation among many newcomers who reacted to the doctors and their interrogation. The immigrants were often reminded of and were scared of persons in uniform in their native country. Eastern European Jews avoided, whenever possible, Russians in uniform, as they often participated in or even perpetrated pogroms. Despite considerable public pressures to exclude the unfit, the doctors at Ellis Island, particularly in comparison to the atmosphere at Angel Island, were generally even-handed, even benevolent, "keepers of the gate" (Parascandola: 7).

In FY 1919, Kerr reported a total of 390,958 individuals processed, comprising 62,253 aliens, 31,534 citizens, and 297,171 crewmembers. The station and its hospitals were kept busy treating venereal disease cases among soldiers. It was the year of the infamous Spanish influenza pandemic, in which New York City suffered 12,562 deaths.

On Ellis Island,

[t]he outbreak preceded in point of time the recurrence of the epidemic throughout the country. There was no evidence that the infections came from abroad. In fact, the bulk of the cases were among the so-called radicals who had just previously been collected together from many parts of the country. By doing so, conditions analogous to those prevailing in the military camps during 1918 were approximated when large numbers of young non-immune were assembled in crowded quarters. An outbreak of respiratory disease was the inevitable result, the infection having in all probability been brought to the station by them. (RG 90, File 219, Box 038)

During the influenza outbreak, 5,978 patients were treated in the hospital, and the labs examined 10,550 specimens and viewed 1,577 x-rays (x-ray equipment having only recently been added to the hospital's equipment). Among the alien immigrants, there were 264 medical certificates issued, mostly for trachoma and venereal disease. Of those, 152 were deported. In December 1919, the outbreak of influenza spread rapidly. One patient a day was diagnosed in October and November; by December, there were fifteen per day. In January 1920, it peaked at fifty-two per day. In February, in tapered to ten per day, and eleven per day in March, finally dying out in April, which saw on average only two per day. The influenza struck aliens, medical officers, immigration officers, and employees working with those in detention (Report of July 22, 1920, by J.W. Kerr, RG 90, File 219, Box 038).

Many of the more than 400 suspected radicals sent to Ellis Island in 1920 were gathered up from thirty-three major cities around the country. The Palmer Raids swept up large numbers: 800 were seized in New England and shipped to Deer Island off Boston, as well as 100 in Philadelphia, 115 in Pittsburgh, 500 in New Jersey, 800 in Detroit, 200 in Chicago, and 100 in Kansas City (Murray: 213–217, 251). Raids were justified by the Espionage Act of 1917. That law was aimed at treason but was interpreted broadly by the attorney general. Fines of $10,000 and twenty years in jail could result from persons' "conveying false reports or false statements with the intent to interfere with the operation or success of the military or naval forces of the United States, or to promote the success of its enemies . . . or attempt to cause insubordination, disloyalty, mutiny, or refusal of duty, in the military or naval forces of the United States . . . or to willfully obstruct recruiting or enlistment service" (cited in Murray: 13–14).

Radicals were deported aboard the *Buford*, popularly called "the Soviet Ark." The *Buford* was an army transport ship, originally launched in 1890 in Ireland as the *Mississippi*. It was purchased by the U.S. army in 1898, becoming the U.S.A.T. (U.S. Army Transport) *Buford*. It was rebuilt in 1900 at the Newport News Shipyard in Virginia and transferred to the navy in New York on the January 14, 1919, being commissioned on January 15 and used to make four round trips carrying cargo and nearly 5,000 troops to France. It was decommissioned in September 1919 and returned to the Army Transport Service (Train, 1979: 172).

Although Attorney General Palmer strenuously tried to deport many radicals, court rulings overturned his attempts. By June 1920, the national hysteria had passed. From November 1919 to January 1920, approximately 5,000 arrest warrants had been issued, of which about 3,000 were actually used. Of the 3,000 warrants used, 2,202 were canceled by Assistant Secretary Post upon review in deportation hearings. Only 559 were upheld and the person involved actually deported, including 35 left over from the *Buford* deportations. As of June 1920, Ellis Island had 591 aliens awaiting deportations, and during the remainder of 1920 and 1921, they were sent in small groups aboard American ships to their native lands. No more "Soviet Arks" sailed into the sunset, and operations at Ellis Island returned to normal.

During 1920, the last full year of operations based on immigration law preceding the enactment of the quota acts, the station at Ellis Island received a total of 333,733 aliens, 95,520 citizens, and 310,666 crewmembers, for a total of 729,914 persons inspected. A report on the certification of excludable diseases issued for July 1, 1920, through December 31, 1920, lists the diseases for which they were issued, fairly illustrative of the array of diseases accounting for exclusions by the 1920s. The traditional and previously feared "deadly contagious" diseases such as bubonic plague, cholera, smallpox and typhus are absent. Generally nonfatal, more characteristically "loathsome" defined diseases predominate, with trachoma continuing to be most often used for exclusion. The one disease still often fatal was tuberculosis (though far less frequently so than a decade earlier). The disease and the number of certificates issued in that six-month period of 1920, ranked order of frequency, were as follows: trachoma 184, trichophytosis 142, venereal 128, favus 73, mental defects 57, insanity/psychopathic inferiority 28, tuberculosis 21 (resulting in three deaths), epilepsy 3, leprosy 1, and framboesia 1 (Kerr Report, RG 90, File 219, Box 038).

In 1921, the Emergency Quota Act was passed, and immigration to the United States and through Ellis Island was dramatically curtailed. The Johnson–Reed Act of 1924 (43 Stat. 153; 8 U.S.C. 201, Document 79, LeMay and Barkan: 148–151) drastically cut the flow. Conditions aboard steamship vessels had been greatly improved, and increasingly vigilant and effective screening and prevention of disease in the major ports of embarkation resulted in greatly reduced incidences of immigrants with contagious diseases arriving at Ellis Island. The need for an island quarantine station was surpassed. After July 1924, only those immigrants held for deportation hearings were physically processed at Ellis Island. The vast majority of the then greatly reduced flow of immigrants arriving at the port of New York were processed aboard ship and never set foot on Ellis Island. Throughout the Great Depression years, when immigration was reduced to a trickle, and through World War II, Ellis Island was essentially an administrative and detention facility. It was closed for good in 1954. Even the immigration records were filed on the island only until 1943, after which time the manifests were handled and filed at the New York Immigration District Office on Manhattan Island (www.members.tripod.com/LAlfano/immig.htm).

SPREADING INNOVATIONS

The volume of immigrants processed through Ellis Island meant that the "doctors at the gates" played an important role, even if no one played a major role in innovations of equipment, devices, or procedures as had the unsung heroes previously described. In its sixty-two years of operation, hundreds of doctors served as medical officers at Ellis Island. None among them achieved the stature of having discovered the cause, or cure, of a disease, nor a treatment innovation for any of the deadly pandemic diseases of the nineteenth century. No Ellis Island doctor was a breakthrough scientist equivalent to a Dr. Robert Koch, or Louis Pasteur, giants of germ theory. None among them was a groundbreaking epidemiologists like John Snow. None developed a new process, as did Dr. Edward Jenner by his use of inoculation to prevent disease. None became notable for a breakthrough in controlling the vector of one of the dreaded killer diseases—no doctors William Gorgas, Walter Reed, George Sternberg, so critically important in defeating yellow fever and malaria. None proved the existence of a bacterium, like doctors Alexandre Yersin and Shibasaburo Kiasota. None of the Ellis Island physicians discovered the DNA of a deadly virus, as had Dr. Jeffrey Taubenberger with the deadly 1918–1919 "Spanish flu virus," arguably the deadliest pandemic in human history.

The doctors at Ellis Island played no critical role in developing or improving new apparatus, as Dr. Joseph Kinyoun did with the Kinyoun–Francis chamber. No doctor at Ellis Island developed an administrative procedure like the rat eradication campaign of Dr. Rupert Blue at Angel Island, nor did any go on to become surgeon general. None among them was instrumental in the very development of the nation's public health service.

At Ellis Island, the more prominent role was that of the commissioner of immigration. Particularly important in that capacity were Joseph Senner, William Williams, Robert Watchorn, and Frederic Howe. Probably the most important position and persons among the station's medical personnel were several of the chief medical officers. Dr. George W. Stoner influenced the physical development and improvement of the physical plant of Ellis Island in important ways, especially with regard to its Contagious Disease Hospital. Others prominent in that capacity were J.W. Kerr, W.C. Billings, Alfred Reed, and J.G. Wilson.

But medical service at Ellis Island involved influence in coping with epidemic disease resulting from its need to process huge volume of immigrants. The influence of Ellis Island's medical staff was felt in other more subtle, but nonetheless important, ways. Service on the medical staff at

Ellis Island carried a degree of prestige. Many of its staff, often in junior roles there at the time, served stints of duty abroad as established by the U.S. M.H.S. and, after 1912, the P.H.S., in the major ports of embarkation in Europe and Asia. That role is exemplified by doctors J. G. Perry, J. W. Kerr, R. A. C. Wollenberg, and H. D. Geddings, all of who served at various times on the staff of Ellis Island and who were posted abroad to ports in Europe or Asia to monitor epidemic outbreaks. Annual fitness reports on the service of the medical personnel were sent to the assistant surgeon general. These reports influenced the decisions of the service about which doctors were to be posted for stints of service at stations abroad, typically when an outbreak of some epidemic warranted sending someone from the service to establish or supervise an "early warning" station there.[7]

Soon after the new facilities were constructed and in operation, in 1903 and 1904, the Bureau of Immigration Services sent out circulars from the Department of Commerce and Labor detailing the procedures being used at Ellis Island for deportation of aliens upon examination by immigration officers in cases of "insane persons, idiots, paupers," and diseased persons who should be certified by a qualified medical officer, setting forth the physical or mental conditions of the alien and giving a professional opinion about whether said condition existed prior to landing in the United States. These procedures were designed to implement the Immigration Act of 1903, which added such conditions to the classes of excludable aliens. Similarly, on November 15, 1904, the Treasury Department sent a letter to the surgeon general of the U.S. M.H.S. regarding a New York state law amending insanity law providing for examinations at the port of New York and ascertaining their methods and procedures for determining the mental conditions of aliens. The New York board recommended that medical officers from the service skilled in mental examinations be stationed at Ellis Island to provide such exams. The methods they developed were later incorporated in a manual that the service provided all immigration stations to guide their methods for such exams (RG 90, File 219, Box 036).

Surgeons from the U.S. M.H.S./P.H.S. regularly attended meetings of the Association of Military Surgeons at which they shared methods and procedures being used at respective hospitals at military bases and at Ellis Island—for example, at meetings held at Atlanta, Georgia, in 1907 and 1908; at Richmond, Virginia, in 1911; at Norfolk, Virginia, in 1907 and 1910; at Buffalo, New York, in 1906; and at Detroit, Michigan, in 1905. Surgeon J.W. Kerr, in a letter dated October 22, 1919, reported on medical officers from Ellis Island attending a meeting in St. Louis, Missouri, of the Association of Military Surgeons on the methods for coping with infectious diseases among U.S. troops during the period when the great

influenza pandemic of 1918–1919 was ravaging military camps throughout the country and was epidemic also at Ellis Island (RG 90, File 114,
Folder 2, Box 16).

Physicians from elsewhere regularly visited Ellis Island to observe its
methods and operations. A letter of January 22, 1905, from G. H. Bryce,
Department of Interior, Canada, sent to Surgeon General Walter Wyman,
thanked him profusely regarding the visit of a Dr. Page, then the chief
medical officer at Quebec, in which they sent medical inspectors to be
temporarily posted at the port of New York to serve the interests of Canadian immigration. In particular, Dr. Stoner was lauded for how he enabled
a Dr. Elliott to take up work at Ellis Island, resulting in "drawing the two
services still closer in the practical work in which they are both engaged"
(RG 90, File 218, Box 036). In 1906, Dr. Sidney Wilgus, then chairman of
the New York state board of alienists, along with several members of his
board, visited Ellis Island to observe their work with respect to medical
exams for the mentally deficient and the insane.

Another important method of spreading influence was the publication
by the P.H.S. of the procedural manuals developed at Ellis Island with
respect to trachoma and to the diagnosis of mental defects. Though these
publications did not spread an innovation on the scale of Dr. Rupert Blue's
manual on the eradication of rats, the prominence of Ellis Island meant
these manuals influenced procedures for these two conditions used at
many other immigrant receiving stations and at public health hospitals not
in the service.

Ellis Island's influence was spread by its medical personnels' attending and speaking at medical conferences and hosting such conferences
at Ellis Island. For instance, on June 12, 1908, Dr. Stoner sent a letter
describing a meeting at Ellis Island with the commissioners of immigration from Boston, Baltimore, and Philadelphia (RG 90, File 218, Box 36).
Yet another example of the latter is detailed in a letter dated July 18, 1908,
from Dr. George W. Stoner to the Surgeon General of the U.S. M.H.S.
regarding such a conference held at Ellis Island and attended by the Commissioner General of Immigration from the Ports at New York, Boston,
Philadelphia, Baltimore, and Montreal, and with a number of medical
officers posted at each of those stations. The agenda of the conference
stressed the detaining for hospital treatment of aliens certified for dangerous or loathsome contagious diseases, with special emphasis on the
length of treatment required and the best methods for the treatment of
trachoma (RG 90, File 218, Box 036).

Trachoma was especially prevalent in eastern Europe, and Dr. Stoner
had been sent, in 1906, to Liverpool and several other ports of embarkation

to investigate and report on the subject. Largely on the strength of his report, trachoma became a leading reason for exclusion as a dangerous and contagious disease. Dr. Stoner recommended treatment of three to four days. His trip was precipitated by an incident in February of 1906, when President Theodore Roosevelt had written two letters regarding the need for improvement in how doctors at Ellis Island conducted eye exams for trachoma. These were written after an incident reported to him by a passenger passing through and processed at Ellis Island, one Dr. Howitt, a medical doctor from Montreal, Canada. He reported observing doctors at Ellis Island examining patients, such as himself, with dirty hands and using instruments not sterilized after each exam, thus being likely "fruitful sources" of carrying the infection from diseased to healthy individuals. President Roosevelt was still urging reforms at Ellis Island with respect to a number of the administrative procedures.[8]

Another conference held at Ellis Island was reported by Dr. Stoner to the surgeon general. He described their role at a February 17, 1912, conference in which they focused on the medical exams given to aliens, with particular reference to the detection of mental health defects (this being just prior to the publication of the manual). The conference was attended by officers from twenty-one ports of entrance. The dominant role played by the Ellis Island station is evident in the report on the number of aliens examined at the more important and sizable of those ports of entrance that year, each of whom sent representatives to the conference at Ellis Island. Whereas Ellis Island examined nearly 750,000 aliens that year, the next most numerous stations were Boston, with just more than 50,000, Philadelphia, with just more than 46,000, and Baltimore, with just more than 23,000. Quebec, by contrast, examined only 17,800 and Angel Island only 10,350. All the other stations in North America examined fewer than 10,000 persons that year. Buffalo, the least of all stations, examined just fewer than 4,000 in 1912. The sheer size and the volume of aliens examined at Ellis Island ensured its prominent role in the conference both thanks to the number of its physicians in attendance and because of the respect accorded them as a result of the volume of inspections they had to process.

The influence of Ellis Island was also spread by visitations from Ellis Island physicians to other stations. A letter dated September 10, 1908, to the surgeon general of the U.S. M.H.S., from Dr. Stoner, then chief medical officer at Ellis Island, reports on his inspection of the immigration work at Black Rock, Buffalo, New York, and at Niagara Falls, New York, regarding their procedures for examination of arriving aliens as to diagnosis of excludable diseases, with particular emphasis on trachoma, and noting the great improvements then being made in the performance at those stations (RG 90, File 219, Box 36).

Sometimes such trips resulted in the sharing of information and procedures, in which the Ellis Island staff learned from the work being done by others as well as influencing those sites as to what procedures were being used at Ellis Island. In a memorandum dated July 15, 1915, sent to the surgeon general by Dr. J. G. Wilson, then assistant surgeon, Wilson reported on work being done at Providence City Hospital on procedures for handling contagious diseases, particularly methods of record keeping at the Boston City Hospital. After his visits to Providence and Boston, and mindful of the ever-present administrative problems of record keeping at a station with the huge volume experienced at Ellis Island, Dr. Wilson urged the P.H.S. to send officers from Ellis Island to Boston and Providence to investigate more fully the methods employed at those respective institutions. On September 14, 1915, Dr. W. C. Billings, then chief medical officer at Ellis Island, sent an extensive report (thirty single-spaced typed pages with a twelve-page appendix of data) to Surgeon General Rupert Blue on methods used at the Providence, Rhode Island, hospital to protect against cross-infections, an ongoing issue of concern at both the general and the contagious-disease hospitals on Ellis Island considering their size of operations at the time (RG 90, File 2855, Box 258).

CONCLUSION

In light of the enormous flow that entered the United States through Ellis Island and the high percentage of that flow relative to immigration to the entire nation, Ellis Island is justifiably considered the most important immigration and quarantine station in the nation's history. Doctors who served at Ellis Island performed remarkably well as a protective barrier against pandemic diseases. They faced cholera, smallpox, typhus, and yellow fever. In the years of the station's operation, no sizable epidemics of any of those deadly diseases broke out on the island or in New York City itself as a result of immigrants' passing undetected through Ellis Island and bringing a pandemic to the city. The largest pandemic with which Ellis Island did struggle—rather ineffectively—was the great influenza of 1918–1919, which took more than 12,000 lives in New York City. But the physicians on service at Ellis Island were no less baffled and defeated by the deadly contagion than were physicians and medical scientists everywhere else in the world. At the time, medical science simply knew too little about viral disease and how it mutated and spread for any doctors or any public health service to adequately cope with the pandemic.

The doctors at Ellis Island were not known for innovation: They developed no new cures, apparata, or administrative processes to cope with pandemics and epidemic outbreaks, other than applying known methods to the task of screening an immigration flow on a thentofore unimagined scale. They did keep themselves apprised of the latest methods, procedures, and approaches in medical science. They developed and applied biological approaches in laboratories that, though primitive by today's standards, were state-of-the-art facilities at the time. That in itself is no small feat.

In many respects the lack of specific or notable innovation reflected two aspects of the story of immigration through Ellis Island: (1) the sheer volume mitigated against the time researchers and administrators needed to develop innovations and (2) the timing of the opening and operation of the Ellis Island station at the very end of the nineteenth century, when the breakthroughs in medical science against pandemic diseases had already been made. What is important for the development of public health in coping with epidemics and pandemics was that it was accomplished at Ellis Island—that public health measures were proven to prevent epidemics from becoming pandemic and that episodes of outbreaks could be mitigated, shortened in duration, and drastically curtailed in their morbidity and mortality rates. Such preventive medicine proved invaluable when confronting a flood of immigration on a scale heretofore unimaginable.

Ellis Island offers insights for the ongoing battle with epidemic disease, whether natural or manmade. Its story and the work of its medical staff demonstrate that the quarantine approach alone is relatively useless in face of the onslaught of a true pandemic (demonstrated so tragically in 1918–1919). The story of Ellis Island shows that quarantine, combined with public health measures, scientific testing in up-to-date labs, and speedy application of the latest in serums, inoculations, and closely supervised, hospital treatment for those who are ill with contagious diseases works. It proves that preventive medicine is the best medicine in confronting epidemics. It shows that an early warning system is invaluable for stopping the worldwide spread of a deadly contagion. It demonstrates that thorough, scientific maritime disinfection, including fumigation of ships and steam and chemical disinfection of baggage, is faster, more efficient, and far more effective than quarantine procedures alone.

Chapter 5

THE NEW ORLEANS STATION

New Orleans presents several parallel experiences to those discussed in the chapters dealing with Angel Island and Ellis Island. But it also saw some important different experiences from those stations. The doctors at New Orleans faced major threats of diseases not commonly faced at those stations. In New Orleans, the tropical disease epidemics of yellow fever and malaria were more prevalent and significant, though like San Francisco and New York, New Orleans also faced pandemics of cholera, smallpox, and influenza. New Orleans, moreover, experienced some important differences in the size, scope, and timing of its immigration flow from that which characterized the patterns at San Francisco and New York. And importantly, too, state doctors at New Orleans played a pioneering role in the innovation of procedures and equipment to battle epidemic outbreaks, perhaps precisely because they faced different threats and much smaller waves of immigration (Holt Report, 1887). The lesser flow of immigration to and through New Orleans afforded them the luxury of such experimentation. As Joseph Logsdon, a leading scholar of immigration through New Orleans, noted:

> New Orleans has an unusual character. It resembles neither southern cities, such as Atlanta and Charleston, nor such northern ones as Boston and Chicago. The unique architecture of its nineteenth century neighborhoods—most still intact—quickly evokes a special sense of place, and a more prolonged stay uncovers a way of life that is neither southern nor northern. To be sure, southern visitors might find some similarity in the climate, the pace of life, and the visible presence of blacks, just as northern visitors might recognize signs of ethnic diversity among the city's white population—Italian fruit stands, a German brewery, Irish politicians, Catholic churches, Latino music, and Jewish synagogues. Yet, for the casual visitor or trained observer, something usually remains strange or foreign about New Orleans (Logsdon: 105).

This strangeness about New Orleans reflects its development while still a French/Spanish colony and before the city and its environs were absorbed by the United States in 1802. That particular historical development forever stamped the city with a Mediterranean flavor not found among its competing port cities on the Atlantic coast.

In the 1790 census, the United States was still overwhelmingly a nation of farmers and frontiersmen, with a population more than 99 percent rural. The country had only two cities having more than 25,000 in population— New York, at 49,401, and Philadelphia, at 28,522 (U.S. Bureau of the Census, 1996). Among its nearly 4 million people, just more than 200,000 were urban dwellers, roughly 0.5 percent. The entire south Atlantic region had just more than 42,000 urban residents. Among the then thirteen states, there were only twenty-four cities—defined as a place having more than 2,500 residents (LeMay, ed., 2013, vol. 1: 47–50). By contrast, New Orleans was then already a city approaching 20,000 in population and had been a sizable city for many years.

As a result of immigration, the total United States' population grew steadily between 1790 and 1860—increasing essentially tenfold, from 3,929,625 to 31,443,321. The population density more than doubled: from 4.5 in 1790 to 10.6 by 1860 (*Statistical Abstract of the U.S.*, 2002, table 1: 8). By 1860, the United States had 392 cities, fifty-eight of which were in the 10,000–25,000 size range, and among the 31 million in total population, more than 6 million were urban dwellers, nearly 20 percent of the total population.

Table 5.1 demonstrates the importance of immigration to that growth. It shows data on immigration from 1820 to 1860, by census years, showing the total population, the total number of immigrants arriving, and the steadily increasing percent of the population that was foreign-born, which by 1860 had reached 13.2 percent.

Table 5.1
Immigration to the United States, 1820–1860

Year	Total U.S. Population	Total Immigrants Arriving	% Foreign-Born
1820	9,638,453	8,385	0.09
1821–1830	12,866,020	49,439	1.11
1831–1840	17,069,453	599,125	3.51
1841–1850	23,191,876	1,713,251	7.39
1851–1860	31,443,321	2,598,214	8.26

Source: Table by author, data from the U.S. Bureau of the Census, Population of States and Counties, 1780–1990. Washington, D.C., Bureau of the Census, 1996.

To place its development within an even broader context, Table 5.2 presents the total U.S. population from 1790 to 2000, by census years, with the percent of that population that was urban and the percent foreign-born. It illustrates clearly the inexorable trend toward increasing urbanization resulting from immigration.

Germany and Ireland were the two countries of origin providing the most immigrants to and through New Orleans before the Civil War. New Orleans is distinctive among other U.S. receiving ports in the number of French- and Spanish-speaking residents when the city was absorbed in 1802 and in the number of immigrants from French- and Spanish-speaking colonies to the country and to New Orleans from 1820 to 1860 (Lewis, 2003).

Table 5.2
Total U.S. Population, Census Year, 1790–2000, %Urban, % F.B.

Census Year	Total Population	Percent Urban	Percent Foreign-Born
1790	3,929,625	5.1	NA
1800	5,308,483	6.1	NA
1810	7239,881	7.3	NA
1820	9,638,453	7.2	NA
1830	12,866,020	8.8	NA
1840	17,069,453	10.8	NA
1850	23,191,876	15.4	9.7
1860	31,443,321	19.8	13.2
1870	38,558,321	25.7	14.4
1880	50,155,783	28.2	13.3
1890	62,947,714	35.1	14.7
1900	75,974,575	39.8	13.6
1910	91,972266	45.7	14.7
1920	105,710,620	51.3	13.2
1930	122,775,046	56.3	11.6
1940	131,669,275	56.7	8.8
1950	150,697,361	64.3	6.9
1960	179,323,175	69.9	5.4
1970	203,302,031	73.6	4.7
1980	226,542,179	73.7	6.2
1990	248,718,301	75.2	7.9
2000	281,421,996	79.0	10.4

Source: U.S. Bureau of the Census. *Population of States and Counties of the U.S., 1790–2000.* Washington, D.C.: U.S. Government Printing Office, 2001.

New Orleans mirrored the rate of U.S. urbanization before 1860. In 1810, the first census taken after the city was incorporated into the United States, its population was 17,242. By the 1860 census, it had grown to 168,675. Table 5.3 shows the population of Orleans Parish (essentially the City of New Orleans) from 1810 to 1990.

As the city of New Orleans and Orleans Parish went, so went the state. Table 5.4 shows the population of Louisiana and the state's total urban and number of foreign-born from 1810 to 1990. Virtually all the foreign-born entered through New Orleans.

Finally, Table 5.5 puts the steady population growth in context with immigration by showing the components of population growth by decades, 1790–2000, and by indicating the rate of net migration by decade and the percent of the total increase specifically attributable to immigration. The dramatic effect of the quota laws and of the Great Depression during the 1930–1940 decade is readily apparent in Table 5.5.

This chapter discusses briefly the history of the immigration to and through New Orleans. There is good reason to say "through" the city. More than any other major eastern port city, immigrants arriving at New Orleans tended to stay for shorter times and to quickly move on to interior destinations than they did elsewhere. Part of the very attractiveness of New Orleans as a port of entry before the Civil War was the comparatively easy access, via river steamboat traffic, for proceeding inland to more attractive destinations for permanent settlement. The chapter covers the establishment of the New Orleans immigration station and the significant role played by the state doctors

Table 5.3
Population of Orleans Parish, Louisiana, 1810–1990

Year	Population	Year	Population
1810	24,522	1910	339,075
1820	41,361	1920	387,075
1830	49,826	1930	458,766
1840	102,193	1940	494,537
1850	119,460	1950	570,445
1860	174,491	1960	627,525
1870	191,418	1970	593,471
1880	216,070	1980	557,515
1890	242,039	1990	496,938
1900	383,104		

Source: U.S. Bureau of the Census. *Population of States and Counties of the U.S., 1790–1990.* Washington, D.C.: U.S. Government Printing Office, 1991.

Table 5.4
Louisiana Total Urban Population, Number of Foreign-Born, 1810–1990

Year	Total Urban	Number of Foreign-Born
1810	17,242	NA
1820	27,176	NA
1830	46,082	NA
1840	105,400	NA
1850	134,470	68,233
1860	185,026	80,975
1870	202,523	61,827
1880	239,390	54,146
1890	283,845	49,747
1900	366,258	52,903
1910	496,576	52,766
1920	628,163	46,427
1930	833,532	30,076
1940	980,439	37,973
1950	1,471,696	29,675
1960	2,060,606	30,557
1970	2,422,175	39,542
1980	2,887,309	85,502
1990	2,871,759	87,407

Source: U.S. Bureau of the Census. *Population of States and Counties of the U.S., 1790–1990.* Washington, D.C.: U.S. Government Printing Office, 1991.

Table 5.5
U.S. Population, Rate of Migration, Immigrants % of Total Increase

Decade	Migration Rate	Immigration % of Total Increase
1790–1799	3.59	11.9
1800–1809	4.19	13.5
1810–1819	3.92	13.7
1820–1829	2.06	7.1
1830–1839	4.77	16.9
1840–1849	8.28	27.0
1850–1859	9.83	32.3
1860–1869	6.26	26.5
1870–1879	5.58	24.2
1880–1889	7.03	30.9
1890–1899	6.19	32.6
1900–1909	6.85	35.3

(*Continued*)

Table 5.5 (*Continued*)

Decade	Migration Rate	Immigration % of Total Increase
1910–1919	2.57	35.3
1920–1929	2.97	20.5
1930–1939	–1.03	–14.0
1940–1949	.34	9.6
1950–1959	1.78	10.4
1960–1969	2.04	16.1
1970–1979	3.80	37.0
1980–1989	2.76	27.9
1990–1999	4.78	42.9

Source: Historical Statistics of the United States, vol. 1, Population, 2006.

serving at the gulf quarantine station in developing germicidal equipment and techniques to cope with epidemics and, before the Civil War, with a considerable immigration flow. After the Civil War, immigration to and through New Orleans tapered off in favor of competing seaports on the Atlantic coast. The chapter also focuses on their role in coping with the tropical disease epidemic outbreaks they faced. Finally, it discusses how they spread the innovations developed at New Orleans to other stations, other cities, and other public health doctors as that field developed from the 1890s into the twentieth century.

A BRIEF HISTORY OF THE CITY AND IMMIGRATION TO AND THROUGH NEW ORLEANS

New Orleans began as a French settlement, founded on May 7, 1718, by the French Mississippi Company. It was named after Philippe d' Orleans, the Duke of Orleans and Regent of France. It was ceded to Spain in 1763 to compensate for the loss of Florida to the British, who also took Louisiana east of the Mississippi River. Spain did not send a governor to take control of the city and its environs until 1766. French and German settlers, who wanted the city returned to French control, forced the governor to flee after less than two years. Spain reasserted control in 1769, sending another governor, though the city was effectively under control of the Spanish garrison located in Cuba (Lewis, 2003).

During its final years as a Spanish colony, New Orleans suffered two massive fires that destroyed most of the city's buildings—in 1788 and in 1794. After these fires, the city was rebuilt in the Spanish style, with more fire-resistant brick buildings, with firewalls, with iron rather than wood balconies, and with open courtyards. Much of this eighteenth-century architecture, so distinctive of "the French Quarter," reflects the Spanish colonial period, exemplified by the St. Louis Cathedral, the Cabildo, and the Presbytere.

In a pattern we will see reflected often during its history, in 1778–1780, New Orleans also suffered epidemic outbreaks of what were essentially pandemic episodes of disease, and migration through the city up the Mississippi River spread the contagion to the interior. In November 1778, smallpox appeared in the Spanish colony of New Orleans, probably brought there by colonists from the Canary Islands.[1] New Orleans was the likely source from which it spread, in 1780, to the Spanish colony in New Mexico and to Mexico City. It moved from New Orleans up-river to the Missouri River, where tribes along the Missouri River likely spread it to the Oglala Sioux, who suffered a devastating epidemic of smallpox in 1779–1780. In the Louisiana colony of Canary Islanders in Galveztown, within a settlement of 404 people, 161 persons died between March 1779 and March 1780. At least half died of smallpox. They likely spread the contagion to the Creek Indians (Fenn: 137, 214, 219, 268; see also Duffy, 1953: 98–99.)

In the 1790s, the sugar industry flourished, and the growth of commerce along the Mississippi River led to the development of New Orleans' international interests. The city became the south Atlantic region's commercial and political center. The construction of levees around Lake Pontchartrain via Bayou St. John, which opened in 1794, further boosted the city's growing commerce and established New Orleans as the most important south Atlantic port city. Indeed, the city was more important for its export traffic during this time period than for its immigrant-receiving status as a port of debarkation.

The population of the city suffered epidemics of yellow fever, typhoid fever, malaria, cholera, and smallpox periodically throughout the nineteenth century (LeMay, 2006, table 2.1: 41, and 2013, vol. 2: 57). City leaders often blamed immigrants for bringing those diseases and epidemic outbreaks with them to the city. In point of fact, however, yellow fever and malaria in particular were by then endemic to the area. In many respects, it was a case of blaming the victims. The economic conditions faced by so many immigrants forced them to settle in neighborhoods that disproportionately suffered from the periodic outbreaks. Immigrants were more likely victims than carriers of these epidemic episodes. Such outbreaks of disease were undoubtedly influenced by the city's notoriously primitive sanitation and lack of public water. As discussed in chapter 2, cholera is spread by feces-contaminated water. Its cause and spread, however, were unknown until the 1880s, so immigrants became convenient targets on whom to lay the blame for the epidemics by city fathers who were unwilling to make the expensive changes necessary to improve basic health conditions.

In an 1832 epidemic of cholera, New Orleans lost an estimated 5,000 lives (Geddes Smith: 18–20, 63). New Orleans again suffered a cholera outbreak in 1848, probably brought to the city aboard vessels from Hamburg and Bremen, as these sites were known sources of the 1848–1849 pandemic at a time when thousands were fleeing the turmoil of the 1848 revolutions (Rosenberg: 105). An especially nasty epidemic of yellow fever struck in 1847, and another significant epidemic was the typhoid fever outbreak during the Civil War, in 1863 (LeMay, 2006: 41). Cholera struck New Orleans again in 1865–1866 (Rosenberg, 1992). Mullan describes a yellow fever epidemic that began in the city in 1877 and soon spread up-river:

> A yellow fever epidemic in New Orleans in 1877 that spread quickly up the Mississippi River valley riveted national attention on quarantine policy and forced congressional action. The Quarantine Act of 1878 was a victory for the Marine Hospital Service, conferring upon it quarantine authority—its first mission beyond the care of merchant seaman in the eighty years of its existence. (25)

In 1795, Spain granted the United States rights to use the city's port facilities. In 1800, Spain and France signed the Treaty of Ildefonso, which returned Louisiana to France. In 1803, Napoleon sold Louisiana to the United States in the Louisiana Purchase. By 1800, the city's population was about 10,000 people, a sizable city for that time anywhere along the east coast of America.

In the first decade of the nineteenth century, immigration of Cuba and French planters from Haiti expanded the city's population. Its cosmopolitan, polyglot population reflected the American, African, French, and Creole–French cultural heritages, especially thanks to the influx of immigrants fleeing the revolution in Haiti in 1804. Haitian refugees, both white and free blacks, arrived in New Orleans. As more and more refugees fled to Louisiana, about 90 percent of them settled in New Orleans. An 1809 migration, for example, brought 2,731 whites, 3,102 free blacks, and 3,226 black slaves to the city. That migration doubled the French-speaking population of New Orleans, and in 1809–1810, thousands more French-speaking refugees came from St. Dominique, fleeing persecution by Cuban officials responding to the French schemes of Bonaparte in Spain.

During the War of 1812, when the city was under martial law, the British tried to capture New Orleans but were defeated by Andrew Jackson's army. The city was attacked by a naval force sent down from the British colony of Halifax, Nova Scotia. The battle took place on January 8, 1812, while the Treaty of Ghent was being negotiated to end the war (it was signed on January 24, 1815) (8 Stat. 218). The battle gave General Jackson his status as "hero of New Orleans" and was the most decisive American victory of the War of 1812. Within an hour, the battle took the life of the British commanding general, Sir Edward Pakenham, who, with eight colonels, were among the 251 British killed and twenty-three wounded (www.historycentral.com/1812/NewOrleans.html).

New Orleans' population doubled again during the 1830s (see Table 5.1). Among the new arrivals to the city were friends of the Marquis de Lafayette, including some who had newly founded the city of Tallahassee, including the nephew of Napoleon Bonaparte, and a large contingent of Creole people. The city's large Gallic community had become a minority by 1820. In the 1830s and 1840s, however, a renewed influx of German and Irish immigrants arrived (Niehaus, 1976; Spletsfoser, 1978). English immigrants arriving in the 1830s simply passed through whenever possible, avoiding settlement in the city, which by then had earned a notorious reputation for sickness, particularly epidemics of yellow fever. This is exemplified by the observation of Rebecca Berland, who with her family arrived at New Orleans in 1831 aboard a sailing packet ship from Liverpool.

No one, except eye-witnesses, can form an adequate idea of the number and variety of vessels there collected, and lining the river for miles in length. New Orleans being the provision market for the West Indies and some of the Southern States, its port is frequented by foreign traders, but by thousands of small craft, often of the rudest construction, on which the settlers in the interior bring down the various produce of their climate and industry. The town itself, from its low marshy situation, is very unhealthy; the yellow fever is an everlasting scourge to its inhabitants, annually carrying off great numbers. As a trading port, New Orleans is the most famous and the best situated of any in America; but whoever values a comfortable climate or a healthy situation, will not, I am sure, choose to reside there. (Berland: 34–35)

Immigrant Berland noted further that on the very next day, the family secured river steamboat passage to St. Louis, arriving there after a twelve-day journey (Ibid.: 40).

By 1840, New Orleans was the wealthiest and third-most populous city in the United States, having a population of just more than 100,000. By 1850, it was the largest city in the entire U.S. South. The surge of Irish into the city, fleeing the potato famine, led to the development of the Know-Nothing Movement in the city and anti-Catholic riots in

New Orleans (LeMay, 2006: 20; see also Soulé, 1961; Beals, 1960; and Ray Billington, 1974).

Another significant immigrant infusion during the 1840–1850 decade was from Italy. By 1850, New Orleans led the nation with its large Italian American population, exceeding even the number of Italians who had settled in New York City (LeMay, 2006: 76; Logsdon: 114–115; and see Taylor, 1971). As we will see more fully, the Italian immigrant neighborhoods were particularly hard hit by the periodic epidemics that struck the city.

The use of natural gas in 1830, the building of the Pontchartrain Railroad in 1830–1831, one of the earliest in the United States, and especially the introduction of the steam cotton press in 1832 all contributed to the rise of New Orleans as the leading city of the U.S. South. The city began its public school system in 1840. Foreign exports in the 1830–1840 decade made it a leading port for international commerce, and the most important Southern port city for exportation. Commerce was further enhanced by the opening of the New Basin Canal, which, as in other cities, was constructed largely using immigrant labor. It enabled shipping of goods from the lake to uptown New Orleans. River boats and steamers joined ocean-sailing vessels in plying a thriving commercial trade.

The city's cultural diversity was boosted by slavery, the quadroon balls, a medley of Latin languages, and a distinctive subculture of the river men. Though still a frontier city of sorts, its seemingly boundless prosperity at the time led to the city's advancement—despite a short setback during the Panic of 1837 (a depression in today's terms). In 1849, Baton Rouge replaced New Orleans as the capital of Louisiana. In 1850, New Orleans was linked to St. Louis and New York City by telegraph. The year 1851 saw the opening of the New Orleans and Jackson Railroad, the first rail outlet northward. It joined what became the Illinois Central Railroad system. Then, in 1854, a western outlet, now called the Southern Pacific Railroad, began. Immigrant laborers were the majority of those who built these railroads westward (LeMay, 1987: 34).

During the 1830s, what was effectively three municipalities made up New Orleans—the French Quarter and Faubourg Treme, the Uptown (upriver from Canal Street), and the Downtown (the rest of the city, from Esplanade Avenue down to the river). They were governed, essentially, as three separate cities for twenty years, with the mayoralty of New Orleans being largely a ceremonial role (Logsdon: 112).

The importance of New Orleans as a financial and commercial center was enhanced when in 1838 the federal government established the U.S. Mint there, a decision by then President Andrew Jackson. The New Orleans Mint produced both silver and gold coinage until 1861, when Confederate

Table 5.6
City of New Orleans Population, 1810–1860

Year	Total Population
1810	17,242
1820	27,176
1830	46,082
1840	102,193
1850	116,375
1860	168,675

Source: U.S. Bureau of the Census. *Statistical Abstract of the United States, 2002.* Washington, D.C.: U.S. Government Printing Office, 2003.

forces took over the building and began minting Confederate money, until it was recaptured by Union forces in 1862.

A massive flood occurred in 1849, leaving about 12,000 residents homeless. It was but one of several floods that plagued the city as portions of the often poorly constructed levees failed. Immigrant labor was essential to their construction and maintenance. Table 5.6 presents the growth in the city's population from 1810 to 1860.

THE NEW ORLEANS STATION

New Orleans' location near the mouth of the Mississippi River provided the city with an important advantage as a port of entry for immigrants because of its access to the then western interior. By 1817, steamboats had begun plying inland waterways as far upriver as Louisville, marking New Orleans as an important gateway to the cheap and fertile interior lands. State officials sent agents to entice European immigrants to the Mississippi Valley, and New Orleans emerged from a backwater colonial outpost into a leading commercial center that was increasingly cosmopolitan (Logsdon: 107).

The key immigration period to New Orleans was 1820 to 1860. During this time there was no official and dedicated station (building) to receive and process immigrants. As was the case at the other ports of entry, immigrants were simply processed on the port's wharfs, and the processing was largely administered by state regulations rather than by the federal government. The federal government did not begin to assert sole control over immigration until 1891 (the act of March 3, which created the Superintendent of Immigration), and by then immigration through New Orleans had begun its decline in size and scope.

During the 1820–1860 boom period of immigration, an estimated 550,000 immigrants streamed through the port. By 1837, New Orleans was second only to New York City as a leading port of entry. Between 1847 (the start of the Irish potato famine-induced flood of Irish immigration to America) and 1857, over 350,000 immigrants jammed the docks of the port, accounting for about 10 percent of all immigrants to the United States and surpassing Boston, Philadelphia, and Baltimore (Conway and Spletstoser, cited in Logsdon: 108). Immigrants coming to New Orleans during this time most often arrived on sailing vessels, typically wood-hulled packet ships. The transatlantic journey usually took three weeks to a month and was often arduous and frequently hazardous. During the sailing ship era, as many as 8–9 percent of emigrants perished during the voyage—by ship-wreck or disease outbreaks during passage (Guillet: 31; Stephen Fox: 6–8).

Immigration to New Orleans virtually ceased during the Civil War. It was reopened after the Civil War, but the annual rate of arrivals after the Civil War rarely exceeded 10,000 and more typically was around 3,000. New Orleans quickly fell behind not only its old mid-Atlantic rivals of Baltimore, Boston, and Philadelphia, but also Galveston and Key West, and even behind the Pacific ports of entry at San Francisco and Hawaii.

During its heyday before the Civil War, immigration to New Orleans was in many ways the result of the city's booming export business. From 1820 to 1860, New Orleans exported agricultural products—increasingly cotton—to Europe. New Orleans trade was somewhat seasonal but was substantial. Ship captains carrying cargo, such as cotton, to European ports such as Liverpool, England; Le Havre, France; and Bremen and Hamburg, Germany, needed cargo for the return trip. They soon dis-covered that carrying immigrants was more profitable than, for example, carrying cheap French wine. As a result, English, German, Irish, and French immigrants provided a good market for ocean passage to New Orleans. Although the trip from northern Europe to New Orleans was a bit longer than to the more northern Atlantic ports, it was typically cheaper (Logsdon: 109). Two English immigrants, who passed through New Orleans in 1831, after a nearly one-month voyage, described why they went from Liverpool to New Orleans:

We were now passengers, in the steerage, on the vessel *Home*, bound for New Orleans. Our reasons for sailing to that port, the most distant in North America, and not in a direct course to the Illinois, were on account of the ready transit we should make thence into the interior up the Mississippi; whereas, by landing at New York, Boston, or Philadelphia, we should have had to cross the Allegheny mountains, and travel a great distance by land, which would have been both very troublesome, on account of our luggage, and very expensive. (Berland: 15)

Ships such as the *Superior, Mary Ann, Nictaux,* and *Elizabeth* plied the transatlantic trade between 1848 and 1860, sailing from Londonderry to New Orleans. Ships such as the *Ernst Moritz Arndt, Teamaker, O. Thigen,* and *Bentine* went from Bremen to New Orleans. The ship *Robert Hex* sailed from Italy to New Orleans in 1861 and the *Anglesea* from Liverpool to New Orleans also in 1861. Packet ships such as the *Kate Dyer,* the *Bark Alice Provost,* and the early steamship *Holino* sailed from Le Havre, France, to New Orleans until interrupted by the Civil War (J.J. Cooke Ships Passenger Lists, 1847–1871). In *Chicago, the Essence of "The Promised Land,"* Swedish immigrant Ulf Beijbom reports, "Of the 1.2 million Swedes who emigrated between 1850 and 1920, approximately every fourth one came from a town." This alters the traditional notion of Swedish emigrants as rural types. Beijbom notes that Swedish emigrants' desire to occupy cities testifies to their importance to the urbanization of the Unites States. The Swedish American Line regularly sailed four steamships, such as the M.S. *Stockholm I,* between Stockholm and New Orleans, in a journey that typically took a week across the icy waters of the Atlantic (cited in Peterson: 8).

Before the Civil War, the fact that river steamship travel to the interior was often faster and cheaper than the land journey from the mid-Atlantic ports gave New Orleans an advantage. River travel by steamboat was not only cheaper, but it was also more dependable. But the Civil War terminated New Orleans's status as a leading port of entry. By the time immigration began again after the war, railroad connections from the mid-Atlantic port cities to St. Louis and points west were operating. The fast and dependable railroad passage to what was then the American frontier, as well as the cheap and abundant lands offered through the Homestead Act, drew immigrants to ports such as Boston, Baltimore, New York, and Philadelphia rather than to New Orleans. Transatlantic shipping lines forged partnerships with those railroads and gained sway over the immigration traffic. Corporate ties to commercial markets in cities such as New York, Boston, and Baltimore, each joined with particular railroad lines. These commercial/transportation partnerships essentially left out New Orleans (Taylor: 76–95). Shipping magnates such as Samuel Cunard, Isambard Brunel, Edward Collins, Robert Dollar, and Clement Griscom transformed the transatlantic crossing. They began with wooden-hulled, sailing packet vessels; transitioned by the 1840s and 1850s to ocean-going steam side-paddle wheelers designed to carry passengers on regularly scheduled service, like the *Great Easterner* and the *Great Westerner*; and developed the steel-hulled, steam-powered early oceangoing liners in the 1860s to 1880s, with each generation of steam liner getting bigger and faster, capable of carrying thousands instead of dozens to at most a few hundred passengers aboard each ship, as had been typical of the pre–Civil War era (Fox, 2001). As Randall Miller notes: "Transportation, then, played a large role in drawing and directing the immigration flow" (128; see also Conway and Spletstoser). Baltimore developed the Baltimore Mail Line with regular transatlantic service between Bremen and Baltimore and in partnership with the Baltimore and Ohio Railroad. The North German Lloyd Company, by 1857, regularly served Baltimore by steam liner. Other lines that provided regular service to Baltimore included the Inman Line and the United States Line (Esslinger: 61–63).

Both Boston and New York City were served on a regular basis by Samuel Cunard's White Star Line—later called the Cunard Line (Fuchs, 1990: 20–21); by the German Hamburg-American Line; by the North German Lloyd Line; by the United States Line; by the Great Western Steamship Line; by the American President's Line; and by the French Liner company Campaigne Generale Transatlantique (Fox). By the 1870s, New Orleans simply could no longer compete (LeMay, "Overview" essay, 2013, vol. 1: 1–22).

As the numbers of immigrants coming to New Orleans declined steadily from the 1870s on, city officials tried to revive the immigrant flow to keep pace with its northern city rivals. Promoters of the New South sent agents to Europe, particularly to Germany, attempting to attract farmers to the state. Louisiana was especially active in its recruitment campaign. Post–Civil War recruitment, however, generated little interest. The very farmers that the southern states most desired were least likely to find the U.S. South's depleted soil and strange climate (compared to northern Europe's) as attractive as the agricultural and economic conditions of the Midwestern states (Miller: 135–136). The inducements generated by business campaigns did not fare much better. As Miller notes:

> Private schemes to foster immigration were more successful if only because state-supported efforts reached such a meager harvest. With mixed success, after 1890, railroad companies sought immigrants to settle their lands, and planters enlisted immigrants to replace or displace black laborers. Failing to persuade German farmers to come, private concerns in Louisiana engaged labor contractors to supply Chinese workers, and later, southern Italians, to work in gangs on large sugar plantations. The labor experiments failed. The Chinese and southern Italians proved as intractable as blacks had been and either fled or were pushed off the plantations. (Miller: 136)

Moreover, in 1891, the federal government took control over the immigration process. The Act of March 3, 1891, Regarding Immigration and the Superintendent of Immigration (28 Stat. 1084; U.S.C. 101), among other provisions, forbade the advertisement for and soliciting of immigrants, increased penalties for landing an illegal alien, created the position of superintendent of immigration, and generally strengthened or specified enforcement processes, thereby establishing the federal government's decisive role in immigration affairs (LeMay, 1987: 58; LeMay and Barkan: 66–70). The superintendent, appointed by the president with the advice and consent of the Senate, served under the secretary of treasury, thereby lodging the immigration service in that department, where it remained until 1903, when the congress moved immigration policy control to the newly established Department of Commerce and Labor (act of February 14, 1903, 32 Stat. 825; 8 U.S.C.; LeMay and Barkan: 89–90). The act of 1891 charged the secretary of the treasury to prescribe rules for inspection along the borders of Canada, including British Columbia, and Mexico and provided for the appointment of federal inspectors of immigration by the Superintendent of Immigration.

Section 8 of the act, cited below, details the work of inspectors and specifically of the U.S. M.H.S. medical personnel:

[U]pon arrival by water at any place within the United States of any alien immigrants, it shall be the duty of the commanding officer and the agents of the steam or sailing vessel by which they came to report the name, nationality, last residence, and destination of every such alien, before any of them are landed, to the proper inspection officers, who shall thereupon go or send competent assistants on board such vessel and there inspect all such aliens, or the inspection officer may order a temporary removal of such aliens for examination at a designated time and place, and then and there detain them until a thorough examination is made. But such removal shall not be considered a landing during the pendency of such examination. The medical examination shall be made by surgeons of the Marine Hospital Service. In cases where the services cannot be obtained without causing unreasonable delay, the inspector may cause an alien to be examined by a civil surgeon and the Secretary of the Treasury shall fix the compensation for such examination. The inspection officers shall have the power to administer oaths, and take and consider testimony touching on the right of any such alien to enter the United States, all of which shall be entered on record . . . . (cited in LeMay and Barkan: 68)

The immigration act of 1891 was soon challenged in the courts, where it quickly made its way to the U.S. Supreme Court, which held the law constitutional in *Nishimura Ekiu v. United States* (January 18, 1892:142 U.S. 651). The justices stressed the sovereignty issue and the power of Congress to set immigration policy and to delegate such powers to service officers (LeMay and Barkan, Document 42: 70–71).

The federal government opened a station in a building specific to those tasks, though ironically, immigration to New Orleans dropped off fairly dramatically soon after the station began processing immigrants. Immigration policy was moved again, in 1940, by executive order of President Franklin D. Roosevelt, which transferred the Immigration and Naturalization Service to the Department of Justice, where it remained until disbanded by the Homeland Security Act of 2002 (Executive Order 8430, June 5, 1940, see LeMay and Barkan: Document 98: 175–177).

Whereas French, German, and Irish immigrants dominated the immigrant wave that came to and through New Orleans before the Civil War, after the war a fairly diverse group of immigrants arrived at the station. New Orleans was one of the few American cities to see a substantial number of immigrants from Spain and Latin America (Logsdon: 114). Regular shipping runs to Cuba and the Caribbean accounts for this flow, for most Spanish entrants stopped in Cuba or a former Spanish colony— a practice that continues to current times, when airline service from Nicaragua, Honduras, Guatemala, and Belize uses the New Orleans airport (Taylor, 1971).

Immigration from Asia continued despite federal restrictions forbidding it (i.e., the Chinese Laborer Exclusion Act of 1882 and its subsequent amendments and increased restrictions in 1885, 1887, 1888, and 1902). These remained in effect until repealed in 1943 (see LeMay and Barkan). Because of these legal restrictions, many Chinese used the port at New Orleans, where it was easier to enter than at the more hostile Angel Island station at San Francisco. Filipinos escaped the exclusionary quota-based laws until 1934, and as many as 2,000 of them settled in New Orleans (Logsdon: 114).

Mediterranean groups also migrated to New Orleans in considerable numbers. Greek immigrants, for example, started the nation's first Greek Orthodox church in New Orleans in 1864. Croatians came in the 1850s to cultivate oysters in the delta and market them in New Orleans. By 1850, Sicilians made New Orleans the site of the largest Italian settlement in the United States, with merchants coming from Palermo, the key depot for citrus fruit from the Mediterranean. Their expertise in fruit handling and merchandising enabled them to expand operations to Central America, where they found different tropical fruits (e.g., bananas) to market (Logsdon: 115). Experienced Sicilian laborers came in the 1870s and 1880s, and between 1890 and 1910, more than 50,000 Sicilians arrived in New Orleans despite violence against them in 1890–1891 (led by the Ku Klux Klan). Even substantial numbers of Sicilians who had come to work on sugar plantations drifted back to New Orleans to establish an industry that dominated the city's truck farming, food wholesaling, and retail grocery businesses. By 1920, for example, nearly half of the city's grocery stores were owned by Sicilians (Logsdon: 115; see also Taylor, 1971). The lack of an industrial economy in the city, with working-class neighborhoods concentrated ethnic enclaves, and the lack of suitable large tracks of land until drainage methods opened up such areas in the twentieth century, meant that German and Sicilian immigrants could and did continue to operate within New Orleans city boundaries bucolic businesses such as truck farms, nurseries, and dairies.

The close mingling of highly diverse immigrant groups contributed to the development of the unique cultural lifestyle that emerged in New Orleans. Anglo-Americans were unable to control the unusual process of acculturation in the city, where by the 1880s ordinary people blended the distinctive cultural way of life of the city by drawing upon traditions from Ireland, Germany, Italy, France, and Spain, but also from places such as Senegal, Angola, China, Haiti, the Philippines, Belize, Cuba, Virginia, and South Carolina (Logsdon: 117–118; Miller: 126–127).

This considerably diverse mixture of immigrant flows was firmly set by the 1880s and by then had established the unique blend that shaped the public cultural life that so characterized New Orleans. The federal government took charge and opened a small station in 1891, essentially in a house building. Immigrants needing to be quarantined were sent to a separate facility for that purpose. Those needing hospitalization were sent to the Marine Hospital 14. But immigration began to drop off by then as well, and the slide continued into the twentieth century. Immigrants comprised about 40 percent of the city's population in 1860, fell to roughly 19 percent in 1880, dropped to 10 percent in 1900, and then dropped again to less than 7 percent in 1920 (Miller: 128). Table 5.7 illustrates that comparative drop-off in immigration through New Orleans by ranking the major ports of entry to the United States and comparing the number of immigrants examined at each for the year 1912.

How the New Orleans station coped with frequent epidemic outbreaks, particularly of yellow fever, and the pioneering efforts made there in developing germicides to enhance the science of "maritime sanitation" programs to replace the previously less effective policy of quarantine, is the focus of this chapter's next section.

Table 5.7
Major Ports of Entry and Number of Aliens Examined, 1912

City/Port	Number of Aliens Examined
New York	749,643
Boston	54,759
Philadelphia	46,857
Baltimore	23,543
Port Townsend, Washington	11,881
San Francisco	10,353
Portland, Maine	7,323
Detroit, Michigan	6,852
Galveston, Texas	5,550
Nogales, Arizona	4,314
Port Tampa, Florida	4,297
New Orleans, Louisiana	4,058
Buffalo, New York	3,936

Source: Table by author, Data from INS Annual Report, February 20, 1912, RG 90, File 219, Box 036.

COPING WITH EPIDEMICS AND PANDEMICS AT NEW ORLEANS

As already mentioned, doctors at New Orleans had to treat immigrants suffering with virtually every communicable disease common in the nineteenth century. The epidemic outbreaks they faced, however, were concentrated in cholera, smallpox, and yellow fever. The prevalence of these diseases in New Orleans, and in the U.S. South more generally, strongly influenced the nature and flow of immigration to and through New Orleans. Cholera and yellow fever epidemics were regular occurrences, for by 1820, these diseases were endemic in the U.S. South, including southern cities (see Cholera files, RG 90, File 397, Box 053).

In the nineteenth century, yellow fever was mostly a southern affliction. New Orleans, as the south's largest city, led the region in health problems. The city experienced yellow fever epidemics in 1817, 1832, 1835, 1837, 1839, 1841, 1847, 1853, 1854, 1855, 1858, 1867, and 1878 (Miller: 132; see also Table 2.1, in LeMay, 2006: 41; and see Carrigan: 339–355). The 1853 epidemic was especially deadly, taking the lives of an estimated 9,000 persons in the city and state. But as Miller notes:

> A host of other endemic diseases added to the city's sorry history of seasonal scourges, as did poor health management, laissez-faire attitudes, and ignorance.

The increasing number and virulence of epidemics in New Orleans after 1830, however, stemmed in part from increased immigration. As large numbers of non-immune immigrants crowded into New Orleans, they became victims of south Louisiana's pestilences. Population growth fed and spread epidemics, which abated only when cold weather came and people left the city. (Miller: 133)

New Orleans, moreover, was slow to adopt preventative measures. Commercial trade interests led civic leaders and businessmen to proclaim the city—despite the prevalent evidence to the contrary—a healthy place. During yellow fever epidemics, they often suppressed information until after the outbreak had spread so far that it could no longer be denied. By then commerce ceased, and all who could afford to do so left the city (Ibid.: 134). City leaders led the "denial" syndrome in the 1853 yellow fever epidemic, which resulted in the death of nearly 9,000 residents of New Orleans, and again in 1878, when the yellow fever outbreak numbered nearly 27,000 cases, with more than 400 deaths (Leavitt: 422–423).

Instead of admitting that the epidemics were endemic, civic leaders and merchants blamed the problems on the immigrants. As Miller puts it:

A brand of "medical Know-Nothingism" emerged whereby immigrants were charged with introducing sickness into the city. Epidemics originated in immigrant wards and raged within them; consequently, opined the worthies of New Orleans, immigrants must be the cause of the disease. . . . The identification of immigrants with epidemics was so often repeated and deeply ingrained that it became an article of faith, even among learned individuals, and persisted to the end of the century. (Miller: 134)

But fear of contracting disease undoubtedly spurred immigrants, as well, to pass on through the city as quickly as was possible if they had the financial means to do so. The city had justifiably earned a frightening reputation among immigrants bound for America. The city's almost regular outbreaks of disease, especially of yellow fever, which came to be known as the newcomers' or immigrants' disease, struck during the tropical heat season from May until October. Immigrant guidebooks and foreign councils alike warned travelers to avoid New Orleans during the season (Conway: 58; Logsdon: 109).

Despite such warnings, thousands of immigrants stranded in the city during the yellow fever season filled the city's hospitals—and cemeteries. Because local leaders wanted a wide open port, they developed only half-hearted efforts for incoming vessels before 1820. After 1820, they turned management of the port to private lessees. Fear of the epidemics, however, did not seem to overcome the attraction of the port as a cheaper port of entry to the interior and as a port where personal handicaps might less likely exclude immigrants from entry than in the more northern port cities (Ibid.: 92–93).

It was not until the terrible outbreak of yellow fever in 1853, which took the lives of about 8,000 in the city—and that was followed in 1854–1855 by another 5,000—which closed the port, that city leaders were finally forced to act. They secured state legislation to set up quarantine stations outside the city and forced ships, particularly those from tropical ports, to stop for health inspections during the yellow fever season. Even then, they delayed construction of on-shore facilities for that purpose until 1859, when the height of the immigration flow to New Orleans was coming to a halt (Ibid.: 128–129).

The endemic nature of yellow fever in New Orleans is evident in that every year between 1817 and 1899, the city experienced some deaths from yellow fever. Table 5.8 lists those years, as well as the number of deaths lost to the disease between 1817 and 1899 in which 400 or more died in that given year. As evident from the table, the nastiest outbreaks were in 1847, 1853–1855, 1858, and 1878, when thousands died each year.

Reacting to the 1853–1854 yellow fever epidemics, the state established the Louisiana State Board of Health by Act 336 of March 15, 1855. The city was unable to protect itself from the frequent epidemic outbreaks (mostly of yellow fever and cholera, but occasionally of malaria as well), nor to maintain a city-established board of health for any length of time, for commercial interests, allied with the local press, overcame efforts to do so. The disastrous 1853 yellow fever epidemic instigated the creation

Table 5.8
Major Yellow Fever Epidemics in New Orleans, 1817–1878

Year	Number of Deaths	Year	Number of Deaths
1817	809	1849	749
1819	2,100	1852	450
1820	400	1853	7,970
1837	442	1854	2,423
1839	452	1855	2,670
1841	504	1858	4,855
1843	487	1867	3,107
1847	2,359	1870	588
1848	808	1878	4,340

Source: Table by author from data in George F. Shrady and Thomas L. Stedman, eds., *Medical Record* v. 62 (1902): 648.

of a sanitary commission of New Orleans, which promptly recommended a city board of health. This action stimulated the state to set up the state board of health to operate a quarantine program for the state (whose population in 1850 was just over half a million). At the time, New Orleans was the third-largest city in the nation, as well as the largest in the state and the U.S. South. The 1855-established state board of health served as the advisor to the New Orleans city council until reorganization, in 1898, when the city established a municipal board of health under the jurisdiction of the state board of health (Freedman: 1,279).

The act to establish the state quarantine allowed the city council one-third representation on the board. Dr. Samuel Choppin, the first state health officer, noted that the theory of the formation of the state board for the purpose of administering the quarantine made it logical to allow the city representation in consideration of its great commercial interests.

After 1877, in reaction to Reconstruction, the city gained a majority of the board's nine members, which it retained until 1898. The quarantine applied to the entire shore of Louisiana along the Gulf of Mexico, and two quarantine stations were located along the coast, one 70 miles south and another 100 miles west (Freedman: 1,280). The lower station, L'Outre, located about 103 miles below the city at an unused outlet of the Mississippi, was used to quarantine infected vessels only. It employed a quarantine tugboat outfitted with disinfecting apparatus to use steam and chemicals (usually bichloride of mercury or sulfur dioxide) whenever a ship was stopped for one of the then three great pestilential diseases: smallpox, cholera, or yellow fever. Dr. C.B. White and Dr. A.W. Perry demonstrated the value of forcing concentrated sulfur dioxide gas into the holds of vessels to disinfect a ship's luggage, baggage and so on (Holt: "An Epitomized Review"). It wasn't until 1916 that Congress approved and appropriated $300,000 for erecting and equipping and otherwise providing a facility designed for a quarantine station at New Orleans (H.R. 12586, March 2, 1916, in RG 90, Box 114, Folder 1205). The Boarding Station was housed in a separate facility on Flood Street, and the station medical director had to frequently communicate with the P.H.S. in Washington, D.C., regarding the assignment of personnel and duties at the Marine Hospital, the Quarantine Station, and the Lower Station (also used for quarantine) between 1923 and 1935 (Folder 1515, Box 114). Dr. George Miller Sternberg organized the Yellow Fever Commission in 1900 (Kaufman, Galishoff, and Savitts, vol. 2: 716–717).

The state board of health was concerned with more than quarantine matters. It gave the mayor and city council input regarding drainage, sanitation in relation to communicable diseases, and violation of the city's sanitary ordinances, the distribution of smallpox vaccinations (after 1898), and the collection of epidemiological data concerning climatology and mortality. Its state health officer, Dr. A. Forster Axson, however, reflecting the idea that yellow fever might not be of external origin, argued that internal sanitary measures in addition to quarantine were necessary. But the largely advisory capacity of the board weakened its effect with respect to epidemics. In its early years of operation, it repeatedly recommended adequate drainage (Annual Reports, 1856, 1857, 1859); the regulation of midwifery and of medical practice (Reports of 1857 and 1860); control by the board of all communicable diseases and sanitation (Reports of 1855, 1857, 1858, 1859, 1860); the practice of pharmacy (Report of 1860); and the broadening of all public health laws (Reports of 1866 and 1882) (Ibid.: 1281).

Doctors Choppin and Axson served until 1860, when they were succeeded by Dr. Nott, the last civilian president of the board until after the Civil War. During the war, General Butler appointed Thomas H. Bache medical director of the Department of the Gulf, as it was then called, in 1862.

Because at the time the cause of yellow fever was unknown, New Orleans–originated epidemics continued to spread up-river. The 1878–1879 epidemic spread from New Orleans to St. Louis, Missouri, aboard the river steamer *A.P. Silver* (*St. Louis Genealogical Society Quarterly* 32, no. 4: 146–148). In that outbreak, more than 27,000 cases were reported, resulting in more than 4,000 deaths (Leavitt: 422–423).

The most persistent opponents of the actions recommended by the state board of health were the New Orleans commercial interests and the press (like at Angel Island in 1900 to 1905). Dr. Joseph Jones, in his annual report of the board for 1882, noted:

> The opponents of the Quarantine System of Louisiana have continually used the press to arouse public indignation and hatred against the Board of Health, and especially against its president, by the cry that the quarantine was destroying the commerce of New Orleans. (cited in Freedman: 1,284)

Table 5.9 lists the presidents of the Louisiana Board of Health from 1855 to 1949.

The impact of Dr. Joseph Jones and Dr. Joseph Holt was especially significant, and their experiences illustrate the effect of federalism in quarantine and health matters. Both of them struggled with local officials and with national agencies. Both had to cope with federal/state funding issues and disputes as well. Both had to fight legal actions in the federal district and the U.S. superior courts, much as with the events at Angel Island. They battled local commercial interests and financial concerns, especially with shipping companies, as did the doctors at Angel Island and Ellis Island.

Table 5.9
Presidents, Louisiana State Board of Health, 1855–1949

Years	Presidents
1855	Samuel Choppin
1856–1859	A. Foster Axson
1860	Charles Delery
1861–1862	G. A. Nott
5/1862–8/1862	Thomas Bache
8/1862–12/1862	Charles R. McCormack
12/1862–4/1866	Richard H. Alexander
4/1866–11/1868	S. A. Smith
11/1868–7/1876	C. D. White
7/1876–5/1877	Felix B. Gaudet
5/1877–1879	Samuel Choppin
1880–1883	Joseph Jones
1884–1887	Joseph Holt
1888–1889	Clement P. Wilkinson
1890–1898	Samuel Rutherford Oliphant
1898–1905	Edmond Souchon
1906–1907	C. H. Iron
1908–1909	D. Harvey Dillon
1910–1928	Oscar Dowling
1929–1940	Joseph A. O'Hara
1940–1942	John H. Musser
1942–1946	David E. Brown
1946–1948	Waldo L. Treuting
1948–1949	William V. Garnier

Source: Table by author from data in Benjamin Freedman, "The Louisiana State Board of Health, Established 1855," *The American Journal of Public Health* 41 (October 1951): 1280–1285.

Dr. Joseph Jones was born in Liberty County, Georgia, on September 6, 1833, and died February 17, 1896. He was a physician and a medical scientist educated at South Carolina College (now the University of South Carolina), who took his B.A. degree from Princeton in 1853 and received an M.D. from the University of Pennsylvania in 1856. From then until 1861, he taught chemistry at Savannah Medical College of Georgia. His work there launched his reputation as a leading student of health conditions in the U.S. South during the nineteenth century. During the Civil War, Dr. Jones served as a Confederate surgeon. He returned to the Medical College of Georgia after the war, in 1865, and then was elected chair of physiology and pathology at the University of Nashville.

In 1868, Dr. Jones moved to New Orleans as chair of chemistry and clinical medicine in the medical department of the University of Louisiana (now Tulane University), where he also served as a visiting physician at Charity Hospital. He studied diseases there and became a leader of the sanitary reform movement in the South, leading a campaign to clean up New Orleans. The most lethal disease he battled was yellow fever, particularly in the form of the deadly epidemic of yellow fever that struck New Orleans in 1878. He was appointed to the Louisiana state board of health in 1877 and became its president in 1880, in which capacity he served until 1883. During that time, he guided New Orleans health reform and, indeed, that of the Mississippi Valley.

Dr. Jones fought for and won the right to collect fees from the shipping lines to pay for the Gulf quarantine system. In 1881, the powerful Morgan Company took the board of health to court, then to the Louisiana Supreme Court, and finally to the U.S. Supreme Court (in 1886). The U.S. Supreme Court upheld the quarantine fees as a legitimate exercise of a state's police power to protect public health. Dr. Jones was among the first medical bacteriologists in the United States.

Dr. Jones' tenure at the Louisiana Board of Health was also notable for a bitter conflict he fought with the national board of health, which had been established on March 3, 1879, largely in response to demands for a national quarantine act in wake of the devastating yellow fever epidemic of 1878. Proponents of the national act argued that state officials could not adequately enforce quarantine policy when a disease, like yellow fever, crossed many state lines as it spread upward and outward from the Mississippi Valley aboard river steamboat traffic and land migrations. Dr. Jones, an ardent believer in states' rights, was the boldest opponent of the national agency's attempts to administer quarantine along the Gulf Coast.

He retired in 1883 to return to teaching and research. During his career, he published more than 100 papers in the leading medical journals of the day. He authored a four-volume set of highly influential medical books, *Medical and Surgical Memoirs*, in 1876 and 1890. Upon his retirement, he was replaced as president of the Louisiana state board of health by Dr. Joseph Holt (Garraty and Carnes: 223–224; Kaufman, Galishoff, and Savitts, vol. 1: 399–400).

Dr. Holt served from 1884 to 1887 and was crucially influential in developing a scientific research program in germicidal agents, processes, and apparata. In 1884, Dr. Holt succeeded in convincing the state of Louisiana to appropriate $30,000 with which he inaugurated his proposed "maritime sanitation" system (Kendall: 764).

Like Dr. Jones, Dr. Holt served as a Confederate army surgeon. He distinguished himself at the Battle of Gettysburg.

During his four years of service in New Orleans, Dr. Joseph Holt, acting on the findings of germ theory advocates in Europe, conducted an elaborate series of experiments to test various chemicals that could be added to steam to disinfect luggage and baggage. He argued that the station should move from a policy of maritime quarantine, as practiced under Dr. Jones and as what was standard policy throughout the nation at that time, to what he termed "maritime sanitation."[2] Dr. Holt defined maritime sanitation as "the application of modern methods suggested by sanitary science and approved by experience in the treatment of all carriers, persons and things traversing the seas."

Holt was reacting, in particular, to the development by Dr. Chamberlain, the disciple of France's pioneering bacteriologist Louis Pasteur, and their groundbreaking work in bacteriology conducted at the Pasteur Institute. As we saw chapter 2, Dr. Chamberlain developed the autoclave. He used this small desktop steam chamber in the laboratory and at surgical hospitals. Chamberlain proved that it would disinfect surgical instruments. By then, the Pasteur Institute had proven that diseases were caused by germs—bacillus—that invaded the human body, and moreover, that a particular bacillus caused a particular human disease. After the particular microorganisms were identified as causing particular communicable diseases—and throughout the 1880s and 1890s they identified dozens of these various bacilli, as described in chapter 2—then "disinfection" and "decontamination" processes could be developed to effectively stop the disease from spreading, and sera could be developed to cure the individual patient, or inoculation procedures could be developed to prevent the disease in the first place.[3]

The Pasteur Institute had shown that steam, under pressure, would kill bacilli. Dr. Holt's pioneering experiments were to identify germicides that could be added to the steam to more effectively and quickly disinfect. He examined virtually every known chemical on the then-known table of chemicals, carefully and scientifically testing their germicidal properties and any side effects they had on clothing, leather luggage, bales of cargo, and so on (Holt Reports of 1887, 1892). New Orleans historian John Kendall said of Dr. Holt:

Dr. Joseph Holt, one of the best known physicians of New Orleans, took charge at what may be considered the most critical period of the warfare against yellow fever, and no man ever espoused a desperate cause with greater courage and determination. (764–765)

After serving for four years, Dr. Holt retired and moved to Portland, Oregon. In 1897, the city of New Orleans established the Holt Cemetery, a potter's field for the poor, in his name and honor.

The New Orleans station developed "disinfection lockers" to decontaminate luggage and baggage from the immigrant-laden ships bringing them to New Orleans. Their design, though effective, was later improved upon by Dr. Kinyoun and others to have less leakage, and for more efficient use to quickly decontaminate entire shiploads of cargo.

Until germ theory was proven, however, and the bacillus causing diseases such as yellow fever and malaria were identified, many in the medical profession clung to the idea that disease resulted from "miasma" or "bad vapours" (Trask: 16–17; see also Friedenberg, and Estes). During the Spanish–American War of 1898, more American soldiers fell to malaria and yellow fever than to battlefield bullets. In part, this was because the concept of a "carrier"—what became known as the vector of the disease—was as yet unknown. Medical practitioners, if not medical scientists, continued to emphasize maritime cleanliness in combating yellow fever. In 1900, then Surgeon General George Stoner advised ship masters that "yellow fever thrives in filth" and that "personal cleanliness and a clean, dry, well-ventilated ship are the best means of protection against the ravages of the disease" (quoted in Trask: 17).

Shortly after Stoner's admonitions, the findings of U.S. Army Major Walter Reed's Yellow Fever Commission's research in Cuba demonstrated that the disease was spread not by human-to-human contact, not by contaminated clothing or bedding, and indeed not by a ship's lack of cleanliness, but rather by the mosquito. In 1901, the U.S. Public Health and Marine Hospital Service applied Reed's findings to a maritime setting, showing that ships were indeed incubators for yellow fever, but not from some sort of "ship's foul vapors," but rather because ships' water casks carried adult mosquitoes and their larvae. Dr. Henry Carter, of the U.S. M.H.S., showed that individuals actually contracted the fever while shipboard when the ship was infested with the infected mosquitoes (Carter, 1902 bulletin).

Dr. Carter was born in 1852. He received his M.D. from the University of Maryland School of Medicine in 1879 and served with the U.S. M.H.S. from 1879 to 1919. He was sent to the Gulf Quarantine Station at Ship Island in 1888 as the service's representative to the U.S. South during the Yellow Fever Campaign in 1899–1906. He has been described as the father of the modern quarantine and is noted for establishing the efficiency of sulphur fumigation and disinfection at ports. His system replaced the previous somewhat arbitrary local and state regulations with a uniform code. Carter directed the first systematic campaign against malaria in the

U.S. South. From 1915 to 1925, he was a member of the Yellow Fever Council and served on the International Health Board of the Rockefeller Foundation (Kaufman, Galishoff, and Savitt: 124).

New Orleans, like most of the U.S. South and, indeed, much of the nation, was struck by the smallpox epidemics of 1898–1903. New Orleans reported 283 cases in 1899, with six deaths, and 1, 468 cases of smallpox in 1900, with 448 deaths (a death rate of 30.5%). Across Mississippi, in 1900, 2,066 cases were reported, with 456 deaths (22%). The U.S. M.H.S. reported 12,000 cases in the U.S. South in 1899, which rose to 15,000 cases by 1900; new cases soared to 39,000 in 1901 (Willrich: 10, 44).

Surgeon General Walter Wyman sent Passed Surgeon Charles P. Wertenbaker, by then the service's leading surgeon on smallpox, to take command of the New Orleans station in 1900. Though this appointment was a "promotion" for Wertenbaker, it was not the promotion he had asked for of the service. He wanted to lead a national anti-smallpox campaign of compulsory vaccination. His idea for a vaccination campaign that would wipe out the disease was not realized until years later (Ibid.: 115).

Dr. J. H. White, of the U.S. M.H.S., and Dr. Wertenbaker, then both stationed at the New Orleans station, were frequently sent during the 1903–1905 campaign against yellow fever to consult with local officials and oversee the campaign's disinfection efforts against the mosquito in Texas (RG 90, Box 169, File 1876, and Box 713, File 1876). Dr. Wertenbaker worked with the local public health commissions in five cities to pass ordinances regarding the screening of cisterns and the treatment of stagnant water supplies to eradicate the mosquito. He sent reports to Surgeon General Wyman and was granted funds out of an "epidemic fund" established by the service to battle the disease all along the Mississippi Coast. He ordered pyrethrum by the hundreds of pounds to battle the epidemics in Eagle Pass, Texas, Laredo, Texas, and so on and dealt regularly with the Louisiana board of health to coordinate the state and federal campaign against yellow fever (RG 90, Box 173, File 1876; see also the assorted yellow fever reports, Box 175). Wertenbaker worked closely with Dr. Edmund Souchon, who in 1903 was the president of the Louisiana board of health and who led the state's "war on the mosquito" (Kaufman, Galishoff, and Savitts: 706). In 1905, Wertenbaker was sent to head the P.H.M.H.S. in Atlanta, Georgia (Box 174).

Yet even after vaccination and mosquito control campaigns proved the value of massive public health campaigns to rid the U.S. South, including New Orleans, of yellow fever and smallpox, support for the "miasma" theory lingered on for some time. Rudolph Matas, a noted surgeon and yellow fever fighter, concluded that "of all the influences that retarded the development of the modern concepts of the infectious and epidemic diseases, the belief in the spontaneous generation of these epidemics out of 'miasms' emanating from decomposing inorganic or dead organic matter . . . was the greatest hinderance" (Matas: 455). And Trask concludes:

> Still, the many contentious issues surrounding yellow fever resulted in the understandably slow acceptance of Reed's findings. Furthermore, Reed's colleagues never identified the pathogen that caused the yellow fever despite their efforts to isolate the virus. This reluctance to accept Reed's findings had tragic consequences. Yellow fever continued to outbreak in the United States until 1905, when, during an epidemic in New Orleans, a well-orchestrated effort eliminated the mosquito-breeding potential of open receptacles and curbed the attack. This eradication campaign, spearheaded by the U.S. Public Health and Hospital Service, marked the last epidemic in America and finally convinced detractors of the validity of the "mosquito theory." (Trask: 18)

The yellow fever epidemic of 1905 may have originated on board a ship. The Quarantine Station at Ship Island, Mississippi, in 1905 found that the steam ship *Hiram* had a yellow fever outbreak that had resulted in two deaths in quarantine (Leavitt: 423). In the 1905 eradication campaign, then U.S. M.H.S. Surgeon Rupert Blue and his assistant, Dr. W. C. Rucker, went to New Orleans to direct the effort. The complexity and the impact of federalism upon the yellow fever campaign that year, the last yellow fever epidemic to strike the United States, is illustrated by Dr. Blue's actions. He battled state and local officials and local businessmen and ship lines. He insisted that the U.S. M.H.S. be paid, by the city of New Orleans, $250,000—in advance—to cover the federal government's expenses in helping to fight the epidemic (Barry: 312).

The service issued a report (*Public Health Reports* 20, no. 32, August 11, 1905) that recommended that to destroy mosquitoes on ship, health officials use sulfur fumigation. They reported it to be highly effective, although they acknowledged that sulfur had "inconveniences." The U.S. M.H.S. (called the Public Health Service after 1912) also recommended the use of powdered leaves of datura (Jimson weed) mixed with saltpeter and burned, one ounce of the mixture to each 200 cubic feet of space in the ship's hold, as a cheap, safe, and effective method for destroying hibernating mosquitoes. Another recommendation was the use of pyrethrum and formaldehyde to dispose of hibernating insects (the latter having less problematic side effects than sulfur). They also recommended that the boarding officials treat all water receptacles with oil—a simple way to kill mosquito larvae—or that they be made insect-proof. For combating mosquitoes on land, they recommended the drainage and flushing of all ditches.

By 1905, with the effectiveness of the eradication approach demonstrated, communities in the U.S. South were finally willing to have boards of health be given military powers to enforce orders to screen, clean up, and drain mosquito breeding sources of stagnant water, as well as to order officials to report suspicious cases of the disease (*St. Louis Medical Review*, August 26, 1905: 182; and "Report by William Gorgas," 1917).

New Orleans was the site of the last outbreak of bubonic plague in the United States, which occurred in July, 1914. The first confirmed reported case was July 25. This episode, which was also an epidemic outbreak, was quickly contained and stopped through the efforts of the U.S. Public Health Service, as it was by then named. Using the lessons that he learned in San Francisco in 1907–1908, then Surgeon General Rupert Blue's "rat eradication" campaign approach was used in New Orleans (RG 90, File 544, Box 065). Rat trapping teams were dispersed, and the National Health Service laboratory in New Orleans conducted research on rats, searching for plague-infected rats. The team, led by Dr. W. C. Rucker, found only twenty-three cases of humans infected and eight-two cases of infected rats. Plague reports by the U.S. Public Health Service issued in 1915 and covering the period from December 26, 1914, to March 26, 1915, demonstrated the effectiveness of that public health campaign in that the outbreak resulted in only ten deaths (RG 90, File 544, Box 67).[4]

Remarkably, Dr. Rucker and the P.H.S. faced legal action against them and the campaign. The rat-proofing ordinances of New Orleans were challenged in the U.S. District Court, Eastern District of Louisiana, in a case (#15207) brought by Mrs. John Kuhlman and four other property owner supplicants of the city, representing 200 property owners who objected to the ordinances. The court upheld the ordinances as valid (Public Health Reports 30, iss. 14–26.)

One would think that after the efficacy of decontamination and disinfection had been proven and demonstrated as better than quarantine, the doctors and hospitals around the country would take heed and adopt the new approach (Tomes, 1998). But well more than a decade after germ theory had been proven, public hospitals were still being planned and built with the "open-air" ward approach—usually called the pavilion plan. In 1893, for example, the Royal Victoria hospital was planned and built in Canada, following the inspiration of Florence Nightingale and other mid-century reformers. Annmarie Adams, in *Medicine by Design*, observes the following:

> At first glance, this reliance on fresh air in an 1893 hospital may seem rather old-fashioned. After all, the germ theory of disease transmission had been

developed decades earlier, illustrating how "animal and human diseases were caused by distinctive species of microorganisms . . . [that] always came from a previous case of exactly the same disease." While many scholars have suggested that the popularity of the pavilion plan hospital waned with the development of the germ theory, this was not necessarily so. Public health historian Nancy Tomes has explained how the germ theory did not immediately displace traditional ways of understanding contagion, such as miasma; rather, as design of the Royal Vic, Johns Hopkins, and many other hospitals illustrates, North America incorporated the new theory into traditional explanations (and existing spatial paradigms) for disease. Pavilion-plan hospitals continued to be built into the 1930s. (Adams: 19)

The new approach, however, did spread, though gradually. And the doctors of the P.H.S., relying upon the experience of those at New Orleans and at Angel and Ellis Islands, did spread the innovations in ideas, in apparata and devices, and in approaches to public health. As more and more vectors of disease were discovered as the carriers of assorted bacilli to humans, the concept of "vector control" of disease replaced simple quarantine procedures. In Dr. Joseph Holt's terms, "maritime sanitation replaced maritime quarantine."

The lessons learned by the bubonic plague outbreak in 1914, however, proved useless in battling the last major scourge that New Orleans—and the nation, and the world—faced in 1918. That scourge has been accurately and suitably described as history's most lethal influenza virus pandemic, which began in an army camp in Kansas, moved east with American troops, and then exploded, killing perhaps as many as an estimated 100 million (conservatively 50 million) people worldwide. It killed more people in twenty-four weeks than AIDS killed in twenty-four years—more in a year than the Black Death killed in a century (Barry, 2005).

Physicians working at the New Orleans naval hospital made the first diagnoses of influenza in any military personnel in the city on September 4, 1918, when forty of forty-two patients admitted had the flu (Barry: 192). As with so many disease outbreaks in New Orleans, the virus followed rail and river traffic into the interior of the continent, from New Orleans up the Mississippi River and into the body of the nation, arriving and breaking out at the Great Lakes Naval station on September 7 and at New London, Connecticut, on September 12. Outbreaks at military camps in Seattle moved east, and from the Great Lakes training station, the epidemic moved to Chicago and from there spread along railroad lines in many directions (Barry: 225).

Rupert Blue knew of the possibility of the influenza's striking the United States. On July 28, 1918, he had rejected a request from Dr. George McCoy, director of the Hygienic Laboratory in Washington, D.C. (run by the service), for a $10,000 grant for pneumonia research to complement efforts of the Rockefeller Institute. But Blue, like most of the medical and medical scientific profession at the time, knew little about the mutation capability of the virus or the possible highly deadly virulence of a mutated influenza strain. Blue had been appointed surgeon general in 1912. When the influenza epidemic reached New Orleans, on September 4, 1918, Blue went there (Barry: 310).

At New Orleans, as at other cities invaded by the virus—Boston, Baltimore, Pittsburgh, Louisville, New York, and many smaller cities— the people first infected suffered the most grievously. Later in the epidemic, even those contracting the illness in the same cities were not dying at the same rate as those who had been infected in the first two to three weeks of the pandemic (Barry: 372).

Surgeon General Blue and the P.H.S. failed to respond quickly to the 1918 emergency. Fearing widespread panic during the war, they agreed to a virtual media blackout about the pandemic. As Barry notes, "In Phoenix, the *Arizona Republican* monitored influenza from a distance. On September 22 . . . it noted the first influenza deaths in New Orleans, two days before the New Orleans daily newspaper, the *Item*, mentioned any deaths in the city" (Barry: 337).

By December 11, 1919, however, Surgeon General Blue and the Public Health Service finally issued a bulletin warning that "influenza has not passed and severe epidemic conditions existed in various parts of the country . . . [and noted] in contrast with earlier stages of the epidemic disease, it now affects many school children; [and that] . . . in Louisiana, the disease again increased in New Orleans" (Barry: 374).

In 1923, the New Orleans station was at Algiers, Louisiana, three miles below the Canal Street Ferry landing on the west bank of the Mississippi River. All activities regarding quarantine as well as the medical inspection of aliens were conducted there (RG 90, Box 115, 1923–1935, Folder 1850). Table 5.10 lists the activities at the station, 1923–1935, along with the chief medical officer in charge for the year.

In 1925, Dr. Williams requested that the Louisiana Board of Health remove the leprosy patients from the Quarantine Hospital to the Louisiana hospital at Carville (Box 114, Folder 1616). In part, Dr. Williams request was made because the station was busy with a cholera outbreak that led to six deaths at the hospital. The epidemic was probably precipitated on board a ship from Cuba, or possibly on a Japanese ship the S.S. *Manila,* then battling the bubonic plague, that arrived in 1926. Surgeon Rucker, then working at the station as its bacteriologist, confirmed the finding of the bacillus of plague (Box 115, File 425).

Table 5.10
Reports of Activities, Medical Officer in Charge, New Orleans Station, 1923–1935

Year	Activities	Officer in Charge
1923	Vessels Inspected: 1992 Crew Examined: 80,091 Passengers Examined: 11,307	C. I. Williams
1924	Vessels Inspected: 2,051 Crew Examined: 80,414 Passengers Examined: 10,609 Vessels Fumigated: NA Rats Recovered: 1,780 Lepersorium Annex: 14 patients	C.I. Williams
1925	Vessels Inspected: 2,343 Crew Examined: 87,571 Passengers Examined: 12,461 Vessels Fumigated: 1,168 Rats Recovered: 1,821	C.I. Williams
1926	Vessels Inspected: 2,102 Crews Examined: 81,797 Passengers Examined: 13,898 Vessels Fumigated: 517 Rats Recovered: 1,852	David Turnipseed
1927	Vessels Inspected: 2,281 Crew Examined: 85,440 Passengers Examined: 14,018 Vessels Fumigated: 482 Rats Recovered: 1,263	D.C. Turnipseed
1928	Vessels Inspected: 2,124 Crew Examined: 85,147 Passengers Examined: 15,266 Vessels Fumigated: 384 Rats Recovered: 2,185	D.C. Turnipseed
1929	Vessels Inspected: 2,255 Crew Examined: 84,918 Passengers Examined: 14,732 Vessels Fumigated: 376 Rats Recovered: 2,198	C. R. Eskey
1930	Vessels Inspected: 2,046 Crew Examined: 78,547 Passengers Examined: 14,520 Vessels Fumigated: 339 Rats Recovered: 2,029	J.G. Wilson

1931	Vessels Inspected: 1,492 Crews Examined: 59,710 Passengers Examined: 12,752 Vessels Fumigated: 205 Rats Recovered: 435	G. T. Liddell
1932	Vessels Inspected: 1,242 Crews Examined: 48,081 Passengers Examined: 9,460 Vessels Fumigated: 140 Rats Recovered: 704	G. T. Liddell
1933	Vessels Inspected: 967 Crews Examined: 38,709 Passengers Examined: 8,018 Vessels Fumigated: 73 Rats Recovered: 257	G. T. Liddell
1934	Vessels Inspected: 901 Crews Examined: 37,530 Passengers Examined: 8,419 Vessels Fumigated: 44 Rats Recovered: 474	C. L. Williams
1935	Vessels Inspected: 1,099 Crews Examined: 43,030 Passengers Examined: 10,034 Vessels Fumigated: 32 Rats Recovered: 171	C. L. Williams

Source: Table by author, data in annual reports, 1923–1935, RG 90, Box 115, F. 1850.

In December 1925, Dr. Williams also requested the transfer of members of crews or passengers suspected of having communicable diseases to be admitted and held for observation and treatment at the Marine Hospital #14 at New Orleans and charging costs for up to twelve cases to masters of vessels who transported such passengers and who should have been able to observe the incidents before transportation (Box 114, File 1725).

In 1923–1925, the station had strained relations between the U.S. P.H.S. and officials of the Port of New Orleans and the U.S. Coast Guard's units in the Gulf of Mexico. In a 1924 letter, for example, the station complained to then Rear Admiral F. C. Billard, U.S. commandant, because the Coast Guard had brought persons found in violation of customs and immigration laws to New Orleans without first having them inspected at the quarantine station (Letter of September 23, 1924, Box 114, Folder 1725).

In 1926, the station reported numerous vessels fumigated with sulphur or cyanide gas and inspected for rat guards. The station used hundreds of pounds of sulphur and cyanide and many pints of sulphuric acid in its anti-rat work (Box 115, Folder 1850).

They also conducted annual "rat trapping" campaigns from the station to trap and kill rats aboard ships or in New Orleans. The station employed two "rat trappers" on its staff (Reports by C.L. Williams, 1926, Box 115, File 520).

During this time, Senior Surgeon C. L. Williams frequently corresponded with then Surgeon General H.S. Cumming, regarding the policy of the Public Health Service (P.H.S., as it was by then known) to use P.H.S. facilities at ports by the Immigration and Naturalization Service for accommodating aliens detained under immigration laws at rates prescribed for detention (Box 114, Folder 950).

In 1929, Surgeon-in-Charge Eskey sent a report on the estimated costs to repair and preserve facilities, and to project new construction costs begun July 1, 1930. The office of the supervising architect recommended construction of new buildings at the station at a cost of $425,000 (Box 112, Folder 245). In June 1929, Eskey reported that an old building at the station had caught fire and burned to the ground (Letter of June 21, 1929, Box 112, Folder 115).

In 1931, T. J. Liddell became surgeon in charge of the New Orleans Station. He had to correct the address to which correspondence was being sent from the Surgeon General's Office to prevent it from being sent to the Lower Quarantine Station or the Boarding Division at the Vernon Street, as apparently frequently happened (letter of September 17, 1930, RG 90, Box 114, Folder 1205). Liddell reported cases of typhus and twelve cases of yellow fever resulting in seven deaths, and in 1931 he reported cases of smallpox at the station (April 9, 1931). Another disease often used for medical certification to prevent immigration was trachoma (Box 113, Folder 425).

The station was closed in 1944 as immigration to and through New Orleans declined so markedly during World War II and the numbers of immigrants could be handled in the city rather than needing the separate Quarantine Station (see RG 90, Domestic Stations, New Orleans Quarantine, 1930–1944, Boxes 52–55; and the Inspections and Investigations file, 1919–1941, New Orleans folders in Boxes 205–212).

SPREADING INNOVATIONS

Among the more rapidly accepted ideas of the germ theory approach, however, was Dr. Holt's experiments with and identification of "germicides." The U.S. M.H.S. and its successor, the P.H.S., quickly adapted the combination of pressurized steam chambers with the mixture of sulfur and, soon after, formaldehyde gas, as maritime decontamination devices. These innovations were spread through reports and medical journal articles by the likes of Dr. George Sternberg in Washington, D.C.; Dr. John Rauch in Chicago; Dr. Joseph Holt in New Orleans; Dr. Joseph Kinyoun; Dr. Rupert Blue in Washington, D.C.; doctors Walter Reed, William Gorgas, and Joseph White; and doctors Joseph Jones and Joseph Holt in Louisiana, describing the methods used in controlling yellow fever through the Yellow Fever Commission, among many others. The books, reports, and manuals they produced on the various epidemics they battled, and on public health campaigns of rat control in bubonic plague epidemics and, soon after, other "mosquito vector control" for yellow fever and malaria, as well as many reports on the design and use of various decontamination devices, soon spread to municipal public health programs.[5]

Dr. Milton Rosenau's authoritative book *Preventive Medicine and Hygiene*, published in 1913, spread the innovations he developed while with the U.S. M.H.S. throughout the nation's developing public health services (Kaufman, Galishoff, and Savitts, vol. 2: 649). Dr. McMullan's authoritative pamphlet on Trachoma diagnosis and treatment was published by the U.S. M.H.S. and became the standard for the disease.

In 1903, the service published its "Book of Instructions for the Medical Examination of Immigration," which also spread innovations throughout the service and from there to local boards of public health, which were becoming increasingly common by the first decade of the 1900s (Box 52, Files 375–397).

Their innovations were advocated and spread by the American Public Health Association. Its 1885 conference, held in Washington, D.C., promoted their ideas and helped develop specialists in the newly developing field of public health. Several of its presidents came from the U.S. M.H.S. backgrounds. The work by John Rauch, of the Health Bureau of Illinois in Chicago, and of Joseph Holt in New Orleans inspired Dr. Frederick Montizambert of Canada, who came to visit them and observed their approaches and procedures, later adopting and adapting their ideas in Canadian stations, first as medical director at the Grosse Ile Immigration and Quarantine Station near Quebec, Canada, and later as the first director general of Canada's Public Health (equivalent to the U.S. surgeon general). Steam decontamination vessels to "disinfect" ships that evidenced contagious disease outbreaks became commonplace by the 1890s.

In Portsmouth, on September 13, 1892, Dr. Holt spoke at the Conference of Medical Officers of Health, giving an address published in the *Journal of the Incorporated Society of Medical Officers of Health* on the "Holt

System Carried Out in the State of Louisiana (5 [October 1892]: 15–16). His address was highly important in influencing the Society of Community Health. Likewise, Dr. Holt addressed the Charity Hospital alumni in 1895, describing the pioneering work done at New Orleans in developing maritime sanitation.

The Angel Island chapter discussed Dr. Kinyoun's "Kinyoun–Francis decontamination tubes," soon used at U.S. stations across the country and, by the turn of the century, across the globe. Similar but smaller devices were developed for municipal hospital use to disinfect bedding from contagious disease wards or hospitals.

Another method of spreading their innovations in practices, procedures, and apparatus was by doctors from one station visiting another station. The New Orleans station, for example, sent Dr. J. H. White to Key West to deal with a smallpox epidemic outbreak in 1896. The U.S. Navy Department and the U.S. Marine Hospital Service enforced a quarantine edict and began a vaccination program. Dr. Porter, the Key West surgeon in charge, completed the tremendous task of a house-to-house inspection and saw that 13,000 of the 16,500 inhabitants were vaccinated. As a direct result of that campaign, during that epidemic outbreak, only one person died of smallpox (Diddle: 14–37).

Likewise, in 1899, Key West battled a yellow fever epidemic at the Marine Hospital, treating army personnel returning from the Spanish–American War. Members of the Florida state board of health and the U.S. M.H.S. were involved. The U.S. M.H.S. sent Dr. A. H. Glennan, a former surgeon during a yellow fever epidemic in 1887, to Key West to make an investigation of an apparent yellow fever outbreak. He concluded that the outbreak was not yellow fever, but probably dengue, which was subsequently confirmed. Between 5,000 and 6,000 persons contracted the disease before the epidemic ended. In 1901, Dr. Porter ordered machinery to disinfect baggage to cope with yellow fever, implementing a "maritime sanitation" approach (Diddle).

The influenza epidemic in 1918, which took a conservatively estimated 50 million lives worldwide, spread throughout the United States. Doctors from the New Orleans station were again sent to help Key West cope with the epidemic outbreak there. Total deaths at Key West numbered fifty-four (Diddle: 31–32).

Another method of spreading the innovations in public health was through internship programs. In 1930, for example, twenty-four institutions were accredited by the American College of Surgeons for internships—many of them Marine Hospitals, including those at New Orleans and at Key West.

CONCLUSION

The Immigration Station at New Orleans, like those at Angel and Ellis Island and at the other major ports on both coasts—and, indeed, at land stations in the Midwest—all had "doctors at the borders" who performed heroically, processing thousands of immigrants, allowing them to enter the country but for the most part serving as effective barriers against the contagious diseases that so often became epidemic or pandemic throughout the nineteenth century. They spread their innovations in the early decades of the twentieth century, serving as pioneers in the development of public health as a specialty field in medicine. Their experiences proved that the public health approach to medicine was invaluable in saving untold thousands of lives. They demonstrated that contagious outbreaks that had once been scourges among humans could, in fact, be controlled and stopped through public health devices and procedures. They proved the value of vaccination in controlling and even preventing some diseases. They demonstrated that "vector control" was the most effective method to manage other contagious epidemics that previously had ravaged thousands during uncontrolled "pestilences." In no small measure thanks to their pioneering work, the diseases that were the scourge of humankind for most of the nineteenth century were conquered or eradicated in the twentieth century.

But their work should serve, as John Barry notes, as a lesson regarding the danger today of bioterrorism. The lessons from battling the great influenza pandemic of 1918–1919 show that a potential pandemic on that scale is highly possible if a mutated virus or even an engineered microorganism is developed as a bioterrorist weapon today. Indeed, his warning is but one of the lessons to be learned that chapter 6 discusses.

The medical scientists discussed in chapter 2 were true heroes in the rise of modern medicine. But the doctors at the immigration stations at Angel Island, at Ellis Island, and at New Orleans were no less heroic, even if largely unsung, in the development and spread of modern medicine and of public health as a specialty field of medicine. Their experiences, described in this volume, offer insights of value today as the United States once again faces an era of mass migration. Chapter 6 is devoted to that topic.

Chapter 6

TEN LESSONS LEARNED

A good reason to study the histories of Angel Island, Ellis Island, and New Orleans is to glean insights from the past—lessons from experience that can help future policymakers and implementers. Any number of such lessons can be drawn, and the careful reader may discern some not discussed here. Largely for concerns of space, the top ten lessons discussed below are drawn from the records and experiences discussed in the previous chapters. They offer insights useful to current immigration policy reform as the U.S. policymakers grapple once again with the issue of mass migration on a scale commensurate with that of the period 1880–1920.

The historical sketches in chapters 3 to 5 demonstrate that with respect to immigration policymaking, both push and pull factors determine the flow of immigration. These factors influence both the size and the composition of the immigration flow—how many attempt to enter for permanent residence, as well as from what countries of origin. They show that policymakers have little direct control over push factors. At best, policymakers can assert indirect influence over push factors through international agreements and economic development aid or humanitarian assistance aimed at developing nations, who today are the major sending countries. Pull factors drawing would-be immigrants to the United States are more responsive to policy enacted to control immigration. All such policy is limited in achieving policy goals. Immigration policies, moreover, often have unanticipated consequences. There are an estimated 20 million refugees worldwide. Many are potential migrants seeking entry to the United States. Many are willing to enter illegally if legal immigration policy prevents their entrance and push factors are compelling. The economy of the United States, a developed economy directly adjacent to a developing economy, has enormous drawing power. Both the northern and southern borders are highly porous, stretching more than 2,000 miles to the south, and more than 3,000 miles to the north. They are ineffective barriers to highly motivated would-be illegal migrants. Of the estimated half-million or more immigrants who annually come to the United States illegally, about 40 percent enter with documents (temporary visas)—that is, as non-immigrants (students, tourists, business visitors, and so on) and then simply overstay and go underground, thereby becoming illegal immigrants. About 60 percent of unauthorized immigrants are undocumented (that is, enter without papers) (see Passel, 2014).

Whatever their legal status, all immigrants travel with microscopic fellow travelers that may be pathogens—the agents of disease outbreaks. In this global age, when the time required for international travel is almost always shorter than the incubation period of an illness, it is all the more challenging to immigration policy and to immigration authorities to stand as barriers against outbreaks of epidemic disease that are potential pandemics. In this period of massive undocumented, and thus uninspected, immigration, the danger posed by such microscopic fellow travelers is greatly increased. In this period of international terrorism, the threat of intentional bioterrorism is all the more serious and difficult to defend against. The lessons drawn from the experiences of these three stations are timely. They are lessons that ought to be of interest to citizens and policymakers alike. They are lessons ignored at our peril.

LESSON 1: A QUESTION OF WHEN, NOT IF

Medical scientists proved beyond doubt the validity of germ theory. Microscopic agents of disease, germs and viruses, are silent travelers accompanying humans as they migrate. We cannot prevent their migration as humans move from place to place. Medical science has shown that when natural agents of disease—pathogens—migrate to new areas and essentially confront a new and "virgin" population (one with little or no immunity), they can cause epidemics with severe morbidity and mortality rates. They become killers on a grand scale. Even diseases we now think of as common childhood illness, such as measles, were and still are deadly when they spread to populations with no natural immunities, as the decimation of American Indians amply illustrates. As one scholar of killer plagues puts it:

> We can be certain that there will be many outbreaks of serious infections. Most will behave as we have seen with hantavirus, Legionnaires disease, Lyme disease, and the various outbreaks of Ebola. People will die locally but the outbreaks will not evolve into epidemics. Less frequently, but with equal certainty, they will become epidemics, and a small minority of these will extend to pandemics. . . . The exact timing of such pandemics cannot

be predicted. But the consequences are all too tragically obvious: there will be great suffering and a great many deaths. . . . How curious that as this fear [of nuclear annihilation] recedes, though it has hardly disappeared, it has been replaced by a renewed fear of the threat from mankind's most ancient enemy, disease causing microbes. (Ryan: 381)

The historical record demonstrates that agents of human disease are often spread through vectors—through mitigating sources of disease commonly referred to as vermin. Among the most common are fleas on rodents. Upon the death of their rodent host, they jump to the next nearby source of blood—usually another rodent, but sometimes a human. Rats are efficient fellow travelers with humans and were and are effective agents for the spread of the plague. The Angel Island chapter documents that plague is now endemic in the wild—that is, among the natural rodent population (rats, field mice, squirrels, and so on) in much of the southwest United States. The lowly but prolific mosquito is an effective vector of malaria and yellow fever. Though we can control the incidence of human transfer of mosquito-borne infections, we simply are unable to eradicate mosquitos. There are too many; they are too dispersed, and they reproduce too quickly and too prolifically. Humanborne lice, another common vermin, are a principle vector for typhus. Water, the necessity for life, is easily contaminated by microscopic life. Humans ingesting contaminated water become victims and carriers of highly contagious and deadly diseases, such as cholera.

The speed and ease with which humans travel today means that human carriers of diseases can quickly spread infection across wide expanses of space. Oceans are no barriers in the day of jet liner traffic. We simply cannot prevent these microscopic fellow travelers from spreading as humans migrate (Kraut; Oldstone). At best, we can only react to their spread to mitigate the incidence of epidemic outbreaks. We can only lessen the duration and intensity of outbreaks and, it is to be hoped, prevent them from developing into pandemics. At best, medical science and immigration policymakers and implementers can reduce the morbidity and mortality rates of epidemic outbreaks. They may control and contain them, but they cannot prevent them from occurring.

In our myopic view, we tend to believe that certain epidemic diseases are events of the distant past. Bubonic plague, cholera, smallpox, typhus, and yellow fever are contagious diseases conquered by modern medicine. They are the stuff of the nineteenth century. Surely they are of little threat today. Experience, such as the recent Ebola pandemic, shows that we delude ourselves with such thinking.

The World Health Organization (WHO) was launched in 1948, then with fifty-five national signatories. Its lofty stated goal was to establish "a state of complete physical, mental, and social well-being and not merely the absence of disease or infirmity" (www.who.int/Mission). The WHO today has 192 member states and regional offices in Africa, the Americas, southeast Asia, Europe, the eastern Mediterranean, and the western Pacific. It has funded campaigns to immunize the world's children against six dreaded diseases that for ages have plagued humankind: diphtheria, tetanus, whooping cough, measles, poliomyelitis, and tuberculosis. Working with the UN's International Children's Emergency Fund (UNICEF) and the UN Educational, Scientific and Cultural Organization (UNESCO), and in close cooperation with organizations like the International Red Cross and the World Bank, and led by experts from the Centers for Disease Control (CDC), the WHO led campaigns of epidemic intervention (Porter: 485–486; LeMay, 2006: 98).

As McNeill concludes, the WHO scored its most notable success in those campaigns when it eradicated smallpox in 1976 (9). A decade earlier, smallpox had infected an estimated 10 million people and had killed 2 million among them in outbreaks occurring within thirty-three countries. Though falling short of eradication, other diseases against which notable strides were made include malaria, tuberculosis, measles, whooping cough, diphtheria, and polio. Yet these diseases still kill millions worldwide every year. One difficulty in coping with these contagions is their uncanny ability to develop resistance to modern bacteriological treatments. Between 1985 and 1991, after having been beaten back to the point where some scientists believed eradication was imminent, tuberculosis made a comeback. Since 1991, in the United States, cases of tuberculosis have increased by 12 percent. In Europe, they have increased by 30 percent. In parts of Africa, where TB and HIV frequently go together, they have increased by 300 percent! In 2006, an estimated 10 million people had active tuberculosis. Today it kills 3 million annually, 95 percent of who reside in developing countries (LeMay, 2006: 99).

Cholera is yet another disease thought to have been nearing eradication that has re-emerged in epidemic proportions. The seventh recorded pandemic eruption of cholera occurred, initially, in Indonesia. It then quickly spread through Asia and Africa, eventually attacking twenty-nine countries in a virulent two-year outbreak. It reached Peru in 1991. From there it spread rapidly through Chile, Colombia, Ecuador, Bolivia, Brazil, Argentina, and Guatemala. As Porter notes, by 1992, it had infected an estimated 1 million globally, including 400,000 persons in Latin America alone, accounting for some 4,000 deaths there (Porter: 491). A mutation of the cholera bacillus led to a new strain of this old enemy, called El Tor. It is believed to have spread to Latin America in the ballast tanks of a ship from China that discharged its pestilential cargo in Peruvian waters, thereby infecting shellfish, lobsters, and fish—and, in turn, humans. El Tor killed quickly, causing massive dehydration from diarrhea. While health officials around the world fought to contain the El Tor pandemic, a new strain of the classic cholera germ, named *Vibrio cholerae* non-01 CT+, emerged in Bangladesh and India. This new germ exhibited "the potential of becoming the agent of an eighth pandemic of human cholera" (Porter: 492).

In 1994, another old enemy, bubonic plague, struck India in a massive outbreak. In 1995, much of the world was struck by the "superbug," methicillin-resistant *Staphylococcus aureus*, known more simply by its acronym, MRSA (Ryan: 115–133). The "staph" germ is very common, carried on the bodies of about a third of the healthy population. It can cause boils and disastrous infection in bone and can be bloodborne. It is among the most common causes of serious hospital infection. The elderly and persons recovering from surgery are at greatest risk. A drug-resistant (hence "superbug") strain of so common a germ gives rise to serious problems, especially in intensive-care facilities. In recent years, another common germ, *pneumococcus*, appears to have acquired resistance to penicillin. A frequent cause of bacterial meningitis in children, it can only be treated with vancomycin, requiring unpleasant injections directly into the spinal canal.

Poliomyelitis had been nearly wiped out. In 1995, the WHO immunized 300 million people. Yet in 1996 it still was reported, with 2,200 cases worldwide. WHO set a goal of 2005 for its eradication but it was unable to achieve that goal. WHO estimates that during the 1980s and 1990s, some 2.5 million children died annually from measles because of the failure to vaccinate. Though its global eradication is projected by 2020, rapid travel to all parts of the globe from persons coming from areas where measles is still endemic poses a very real hazard to susceptible people in distant lands. WHO indicates that it still infects 40 million children and kills about 1 million per year (Oldstone: 88–89).

Viral mutation is even more frequent than is germal. The experience with the pandemic of the "great influenza" of 1918–1919 shows how deadly such a pandemic can become. That particular mutation caused a pandemic estimated to have killed 20–50 million globally, including an estimated 500,000 in the United States (Kolata, 1993; Davies, 2000; Getz, 2000; and Barry, 2005). It was a virulent mutation that remained a medical mystery until 2005, when its genetic code was finally deciphered by Dr. Jeffrey Taubenberger of the Armed Forces Institute of Pathology. As we have seen, it was spread by troop movements during World War I.

The Vietnam War spread outbreaks of malaria in the late 1960s. After the first Gulf War, in 1991, puzzling symptoms of illness among returning soldiers became known as the Gulf War Syndrome. Medical scientists have yet to determine its nature. Recent and current conflict in the Mideast could be the proximate cause for the spread of some other viral infection. DNA research into viruses holds great promise for medical science's battle against future pandemics.

Medical scientists fear the return of some similarly lethal influenza virus. The first major change in the flu virus that caused an influenza pandemic (though far less lethal than that of 1918–1919) occurred in 1957–1958. Another was the Hong Kong flu of 1968.

The AIDS pandemic continues to spread. It illustrates how difficult it is to develop a vaccine against viral diseases that mutate rapidly and affect the immune system of the body, the natural first barrier against infectious disease. By 1996, AIDS killed an estimated 1.39 million people. AIDS first appeared in Africa at the same time when WHO was eradicating smallpox. That may be more than coincidental. During the 1970s campaign to eradicate smallpox, WHO teams reused needles fifty to sixty times. Live vaccines, such as smallpox, directly provoke the immune system and can awake sleeping giants such as viruses (LeMay, 2007: 100). Dr. Nancy Cox, of the Atlanta CDC, keeps an eye on flu outbreaks around the world. She identifies certain conditions under which a flu pandemic could arise: The DNA of the flu virus must mutate and change sufficiently that people around the world have little immunity to the new strain; the new strain must be sturdy and contagious, capable of traveling easily from person to person; and finally, it must reproduce well in epithelial cells. A new flu strain meeting those conditions could produce a pandemic killer on the scale of the 1918–1919 pandemic. That is certainly the basis for the high level of fear aroused by the swine flu pandemic outbreak of April 2009, which infected thousands worldwide and killed hundreds.

Among emerging and widely feared viruses is the avian flu, commonly called bird flu. It has spread from Asia to western Europe and has been found among dead birds in the United States. The twenty-eight–nation European Union (EU) announced in February 2006 that it had detected the deadly H5N1 strain of the virus in dead swans. The strain is pandemic among domestic fowl in much of Asia. Because it has obviously moved to birds in the wild, it is in all the more danger of traveling around the world with the migration of those birds. The avian flu strain infected several hundreds of people, mostly in Asia, and killed close to one hundred. It has raised medical concern, and economically it ravaged poultry stock across

Asia (millions of domestic fowl were killed in the effort to stop its spread, with limited success). The infection seems to spread only from birds to humans, and only when humans have close and sustained contact with infected birds. But should the strain mutate so that it can be spread directly from human to human carriers, it could become a devastating pandemic. Medical science does not yet clearly understand how viral mutation occurs ("Scientists Must Wing It on Future of Avian Flu," 2005).

Epidemiologists warn of an inevitable pandemic on the scale of the great influenza of 1918–1919. "Warning" episodes include the HIV/AIDs pandemic, the SARS virus epidemic in 2002, the Ebola hemorrhagic fever outbreak in 2009 and again in 2014, a new strain of Lyme disease, and the April 2009 swine flu pandemic (Walters: 148–151; Ryan: 13; *Time Magazine*, 2014).

Of particular concern with respect to the massive rate of unauthorized immigration today is the potential for its use by international terrorist organizations to intentionally spread infectious diseases as agents of bioterrorism. Richard Preston, in his book *The Hot Zone* (1994), discusses the new viral diseases that spread naturally. He offers a chilling fictional account of bioterrorism in *The Cobra Event* (1997). Though fictional, the latter is based on real science and portrays a very plausible scenario. The Center for Disease Control (CDC) has identified a number of diseases as potential bioterrorism threats: anthrax, botulism, *Chlamydia psittaci*, cholera, Ebola virus hemorrhagic fever, plague (*Yersenia pestis*), E. coli 015H7, food safety threats (for example, various salmonella species), lassa fever, Marburg virus hemorrhagic fever, Q fever, ricin toxin, smallpox (*Viriola major*), and typhoid fever.

Dr. D. A. Henderson, first director of the CDC's Smallpox Eradication Program and later director of WHO's global smallpox eradication program, became founder of the Center for Civilian Biodefense Strategies (Etheridge, 1992: 189). In 2001, he was named director of the Office of Public Health Preparedness (OPHP) in the United States Department of Health and Human Services (HHS). OPHP was established after the anthrax attack via the U.S. Postal Service in November 2001. OPHP was created to defend against bioterrorism, the danger of which is very real, not science fiction. The extraordinary potential of bioweapons has long been recognized by the U.S. military. During World War II, the U.S. Army experimented with bioweapons and concocted a botulinum toxin so potent that one pound of it, if expertly dispersed, could kill 1 billion people. The botulinum toxin is the most lethal compound known. It is 15,000 times more lethal than nerve gas and 100,000 times more so than the sarin toxin used in the 1995 Tokyo subway terrorist attack. If properly aerosolized, one gram could kill 1.5 million people. Ricin, another toxin, extracted from castor beans, can be aerosolized. If breathed in or ingested, it kills through severe respiratory distress in a matter of a few days, and it has no known treatment (Bertolli and Forkiotis: 8).

Dr. Henderson was among the leaders of the CDC/WHO team that helped eradicate smallpox, and he knows the virus better than almost anyone else. He sees it as potentially one of the deadliest bioterrorism agents. Today the virus is sequestered in two facilities sanctioned by the WHO, the CDC in Atlanta, and in Novosibirsk, Russia, at the State Center of Virology and Technology. WHO approved the destruction of all other smallpox stock, allowing these two approved sites for scientific study to develop antiviral therapies, vaccines, and rapid diagnostic and analytic tools. Dr. Henderson, however, opposes maintaining even the two stocks of smallpox, arguing that there is little scientific insight that cannot be gained using other orthopoxviruses. He serves as a distinguished scholar at the Center for Biosecurity of the UPMC at the University of Pittsburgh. He is dean emeritus of the Johns Hopkins School of Public Health and the Founding Director, in 1998, of its Biodefense Strategies program, and from 2001–2003 was the principle science advisor for public health emergency preparedness to the secretary of health and human services. He was an associate director of the Office of Policy, Executive Office of the President and in 2002 received the Presidential Medal of Freedom (www.upmc-biosecurity.org). His recommendations simply cannot be ignored.

Smallpox is considered one of the most dangerous of the top fifty bio-weapon pathogens, only thirteen of which have vaccines or treatments. It typically kills about 30 percent of its unvaccinated victims, and in the case of an epidemic outbreak among virgin-soil population, it is known to have killed as many as 50 percent. Smallpox spreads rapidly, radiating in ever-widening waves. In the first wave, every infected person infects ten to fifteen more, each of whom—unless quarantined—does the same. If the initial or first generation of infected victims numbered 200 to 300 persons, the next would be 2,000 to 3,000, and so on, if the population is not rapidly vaccinated and the sick isolated. Smallpox immunity wanes after about a decade. Because the last vaccinated persons in the United States received the shots in 1972, and worldwide the last vaccination campaign ended in 1976, virtually all the world's population is now virgin soil. According to Drexler, there is less immunity to smallpox today than ever before in human history (239–240).

Smallpox has been menacing humanity since at least 1000 BC (the mummy of Ramses V shows evidence of smallpox). In the 1990s, U.S. intelligence agencies reportedly suspected that the virus was in less secure, less friendly hands (North Korea, Iraq, al Qaeda). In 1972, a smallpox aerosol release indicated that either an accidental or intentional (test-run) incident had occurred. A former Soviet Union weaponized or genetically altered form of the deadly virus was reportedly transported to Iraq in 1990 (Drexler: 238; LeMay, 2006: 103).

Of particular threat would be bioterrorists manipulating several deadly agents, like those listed above, so that they work together, one enabling its ease of rapid spread (its morbidity rate), and another increasing its lethality—its mortality rate (Drexler: 242–243). In 2001, an accidental discovery by Australian researchers proved the possibility. They were attempting to make a mouse contraceptive for pest control. They inserted into a mouse-pox virus a gene that makes a large quantity of interleukin-4, a molecule produced naturally in mice and humans. Their "designer virus" crippled the immune system, and 100 percent of the mice died. The new virus resisted vaccination. In 1998, Russian scientists inserted genes from a harmless bacterium into anthrax bacterium and inadvertently created a new form of anthrax that was resistant to both penicillin and vaccines (Drexler: 243).

The Soviet bioweapons program was experimenting with combining small-pox with Ebola hemorrhagic fever virus or Venezuelan equine encephalitis virus. Such a genetically altered or "engineered" virus is called a "chimera," after the Greek mythological creature that had the head of a lion, the torso of a she-goat, and the tail of the dragon. "This same civilian technology is theoretically able to make this pox virus [the mouse-pox virus] deadly to humans as well. This is an example of the availability of genetic technology that could very well be used utilized by unfriendly forces" (Bertolli and Forkiotis: 9).

"Agro-terrorists" could target agricultural crops or animals. The increasing centralization and globalization of the food supply renders it vulnerable to attack at numerous points along the chain. Three multinational corporations process about half of all U.S. meat. A planned attack of foot-and-mouth disease, the highly contagious infection that shook the British and European livestock industry in 2001, could cripple the U.S. meat industry. Contamination of seed supplies with spores of soybean rust, for example, would have global repercussions, for the United States raises about half of the world's soybean crop. From wheat or rice rust, to the intentional spread of avian flu among poultry, the potential of agroterrorism is considerable.

LESSON 2: POLITICAL EXIGENCIES TEND TO TRUMP MEDICAL ADVICE

The needs of local politics, politicians, and economic concerns distort perspectives. As the old saying has it, all politics is local. Call it wishful thinking, or the head-in-the-sand effect, but policymakers who ought to know better and who have initial political power in the case of an epidemic outbreak are often the most reluctant to recognize and admit it even when the disease is staring them in the face and killing persons they are charged to protect.

The political leadership of San Francisco too long refused to believe the scientific evidence of Dr. Joseph Kinyoun that the bubonic plague had erupted there in 1900 (Chase, 2004; Shah, 2011). Like the fictional chamber of commerce members in the film *Jaws,* who refused to publicize a great white shark's infestation of local waters, attacking and killing people, for fear of how it would hurt the local economy by halting tourism, so, too, did the real-life businessmen of the city by the bay attack and vilify Dr. Kinyoun rather than admit the reality of a plague epidemic. It was easier to attack the messenger than to face openly the bad news he bore. New Orleans city officials, for decades, denied that yellow fever and smallpox were endemic in the city, as they were in much of the U.S. South.

World War I exigencies dictated the censorship of news about the beginnings of the great influenza of 1918. Even after medical scientists and public health officers, and even a few army medical officers, urged a halt in the deployment of recruits to military camps to avoid spreading the influenza outbreak, and even long after the death rate skyrocketed among them, troops were moved all over the world. Military necessity overpowered medical advice. What began as an epidemic at one military camp in Kansas became, in a matter of months, the deadliest pandemic in human history (Barry, 2005).

Long after the "Spanish flu" epidemic was known to be spread at military camps by bringing together large numbers of persons from many places and confining them to close quarters, the hysteria of the "Red Scare" overcame common sense, and thousands of radicals were rounded up, hundreds herded onto Ellis Island to await deportation hearings in crowded detention facilities. That policy resulted in the epidemic outbreak that occurred at Ellis Island and in New York City.

Even before medical science proved the validity of germ theory, doctors were aware that epidemics of contagious disease spread faster by close proximity. When the quarantine stations at Grosse Isle and at Angel Island were first being built, and when quarantine was the only recognized policy to cope with epidemics, the medical officers advocated placing hospitals away from troops and from other noninfected immigrants. But when initially building the immigration stations there, the need to save time and money resulted in facilities in close proximity. Thousands died on Grosse Isle, at least partially as a result.

The simplicity of that lesson, amply demonstrated at all three island stations, did not seem to make it any easier to learn or accept. National government policymakers ignored that lesson to save money, to save face, or in the name of national security. The government of the former Soviet Union hid the truth about the Chernobyl disaster rather than admit to the world its failure to prevent the disaster, and many died of radiation poisoning as a result. For months the government of China hid the existence of avian flu, and the world lost precious time when other countries could have been alerted and forearmed. Nearly a hundred lives were lost to the disease, undoubtedly including some who could and would have avoided that fate if preventative measures had been enforced against the spreading avian flu pandemic.

Myopia is commonplace. Government policymakers seem prone to dream up reasons to suppress the truth rather than to admit an epidemic. They want to avoid panic. They need to prevent hysteria. They need time to be absolutely sure before they will spend millions on what might turn out to be a false alarm. The reasons justifying inaction are legion. The deaths that result from inaction and delay are all too real and all too many.

Lesson 1 tells us that a future epidemic is inevitable. Lesson 2 tells us that governmental policymakers tend to ignore the inevitable until some time after it has arrived. It suggests why some future epidemic will become pandemic. It suggests that original outbreak will be hidden, lied about, and explained away, the truth about the outbreak, about its very nature, suppressed until the epidemic has spread beyond the boundaries of the original outbreak and developed into a pandemic.

LESSON 3: PREVENTIVE MEDICINE IS BEST

The history of these quarantine stations shows that preventive medicine is best. It is better in terms of lives saved and of costs to taxpayers to prevent an outbreak's occurrence than to treat persons after they have contracted a contagious disease. Public health efforts save many more lives by prevention than do heroic doctors dramatically saving the life of a patient on the "deathbed."

These histories demonstrate the importance of understanding the cause of contagious diseases. A clear understanding of the nature of the illness enables public health practitioners to discern its cycle. As in any war, the adage "know thy enemy" is paramount. Success in battle depends on attacking the enemy at their weakest point. That is no less true in the battle with epidemic and pandemic disease. For the pandemics reviewed here, attacking the disease by intervention in the natural cycle of the disease, by eradication or control of the vector, was the most effective and cost-efficient approach.

The "ship-fever" pandemic of 1847 cost 10,000 lives. Medical practitioners had not yet understood the role played by human lice in spreading the disease. After the nature of the typhoid cycle was understood and the vermin vector identified, it was relatively simple to avoid epidemic outbreaks by killing the vermin. Developing steam and chemical disinfection chambers was relatively cheap, certainly so in comparison with treating tens of thousands of patients suffering from typhoid fever. Easier still was the simple administrative procedure of mandating delousing showers to kill the vermin. Fumigation of ship's holds and cargoes to eradicate vermin such as rats before they could debark was the cheapest, fastest, and most effective method to cope with the spread of plague (Sevigny, 1995b; Etheridge, 1992; Drexler, 2002; Porter, 1999).

Actions taken at Angel Island, Ellis Island, and, later, New Orleans proved that rat surveys and eradication campaigns prevented the plague from spreading and quickly stopped an epidemic in place. They faced epidemics but prevented them from developing into pandemics. The Public Health Service used its manual on rat eradication to broadcast broadly its effectiveness. The Public Health Service proved the value of public health campaigns. Typhus and cholera still exist, are yet endemic in some areas, but fumigation and delousing have rendered them controllable. In the 1870s, epidemics of smallpox, typhus, and cholera took hundreds of lives in New York City, but by the first decade of 1900, they took mere dozens of lives, and by 1920 those diseases no longer occurred in epidemic episodes. Massive and compulsory vaccination programs, implemented as part of public health campaigns and led by the Public Health Service, essentially wiped out smallpox in the United States by 1970 (Etheridge, 1992; Porter, 1999).

Public health campaigns to wipe out mosquito carriers of yellow fever, and more recently of malaria, proved highly effective, clearly the most efficient method to cope with epidemics of those diseases that until the twentieth century had been scourges on mankind and the source of periodic pandemics. Eradicate the mosquito from locations near dense human habitation, and you effectively stop the epidemic nature of the disease. In 1942, Dr. Joseph Mountain, who directed the P.H.S.'s State Services Division, had a plan for dealing with the emergency situation that World War II so clearly posed with respect to the likelihood of malaria epidemics among troops stationed in the south. He proposed a national organization to keep malaria-free some 600 military bases and essential war production industrial plants in the U.S. South. Those plans led to the establishment of the

Malaria Control in War Areas (MCWA) division within the P.H.S., from which evolved into establishment of the federal Communicable Disease Center in 1946, now known as the Centers for Disease Control and Prevention (CDC). In 1945, DDT was developed and demonstrated effective against the mosquito—a cheap larvicide costing a fraction to spread per acre as did fuel oil, which had previously been used in mosquito-control campaigns against yellow fever. It was only years later that the unanticipated consequences of the widespread use of DDT in related health-issue costs became known. In 1946, sixty-eight counties in nine states participated in a campaign that sprayed DDT at over 600,000 homes. More than 1 million homes were sprayed in 1947 (Etheridge: 11).

Immunization, the prevention of epidemic disease by inoculation to induce immunity, is even more effective. Though expensive, massive inoculation campaigns are still the most cost-effective way to cope with some diseases. To date, only smallpox has been eradicated globally through immunization. Immigration stations and their quarantine hospitals were among the first public health efforts to mandate vaccination of large numbers. Learning from those efforts, the U.S. government through the CDC, in conjunction with the World Health Organization, other governments, and a few non-governmental organizations (NGOs) that assisted with funding, developed the administrative processes to launch a global vaccination campaign. Its smallpox campaign, fully successful in 1976 and at a cost only of several hundred million dollars, proved that a highly contagious and deadly disease could be fully eradicated. The U.S. M.H.S., now the U.S. Public Health Service (P.H.S.), developed a host of sera and toxins to vaccinate against diseases, some to immunize, some to effectively treat cases of contagious diseases. In the 1960s, the CDC managed the P.H.S.'s tuberculosis control program, an effort in which many state and local public health organizations vigorously fought tuberculosis. Then, in 1966, the CDC launched its most ambitious and triumphant project, the eradication of smallpox through immunization. In a second phase, after success of the smallpox campaign had demonstrated the worthiness of a global immunization of children approach, the CDC targeted measles (Etheridge: 153).

Sterilization is a simple method to fight infections and contagious diseases. After germ theory was understood, proven, and broadly taught to medical practitioners, the simple procedural safeguard of sterilization in hospitals and clinics became standard practice. The contagious disease hospitals at Angel Island, Ellis Island, and New Orleans were among the earliest practitioners of sterilization, models for public health services all over the world. They were instrumental in the development of the public health approach to medicine. Their labs were among the first to demonstrate on a wide scale the effectiveness of bacteriology in medicine and of the development of germicidal agents to enhance decontamination efforts. Their influence spread from quarantine hospitals to public health hospitals in municipalities across the country and, ultimately, to the general practice of medicine.

LESSON 4: MISSION COMPLEXITY HAMPERS EFFECTIVE RESPONSE

A factor of any bureaucratic organization that influences its effectiveness has been referred to as "mission complexity."[1] Administrative problems develop when a bureaucracy tries to do too much and too varied an array of tasks. As the U.S. M.H.S. morphed into the Public Health Service from the mid-1880s through the 1920s, it undertook an astonishing spectrum of tasks. It was crucial in developing the public health service approach. It played an effective and critically important role as primary barrier against outbreaks of pandemic episodes through its management of the quarantine station operations at an array of stations in the United States and abroad.

Its mission complexity is clearly evident. Consider that by the 1880s, the service was managing and operating a substantial string of hospitals, both general and contagious disease hospitals, at numerous stations across the country. It provided medical services for merchant seaman, federal prisoners, coast guardsmen, lepers, and narcotic addicts. It conducted medical examinations for immigrants, federal employees, and longshoremen. The P.H.S. administered public health grants to states and conducted venereal disease and tuberculosis-control programs. It administered the Biologics Control Act, the cancer program, and intramural research at the National Institute of Health. It conducted epidemiology studies of cancer in various hospitals around the country. It developed and ran biological laboratories at a national site (the NIH) and at all of its immigration stations. It developed and carried out basic biological research in all the labs it operated to test for and confirm the diagnosis of various contagious diseases. It developed research programs for sera and toxins to treat infectious diseases as well as managing contracts with numerous private businesses to develop sera and toxins. The P.H.S. tested and approved sera and toxins and inspected facilities developing them. It tested food additives that might pose dangers to public health. It ran extensive public education efforts to inform citizens about numerous infectious diseases and popularized simple measures the public could take to protect against and reduce the spread of contagious disease. It set up administrative procedures at ports in many nations abroad and across the country to monitor epidemic disease episodes around the world and across the nation to serve as an early warning system about epidemic disease outbreaks. It published manuals for its doctors and for other public health care professionals on effective treatments and procedures to cope with a wide variety of infectious diseases. The P.H.S. organized and ran extensive rat eradication campaigns. It developed and administered extensive inoculation campaigns and efforts. It spread knowledge within the medical profession on the importance of sterilization procedures. The service developed and improved on the design of various devices and apparatus to disinfect and fumigate against vermin, purchased those devices and promoted their use at stations, and at hospitals and the major ports of embarkation around the world. It virtually invented the concept and the practice of vector control. A complex mission indeed (Mullan, 1989; Kohn, 1995)!

The tragedy in 1847 at Grosse Ille in Canada, in which 10,000 persons lost their lives to the typhus pandemic before the development of scientific maritime decontamination devices and procedures, illustrates the importance of the quarantine hospitals and labs in demonstrating the validity of germ theory and the value of its application to modern medicine. The success in controlling the plague epidemic in San Francisco in the early 1900s proved the value of the rat eradication campaign and was critically important to the very development of the Public Health Service, as well as to the appointment of Dr. Rupert Blue as surgeon general of the United States.

Yet that mission complexity was, without question, a factor in its inability to cope adequately with the great influenza pandemic of 1918–1919. When the epidemic erupted, the P.H.S. frantically tried to develop a serum to treat victims. Research scientists strove heroically to understand this new viral infection that was so puzzling and so quickly lethal. But as an organization leading the battle, the P.H.S. was inundated with cases at hospitals it operated across the nation. It struggled simply to provide doctors and nurses to cope with the pandemic. At first, wartime censorship prevented the P.H.S. from conducting a public education campaign to inform the public about what measures could prevent the spread of the "Spanish influenza." By mid-1919, it launched an effort to do so, but the advice was too little, too late, and next to useless in its suggestions. The P.H.S. simply tried to do too much too quickly under the additional stress of wartime constraints and in the face of a baffling pandemic that stubbornly defied the best that medical science offered at the time. It had never before faced a flu virus with the morbidity and mortality rate of the 1918 mutation. Though medical science was beginning to understand the basics of germs and how they caused diseases and the role they played in the spread of contagious diseases, it did not yet understand well the role of the virus. It understood even less about the incredible ability of the virus to mutate. Its efforts were futile in the face of this most deadly of pandemics. In hindsight, the pandemic seems inevitable, but mission complexity was a factor in its extraordinary global lethality (Barry: 299–300).

The P.H.S. learned an important lesson from that tragic experience. Its mission complexity was reduced as it gradually "spun off" responsibilities and as other organizations, both public and private, took on some of its pioneering responsibilities. In 1906 the federal government created the Food, Drug, and Insecticide Administration to administer the Food and Drugs Act of June 30, 1906. That act was passed to protect the consuming public from misbranded or adulterated food, drugs, naval stores, insecticides and fungicides, and the honest producer against enforced competition with such commodities—later becoming the FDA (Weber: 36).

In 1946, the P.H.S. established the Communicable Disease Center that in 1968 morphed into the National Communicable Disease Center and eventually into today's Centers for Disease Control and Prevention (CDC). These took over malaria control and typhus work, and linked epidemiology in CDC labs to training and education. The scope of the CDC's work expanded from its original emphasis on tropical diseases with insect vectors to ones with zoological origin: malaria, amebiasis, the schistosomiasis, hookworm disease, filariasis, yellow fever, dengue, certain neurovirologic disorders, various forms of typhus and plague, sand-fly fever, and diverse diarrheas and dysenteries. The CDC supplied state and local health units with the support they needed to cope with communicable diseases, although that role developed slowly and sometimes in opposition from other better-established wings of the P.H.S. that resented the intrusion of the newcomer (the CDC). In 1948 the National Institutes of Health did basic research, and the CDC was given responsibility to help states recognize and control communicable diseases. The lines of responsibility were blurred, however, as the National Microbiological Institute served as reference serologists and entomologists and used field work to support and clarify laboratory work. At the CDC, in contrast, its primary role was to control disease, but bench work was necessary to back that up (Etheridge: 30).

With the outbreak of the Cold War in the 1950s, and the military's biological warfare programs, the CDC increasingly became disease detectives. In the mid-1950s, the increasing incidence of poliomyelitis and the Asian flu pandemic of 1957 moved the CDC, in a five-year period, from a position of relative obscurity in public health to one taking major responsibilities for epidemic control.

With the establishment of the United Nations and through it the World Health Organization, much of the global monitoring of pandemic and epidemic disease efforts shifted to WHO, which worked in conjunction with CDCs to establish an international system with more than 100 stations around the world to monitor epidemics and to help administer its campaigns to eradicate contagious diseases such as smallpox, diphtheria, tetanus, whooping cough, measles, poliomyelitis, and tuberculosis.

Rather than one agency trying to do basically all things, numerous agencies—public and private, including research conducted by NGOs organized on the basis of specific diseases—took up parts of the struggle to research, prevent, control, treat, or monitor the various epidemic and especially the deadly contagious diseases. That diversification of effort became all the more important as global monitoring stations watch for newly emerging variants of the influenza virus and for the return of well-known types, and the appearance of the hemorrhagic fevers and HIV, which challenge a new generation of microbe hunters as did smallpox, poliomyelitis, measles virus, and yellow fever the medical researchers already discussed (Oldstone: 191).

LESSON 5: AS MAN ADAPTS TO NATURE, NATURE ADAPTS TO MAN

Microscopic life is rich in its diversity, incredibly prolific in its ability to reproduce, and utterly fantastic in its adaptability. The bacterium is the most common life-form on earth. Modern science has found microscopic life miles deep in the oceans, where no light penetrates and where the pressure is incredible. Scientists have found them living where there is no oxygen. Some forms of microbes withstand vast extremes of temperatures. Scientists have discovered microbes in the frozen tundra of Antarctica and in the most scorching and arid deserts on earth. Scientists in labs have cultured microbes from fossil samples that seem to have survived in dormancy for millions of years.

As medical science unlocked some of nature's secrets and developed sera and other bacteriological tools to fight disease, the organizations of modern medicine developed increasingly elaborate practices and methods to cope with epidemics. Local public health programs were assisted by national programs, and then even multinational/international programs. After World War II, modern medical science dared to dream of, and organized to fund and administer, ambitious programs whose goal was no less than the global eradication of pandemic disease. When the WHO, and importantly, the CDCs eradicated smallpox in 1976, many dreamed of the similar defeat of most other pandemic disease that for much of human history had been scourges periodically becoming pandemics killing thousands, even millions, of people. WHO then launched eradication campaigns against diphtheria, tetanus, whooping cough, measles, poliomyelitis, and tuberculosis.

That optimism faded when confronted with the reality of how difficult an enemy microscopic life was to battle and defeat. Mankind learned that even as we adapted to nature and developed increasingly ingenious methods to manipulate and control it, germs and viruses proved even more adept at adapting to mankind's efforts. Germs and viruses developed drug resistance to the germicides that humans concocted. They mutated into new strains that defied human effort to eradicate them.

The Institute of Medicine at the National Academy of Sciences noted:

> Today's outlook with regard to microbial threats to health is bleak on a number of fronts . . . . Pathogens—old and new—have ingenious ways of adapting to and breaching our armamentarium of defenses. We must also understand that factors in society, the environment, and our global interconnectedness actually increase the likelihood of the ongoing emergence and spread of infectious disease. (Walters: 147)

Many epidemiologists warn that a pandemic as lethal as the great influenza will arise from among a number of newly emerging pathogens that medical science continues to identify. When it was first discovered, many feared that HIV/AIDS would be the source of such a pandemic. Though it has killed in the millions to date, its rate does not portend global deaths on the scale of the 1918–1919 pandemic. In 2001, another previously unknown virus struck in the form of severe acute respiratory syndrome, or SARS. The WHO considered SARS "the first severe and easily transmissible new disease to emerge in the 21st century." It joined a list of newly emerging epidemic diseases: HIV/AIDS, Ebola hemorrhagic fever, Lyme disease, and the like. The WHO sent the director of its Western Pacific Region to investigate the new disease. On March 12, 2001, the WHO declared it a virus that was a "world-wide heath threat." The virus seemed to kill about 7 percent of those infected. At that rate, if it spread in China, where one in ten could become infected, its death toll would exceed 30 million, on the scale of the Spanish influenza. A SARS outbreak in Hong Kong, though fortunately contained rather quickly, was found to have a death toll of 15 percent among those younger than 60 and more than 45 percent among those older than 60 (Walters: 148–150).

There is a bewildering list of newly emerging pathogens. "In the fall of 1999, the list of identified arboviruses numbered 538. Of this list, those known to cause human disease ran to 110" (Drexler: 38).

Table 6.1 presents a list with but a sample of the new viruses, viral strains, and new germs that have emerged since the 1930s, along with where they are most commonly endemic and the known or suspected vector carrier

Table 6.1
Emerging Pathogens Worldwide, 1930–Present

Year Identified	Name	Origin/Infection Location	Vector
1933	Eastern Equine Encephalitis Virus	N. America/ S. America/ Caribbean	Wild birds/ mosquito
1943	California Encephalitis Virus	Western U.S. and Canada	Rodents/mosquito
1950	Hantaan Virus	Asia/E. Europe	Rodents
1956	Chikungunya Virus	Tropical Africa/ Asia	Primate to human, via mosquito
1957	Kyasanur Forest Virus	Asia/India	Rodents/bat/tick
1958	Junin Virus	S. America/ Argentina	Rodents
1960	La Cross Encephalitis Virus	Canada/Alaska/ Eastern U.S./ Western U.S./ Europe/Finland/ East Africa	Chipmunk/squirrel/ mosquito/domestic animals (rabbits)
1966	Machupo Virus	S. America (Bolivia)	Unknown/primates suspected
1967	Marburg Virus	Germany/ E. Africa	Primates
1970	Lassa Virus	Africa	Rodent
1973	Rotaviruses	Developing countries	Unknown/ coevolving with humans, fecal–oral
1974	Parvovirus B19	Global	Unknown, coevolving with humans
1976	Ebola Sudan Virus	Africa (Sudan)	Unknown animal source
1976	Ebola Zaire Virus	Africa (Zaire)	Unknown
1977	Seoul Virus	Asia/Europe	Rodents
1980	Human T-lymphotropic Virus (HTLV-1)	Central Africa/ Caribbean/ NE South America	Primates/now coevolving with humans
1983	Human Immunodeficiency Virus-1 (HIV-1)	West Africa	African primate

(Continued)

Table 6.1 (*Continued*)

Year Identified	Name	Origin/Infection Location	Vector
1986	Human Herpesvirus-6 (HHV-6)	Global	Unknown/ coevolving with humans
1988	Hepatitis E Virus	Tropics of Asia, Africa, S. America	Unknown, coevolving with humans
1989	Hepatitis C Virus	Global	Primate?
1989	Ebola Reston Virus	Asia/Philippines	Unknown
1991	Guanarito Virus	S. America	Rodent
1993	Sin Nombre Hantavirus	SW United States	Rodents
1994	Ebola Gabon	Gabon, Africa	Unknown
1995	Human Herpes Virus-8	Global	Unknown
1995/1996	Argentinean Hantavirus	Argentina	Person-to-person?
1996	Ebola Gabon	South Africa	Chimpanzees

Year	Emerging Bacteria
1975	Lyme disease (*Borrelia burgdorferi*)
1976	Legionnaire's disease (*Legionella pneumophila*)
	Acute and chronic diarrhea (*Cryptosporidium parvum*)
1977	Bowel infection (*Campylobacter jejuni*)
1978	Toxic shock syndrome (*Staphylococcus aureus*)
1982	Hemorrhagic colitis
	Hemolytic uremic syndrome
1983	Cat scratch disease (*Afipia felis*)
	Peptic ulcer disease (*Helicobacter pylori*)
1984	Persistent diarrhea (*Enterocytozoon bieneusi*)
1985	Persistent diarrhea (*Cyclospora cayetanensis*)
1991	Atypical babesiosis (new species of Babesia)
1992	Seventh pandemic of cholera (*Vibrio cholerae* 0139)
1993	Cat scratch disease (*Bartonella henselae*)
1994	Flesh-eating bug (*Beta hemolytic streptococcus*)

Year	Emerging Protozoa
1991	Conjunctivitis, disseminated disease (*Encephalitozoon hellem*)
1992	Disseminated disease (*Encephalitozoon cuniculi*)

Source: Table by author, adapted from appendix, Frank Ryan, *Tracking the New Killer Plagues*, Boston: Little, Brown and Company, 1997.

of each. Some of these new viral agents are especially worrisome, because epidemiologists have yet been unable to determine their origin or the vector or carrier. The Sin Nombre virus, for example, suddenly appeared on the Navajo reservation in New Mexico. It killed several natives and eventually was identified as a new form of hantaan virus. Previously, that virus was located in Europe and caused kidney and liver failure (Walters: 113–126). Sin Nombre took some time to diagnose, because it appeared suddenly in New Mexico among victims who had no known travel to or contact with Europe. More puzzling still, the Sin Nombre (No Name) virus caused pulmonary disease, attacking the respiratory system rather than the kidneys or liver (Peters and Olshaker: 7–40). Other newly emerging pathogens are frightening in the speed with which they are spreading. The West Nile virus, for example, assisted by migrating birds, international travel, and perhaps climate changes resulting from global warming has begun spreading from west Africa to become a global threat, spreading "[l]ike a smoke plume swept into a wind" (Walters: 146).

Some of the new viruses are of special concern because they are highly lethal. The eastern equine encephalitis virus, for example, kills more than 30 percent of its victims by acute infection of the brain and central nervous system. The hantaan viruses are another highly lethal pathogen. And then there are the many types of hemorrhagic fever virus that exhibit high lethality: Junin virus, Machupo virus, Marburg virus, Lassa virus, the various strains of Ebola (Sudan, Zaire, etc.) virus, the Seoul virus, Sin Nombre virus, and Sabia virus. Until fairly recently, AIDS was nearly always fatal and almost untreatable, because it attacked the human immune system itself (AIDS is the disease caused by the human immunodeficiency virus, or HIV as it is commonly known).

Some are especially scary (although less lethal) because of the nature of their symptoms and the difficulty medical science has to treat them. An example of that type is one among the new "superbug" pathogens of emerging bacteria, the so-called "flesh-eating bug" that emerged in 1994.

Still others are yet so puzzling because they have no known origin or animal host, or their vectors are uncertain. Examples of these include Mayaro virus (identified in 1954), O'nyong-nyong virus (1959), La Cross encephalitis (1960), rotaviruses (1973), parvovirus B19 (1974), the various Ebola virus (whose suspected animal hosts are primates), human herpesvirus-6 and human herpesvirus-8, and the hepatitis E virus.

LESSON 6: WE HAVE MET THE ENEMY, AND HE IS US

With apologies to Pogo, a sixth lesson is closely related to lesson 5. Germs and virus adapt to human intervention and to human behavior. Patterns of human behavior contribute significantly to the development and spread of disease. Human culture and customs are closely linked to disease cycles. Human intervention in nature, through widespread agriculture, for example, and through massive inroads into the rain forests to support ever more and larger urban habitation centers, disturbs the natural environment in ways that seem to spread the incidence of human disease and contribute to the emergence of new diseases, which may have been endemic for ages but have rarely infected human beings. One of the strongest aspects of human culture, religious beliefs, sometimes obstructs good medical practices designed to prevent the spread of diseases or delays or even stops outright basic research against them.

Take, for example, human sex practices. Long after AIDS was identified and shown to be transmitted from human to human through intimate sexual contact, and long after rather simple and inexpensive "safe sex" methods were demonstrated effective against the spread of HIV/AIDS, millions of people continue to have unprotected sex. Millions have died from AIDS, yet humans persist in having unsafe sex (unprotected by use of a condom, for instance; or through a sexual practice known to be more likely to spread the infection—through oral or anal sex, for example). Incredibly, countless persons known to be HIV-infected and therefore carriers of AIDS continue to practice unsafe, unprotected sex. Some religious movements still oppose safe sex education campaigns and condom distribution programs among teens (see Shilts, 2007; Hayes, 1998; Kraut, 1994).

The experiences at the three stations discussed here have shown how cheap and rather simple hygiene practices can effectively prevent the contamination of water so crucial in the life cycle of a highly contagious and deadly disease like cholera. The case of the rather basic hygiene experiments in Manila, the Philippines, in the early 1900s, as described in chapter 2, proved that the sources of cholera can be easily eliminated. The simple steps and measures are detailed in an early 1900 U.S. M.H.S. report (RG 90, File 397, Box 053). Yet despite the knowledge and ready availability of simple and cheap methods to prevent contamination or to decontaminate water supplies, cholera remains endemic in many developing countries. Mankind continues to spread cholera around the world, generally from the developing world to locations in the developed world, either as human carriers of cholera infection or as ready transporters of contaminates from the developing world to elsewhere. The seventh cholera pandemic was carried from Asia to Latin America in contaminated bilge or ballast water and foolishly dumped in coastal waters, resulting in the spread of cholera in modern times to infect more than 1 million and cause the needless death of many thousands.

We know that bubonic plague is spread by rodent fleas. Like cholera, bubonic plague is endemic in many parts of the world, which therefore remain a potential source for epidemic outbreaks. Yet we launch rodent eradication efforts only after pandemic episodes, rather than preemptively. We are willing to spend billions on preemptive war but seem unwilling to spend millions on preemptive preventive medicine—for example, on vector control efforts among common rodents in rural or wilderness areas where bubonic plague is endemic.

Since the turn of the twentieth century, we have known that typhus is spread by human lice. Yet by the first decades of the twenty-first century, thousands if not millions of humans fail to use even the most basic of hygiene practices that would easily and cheaply kill lice. Although typhus epidemics are rare today, because mankind does employ prophylactic measures when typhoid fever cases emerge, if a mutation should occur in the typhus bacillus, the potential for a renewed epidemic of that age-old enemy is possible.

We know many contagious diseases are spread when humans congregate in close proximity and high density and bring together large numbers of persons from distant places of origin where their natural immunities are quite varied. Yet we persist in essentially creating virgin populations in military camps. Not even the warning experience of history's most deadly pandemic seems to have taught us the danger of that human folly. The need to wage war and the military necessity of camps to train and assemble large numbers of troops seems to be more important than preventing another deadly pandemic. And so another such episode is highly likely, if not inevitable, as many medical scientists believe.

Religious beliefs hamper attempts to control the spread of HIV/AIDS. Venereal disease continues to be epidemic, particularly among teenagers. Without question, that sad fact is partly because some religious beliefs and movements oppose public education efforts aimed at promoting safe sex practices. They have undermined, and sometimes prevented outright, public funding of condom distribution. Religious beliefs influence public policy about basic genetic research and some stem-cell research, which hold potential for breakthrough therapies for any number of diseases.

Medical science itself is susceptible to manipulation by humans who actively develop biological agents as weapons. We may have eradicated the smallpox virus "in nature," but we keep it in labs. Its potential for being adapted for bioterrorism is quite real. Only *human behavior* accounts for biological weapons, biological warfare, and biological terrorism. Germs and viruses mutate naturally, and humans, in a very real sense, are in constant warfare with them when those mutations result in the germ or virus becoming infectious human diseases, but the next pandemic on a scale akin to the great influenza of 1918–1919 may be the result of bioterrorism rather than from natural development. That reality leads us to our next lesson.

LESSON 7: THE SPECIAL THREAT OF BIOTERRORISM

Ushering in the twenty-first century, 2001 proved to be a wake-up year in the United States when it came to the threat of bioterrorism.[2] The attacks of September 11, 2001, on the Twin Towers of the World Trade Center in New York City and the Pentagon in Washington, D.C., followed closely by the anthrax bioterrorist attack on Congress via the U.S. Postal Service, issued that wake-up call. Before those events, the Department of Defense (DoD) had developed defenses against biological warfare focused primarily on the U.S. military itself, on the troops and U.S. military bases—mostly those abroad. DoD plans focused little or none at all on the general civilian population, nor on domestic terrorist attacks. International terrorism was seen as something that happened "over there," not at home. In response to 9/11 and the anthrax terrorist attacks, the federal government established the Office of Public Health Preparedness, housed within the Department of Health and Human Services (HHS) and directed by Dr. D. A. Henderson.

Among the first acts of the new office was to release, by early December, 2001, a list of microbial pathogens considered to be the most likely threats from biological terrorism aimed at the civilian population. That list is presented in Table 6.2. The civilian population as the target of such agents required a different approach than did the defense of troops in combat situations. The former include people of all ages and health status. The means of delivery are likely to be different. The possibility that such attacks might be aimed simultaneously at numerous urban centers of population dictated the need for HHS and the Department of Homeland Security (DHS) to develop partnerships with state and local governments and their first responders (police, fire, local public health departments, hospitals). Even if an attack is aimed at only one large urban area, it is considered highly likely that the disease outbreak would be of such a magnitude as to overwhelm the effective response capabilities of local medical and public health professionals. This required the federal government to provide protective and responsive measures for the affected populations. The following section describes several approaches developed by OPHP to deal with the effects of biological, chemical, and similar terrorist acts ("The Science of Bioterrorism: HHS Preparedness," www.house.gov/science/full/dec05/henerson.htm).

Table 6.2
Critical Pathogen Agents

Category A Agents	Category B Agents
Variola major (Smallpox)	*Coxiella burnetii* (Q fever)
Bacillus anthracis (anthrax)	Brucella species (brucellosis)
Yersinia pestis (plague)	Brucella species (brucellosis)
Clostridium botulinum toxin	Alphaviruses
(botulism)	–Venezuelan encephalomyelitis
Francisella tularensis (tulararemia)	–Eastern/western equine
	encephalomyelitis
Filoviruses	Food or Waterborne Pathogens
–Ebola hemorrhagic fever	(B Subset)
–Marburg hemorrhagic fever	–Salmonella species
	–Shigella dysenteriae
Arenaviruses	
–Lassa (Lassa fever)	–Escherichia coli 0157:H7
–Junin (Argentine hemorrhagic fever)	–Vibrio cholerae
–Related viruses	–Cryptosporidium parvum

Category C Agents
–Nipah virus
–Hantavirus
–Tickborne hemorrhagic
fever viruses
–Yellow fever
–Multidrug-resistant
tuberculosis

Category A agents are easily disseminated or transmitted person-to-person, have high mortality and major public health effects, can cause panic and social disruption, and require special action for public health preparedness.

Category B agents are moderately easy to disseminate; cause moderate morbidity and low mortality, and require special enhancements of CDC's diagnostic capacity and enhanced disease surveillance.

Category C agents are emerging pathogens that could be engineered for mass dissemination because of their availability, ease of production and dissemination, and potential for high morbidity and mortality with special health effects.

Source: Table by author, adapted from appendix of critical biological agents, D. A. Henderson, www. house.gov/science/full/dec05/henderson.htm, and from information from Frank Ryan, *Tracking the New Killer Plagues*, Boston: Little, Brown and Company, 1997.

Of particular concern is the possibility that bioterrorists might combine more than one agent in an attack. That possibility is not far-fetched. In Africa, TB and HIV/AIDS combine as health threats to the many hundreds of thousands of victims. Some of the biological agents presented in Table 6.2 are categorized as high-priority organisms because (1) they can be easily disseminated or transmitted person-to-person, (2) they cause high mortality, and (3) they have the potential for high morbidity—that is, for a major public health effect that might cause widespread public panic (always a goal of terrorism) and social disruption. A bioengineered virus having the characteristics of smallpox and Ebola or Marburg hemorrhagic fever, for example, would be an awesome bioweapon. The OPHP lists six emerging pathogens that could form the basis of such a bioengineered agent because of their availability, ease of production and dissemination, potential for high morbidity and mortality, and potential for major health effect.

In 1995, HHS developed a Metropolitan Medical Response System through its Office of Emergency Preparedness. This system of contractual relationships with existing state and local response agencies aims at responding to natural disease outbreaks or serious health risks after natural disasters beyond the capacity of the local resources of emergency management, medical and health care providers, public health departments, law enforcement, fire departments, EMS services, and national guard units. The MMRS is designed to link all those resources with HHS teams to provide an integrated, unified response to a mass casualty event. By September 2001, the OEP had contractual links with ninety-seven municipalities to develop MMRSs. After the attacks in September and November of 2001, that system was expanded to add twenty-five additional cities and to incorporate bioterrorism planning and response to the MMRS ("The Science of Bioterrorism," Henderson, 2005; see also Ryan, 1997).

HHS uses the OEP to manage a National Disaster Medical System (NDMS) in partnership with the DOD, the Department of Veterans Affairs (VA), the Federal Emergency Management Administration (FEMA), and the Public Health Service Commissioned Corps Readiness Force. Depending on the severity of a national disaster event (natural or manmade), the NDMS can be activated to assist in an event by providing additional services to aid disaster victims. The NDMS comprises more than 7,000 volunteer health and support professionals capable of being deployed anywhere in the United States when called on to respond to an event that overwhelms the local response team, many of whom are likely to have been incapacitated.

In response to the events of 2001, HHS created the OPHP. The OPHP and HHS work with the VA, one of the largest purchasers of pharmaceuticals and medical supplies in the world, which means that the VA has enormous buying power. They set up a National Pharmaceutical Stockpile of antibiotics, antidotes, vaccines, and medical material to respond rapidly to an event to prevent further spread of a disease resulting from a terrorist threat agent. The NPS supplemented the types of material in its stockpile specifically as a result of the September 11, 2001, events, so it is now an "all-hazards" supply. It has stockpiles of 600 tons and plans to enable accelerated production of vaccines and antibiotics for those areas most critical to responding to bioterrorism, including more than $500 million dollars allocated to speed the development and purchase of smallpox vaccine.

HHS and the CDC developed an Agency for Toxic Substances and Disease Registry (ATSDR) to identify and clean up contaminated facilities. It refined methods of environmental sampling to assess whether contamination, such as an anthrax event, had occurred, and developed recommendations to conduct environmental sampling and cleanup and to better protect first responders, investigators, and cleanup personnel. These were broadly disseminated to federal, state, and local health and environmental agencies and are posted on a CDC bioterrorism website.

LESSON 8: THE IMPORTANCE OF AN EARLY WARNING SYSTEM

Earlier chapters discussed how the U.S. M.H.S. and then the P.H.S. developed and depended on a host of U.S. state department counselor offices posted in the countries that had major ports of embarkation around the world to monitor events in those countries for any suspected outbreaks of epidemics. In the U.S. M.H.S,. an effort was made to establish, in essence, an early warning system. Monitoring officials warned the offices of the secretary of state, the surgeon general of the United States, and the immigration stations at the ports of entry to which any potentially contaminated vessels might be bound. They established an informal but important early warning system. An early warning system is all the more important now in light of the speed and ease of international travel today, which quite simply shrinks the world to a global village.

The threat of bioterrorism indicates the danger of biological pathogens' being intentionally disseminated—it increases the need for an early warning system. Unless we are forewarned and prepared to respond quickly to an attack, an event of that nature could precipitate an epidemic episode, the intent of bioterrorists. Depending on the nature of the agent in such an attack, if not quickly and effectively responded to, it could start a pandemic.

Likewise, the 2014 outbreak of Ebola in Africa demonstrated the need for nations of the developed world—most important, the United States—to help combat, control, and contain those epidemics in situ before they spread more widely to the rest of the world. Those epidemics reminded us, as well, of the need to develop protocols to contain Ebola when it inevitably spreads cases to the United States, as it did so recently. We cannot prevent cases from migrating to the United States, but we can contain them from becoming epidemics here.

The massiveness of current illegal immigration increases the likelihood of a natural outbreak of disease from one of the newly emerging viruses or the re-emergent epidemic disease strains that are today referred to as "superbugs" because of their resistance to multiple vaccines and antibiotic therapies. Historical analysis amply demonstrates how difficult, if not impossible, it is to deal effectively with illegal immigration flow (LeMay, 2007). Illegal immigrants tend to travel from developing nations, where those strains of disease are still endemic and from which the re-emergent and newly emerging strains of pathogens are most likely to arise, to populations in the developed world, often all the more susceptible today because natural immunity has been lost or dissipated. Today illegal immigrants travel with speed. Where they relocate is no longer confined to and concentrated within six or ten "gateway" states.[3] The dispersal of illegal immigrants in the United States is far wider than ever before—nearly nationwide. Migration for permanent resettlement—both legal and illegal—is widely dispersed among developed countries. Those facts establish the need for an effective global early warning system.

In part a response to the problem, a major NGO effort was launched in 2008 by Google.org, a philanthropic arm of Google.com. It seeks to identify "hot spots" of emerging threats from infectious diseases and has established and funded a "predict and prevent" effort using information and technology to empower a global system of local communities to predict and prevent emerging threats ("Global Initiatives," www.google.org).

The CDC established a system of epidemiology laboratories collectively forming a surveillance system. It established the Health Alert Network—a nationwide electronic communication system. It established teams of expert epidemiologists who could be sent to states and cities to help them respond quickly to infectious disease outbreaks and other public risks. The CDC has a staff of more than 100 specially trained anti-terrorist experts in epidemiology, surveillance, secure communications, and laboratory diagnostics (Henderson: 5). It awarded more than $130 million in cooperative agreements to fifty states, one territory, and four major metropolitan health departments for preparedness planning and readiness assessment, epidemiology and surveillance, improved laboratory capacity for biological or chemical agents, and the aforementioned Health Alert Network, in which the federal government funded at least one epidemiologist position in every state who was trained in the CDC's Epidemic Intelligence Service program.

The CDC and HHS created the Agency for Toxic Substance and Disease Registry (ATSDR) after the anthrax terrorist incident in November 2001. The CDC, ATSDR, and Occupational Safety and Health Administration (OSHA) have developed exposure limits for fumigants, as well as detection methods to determine when any residual fumigant is below established limits. After buildings are cleaned and after cleaning environmental sampling is conducted, the CDC and ATSDR provide technical input to the incident command and other experts to determine when a building is safe and ready for re-entry.

The FDA has the Center for Biologics Evaluation Research (CBER). It provides regulatory guidance to the DOD, CDC, and others conducting studies to develop new vaccines and drugs and to screen new and unusual ideas for developing products to treat diseases and to develop new diagnostic tools. According to Henderson, biowarfare defense vaccines and drugs undergo the same FDA review process as any other vaccines or drugs (8).

Public health programs have come a long way. In the 1890s, their staffs often wore no protective gear, sometime dressed simply in smocks or coveralls that could be easily washed but that provided no barrier against contamination. By 1918–1919, medical personnel were wearing gauze masks, which had proven effective against the spread of some germs (those contained in saliva, for example) but that were unfortunately far too porous to be effective against the airborne mutated influenza virus. Today, medical scientists studying or combating proven or suspected outbreaks of highly contagious and deadly diseases wear biohazard suits that effectively encase them in sealed atmospheres.

LESSON 9: THE NECESSITY FOR INTERNATIONAL COOPERATION TO FACE A GLOBAL THREAT

The tragedies of the epidemics that occurred at Angel Island, Ellis Island, and New Orleans showed the value of and the need for international cooperation when facing pandemic diseases. Initially the U.S. M.H.S., and then its successor, the P.H.S., established cooperation with the governments of all sending countries to monitor and respond to pandemic diseases. This patchwork of ad hoc arrangements provided some measure of early warning and eventually inspired many countries to enhance their public health efforts. The governments of some countries, however, hid the fact that epidemic diseases raged in their territories. The ad hoc nature of these arrangements resulted in gaps and sometimes failures to forewarn the P.H.S. of vessels whose passengers or crews were likely infected.

As a result, after World War I, the international community organized the League of Nations, which in turn, established one of the first public or governmental systems for international cooperation to confront pandemic diseases. After World War II, the international community went further by establishing the United Nations, with its ancillary agencies of international cooperation regarding threats to world health: WHO, UNESCO, UNICEF, and the United Nations High Commission for Refugees (UNHCR). The UN works closely with international NGOs, such as the International Red Cross. Collectively, these agencies and organizations form an *international* system for the purpose of early warning about epidemic threats and to fund international efforts to eradicate diseases, such as the worldwide campaigns to vaccinate children against smallpox, measles, whooping cough, polio, and so on.

This international system of cooperation helps various governments fund basic research to study newly emerging viral and bacteriological disease threats to the international community and to world health. "The WHO is now *the* organization that monitors the global threat of infections; that initiates and coordinates responses to such a threat" (Ryan: 149, emphasis mine). Although that role is critically important, it must be noted that WHO operates no diagnostic laboratories of its own. It relies on the charity and interest of a global network of collaborating scientists and their laboratories, funded by national governments.

Given the effects of push factors that underlie international migration and contribute to mass refugee movements, which contribute to the threat of an epidemic disease outbreak's becoming pandemic, the system of international cooperation continues to be vitally important. Massive legal and illegal immigration increases the threat of a pandemic. Because the threat is global, the response must also be global. The eradication of smallpox demonstrated that collectively the world community could raise sufficient funds to mount a global eradication campaign. The success of the campaign demonstrated what such cooperation could accomplish (Etheridge: 188–210).

The existence of a system of more than 100 laboratories around the world to monitor and study pandemic health threats is vitally important to preparedness. Only the cooperative work of this system of research facilities can sufficiently increase human knowledge about new pathogens about which we now have limited knowledge. This system is vital to increased knowledge of how such pathogens might be artificially dispersed (to protect against international bioterrorism). Newly emerging pathogens, and the re-emergence of more drug resistant strains of old enemies, underscore the need for international cooperation. Only an international response can confront international terrorism and bioterrorism.

The CDC's work with and through the WHO in the smallpox and measles eradication projects demonstrates the effectiveness of piggybacking one immunization effort with another. In most of Africa, measles is a greater threat than smallpox. On the African continent, throughout much of the 20th century, measles killed 10 percent or more of children before their fifth birthday. Great inroads toward eradication have been made by combining the efforts of the CDC, the WHO, the Agency for International Development (AID), and Epidemic Intelligence Service (EIS) epidemiologists. For a relatively small additional cost, measles was greatly curbed as smallpox was eradicated from west and central Africa as part of the global smallpox eradication program (Etheridge: 192–193).

Cooperating in the effort were then otherwise Cold War rivals (the United States and the former Soviet Union), who contributed hundreds of millions of dollars and donated millions of doses of smallpox vaccine. The smallpox eradication campaign showed that the WHO surveillance system was key to success in eradicating smallpox.

By 1980, the WHO funded the first global EIS program, begun with the cooperation of the World Bank, the AID, the Food and Agriculture Organization, and various regional health groups. The CDC supplied epidemiologists who ultimately trained scientists in other countries to achieve self-sufficiency. EIS programs were established in Thailand, Indonesia, Mexico, Taiwan, and Saudi Arabia. Within five or six years, the CDC's epidemiologist was moved out of the country, and the program stood on its own. In the 1980s, the CDC set up international efforts in various refugee camps (beginning in Kampuchea), and CDC teams identified the principal causes of death and severe illness among refugees in the camps and initiated appropriate treatments and preventive measures. The Kampuchea experience was followed by a similar undertaking in Somalia. Between 1980 and 1983, the CDC used the surveillance program to make humanitarian efforts effective and proved its value to the WHO and the UN's refugee relief programs (Etheridge: 286–287).

The measles immunization program was expensive, but it attracted the resources and commitment of several international organizations that made the effort possible: the World Bank, the Rockefeller Foundation, the United Nations Development Programme (UNDP), and the United Nations International Children's Emergency Fund (UNICEF). Collectively, they organized the Task Force on Child Survival. They attracted the commitment of Rotary International, persuaded by Dr. Albert Sabin to provide any country in the world with the polio vaccine it needed for five years. Rotary International committed to raise $180 million to the effort but in four years raised $240 million and provided the catalyst toward the global effort at polio eradication (Etheridge: 293–294).

Today, trachoma is being targeted by a similar type program launched by Lions Clubs International (its Campaign Sight First II), the largest NGO and a partner with the UN's WHO. Lions International raised nearly $210 million, a substantial portion of which will be aimed at eradication of trachoma.

LESSON 10: PLAN TO SUCCEED, OR PLAN ON FAILING

The historical experiences at the three islands illustrate, tragically, what can happen when officials have not planned for epidemic disease outbreaks. In 1847, immigration officials simply did not know enough about typhus to plan well for that disastrous outbreak. The size and deadliness of the 1847 typhoid pandemic cost more than 10,000 lives, in no small measure as a result of that lack of planning. At Angel Island, Dr. Joseph Kinyoun had no real plan to deal with the epidemic of bubonic plague. Hundreds of lives were lost there before Dr. Rupert Blue developed the rat eradication plan that eventually stopped the epidemic. Doctors at Ellis Island, as at every immigration station and military camp across the country, had no plan to deal with an influenza pandemic that turned so terribly lethal so quickly and so pervasively. No one understood the mutation of the flu virus sufficiently well to plan measures to prevent or even slow down the pandemic. Without plans, they were powerless in the face of the relentless march of the disease across the nation, from military camps to the civilian population, in city after city.

But medical science learned about the complexity of the threat of pandemic disease. Epidemiologists learned about the cycles of these diseases, and that pandemics are complex social phenomena as well as health crises. They learned that the complexity of epidemic outbreaks requires careful and comprehensive planning. Medical personnel, health professionals, and fire and police first responders have to be trained in advance to cope with particular epidemics. Epidemiologists need to train doctors to recognize the outbreak quickly. Vaccines and appropriate antibiotic supplies need to be developed and stockpiled, ready for distribution. Planning is needed for efficient dissemination of those supplies. Only carefully planned campaigns have a chance at success in the face of the threat from pandemic diseases.

The CDC responded to this need in several ways. It has prepared smallpox response team guides that it has provided to every department of health in every U.S. state and to every embassy mission. Months of local planning in many of the states established detailed courses of action for the all-volunteer response teams. Teams were constituted, as their name implies, to react to the threat of a smallpox terrorist attack (after the 9/11 attacks and the anthrax incident in 2001). The detailed plans they developed could be applied to other epidemic disease outbreaks, from bioterrorism or from naturally emerging incidents (Bertolli and Forkiotis: 7).

The success of the smallpox eradication campaign reveals what careful planning can accomplish. The CDC worked out a master plan, and convinced—and got the approval of—a host of participating agencies before the program began. Governments had to approve the enormous funding. The U.S. Congress had to be convinced of the value of preventive measures—that sufficient American lives and American children would be saved by massive, global immunization of children in far-off Africa and Asia to justify allocation of $300 million to the effort. A smallpox eradication team had to be assembled at the CDC in Atlanta, Georgia. Millions of doses of smallpox vaccine had to be created, stored, and distributed, including by convincing officials in the Soviet Union to join in the effort. At the time, WHO reported 131,418 cases of smallpox, but the real figure was more like 10–15 million cases. WHO planned on vaccination of 80 percent of children in western Nigeria, at the start of the campaign, anticipating that improved surveillance would finish the effort. Religious opposition had to be overcome (in the local language, the word for smallpox was the same as the name of the local earth god, and people were at first incensed that foreign doctors were coming to make war on their deity). But careful planning, and continuing development of the master plan as various parts were accomplished, resulted in global eradication.

The lesson learned as to the need for elaborate planning is certainly evident with respect to the threat of bioterrorism. In the United States the NIH's bioterrorism research program involves both short- and long-term research targeted at the development, evaluation, and approval of diagnostics, therapies and vaccines needed to control infections caused by microbes with potential for use as biological weapons, focused primarily on the threats by anthrax and smallpox, but increasingly on other newly emerging pathogens as well. Careful collaboration with other federal agencies has been developed. New vaccines are being developed and tested. Through interagency agreements, the National Institute of Allergy and Infectious Diseases (NIAID), which spearheads national planning efforts, collaborates with the Department of Defense's U.S. Army Medical Research Institute of Infectious Diseases to develop a new vaccine using recombinant protective antigen vaccine to protect all ages of the American public, including military personnel. The CDC, FCA, and DoD work with the NIH to refine standard serological tests on the effectiveness of anthrax vaccines.

National research has been substantially expanded since 2002, and NIAID has solicited from the scientific community's research proposals on anthrax and other bacteriological pathogens to encourage research toward better diagnosis, prevention, and treatment. The molecular mechanisms involved in the germination of anthrax spores in vivo have been used to develop novel and promising post-attack strategies that promise to be more effective than the widespread use of antimicrobial drugs not specific to anthrax and that must be given to large groups of exposed individuals, inadvertently promoting the development of antibiotic-resistant strains of other bacteria. NIAID and the Office of Naval Research are working to sequence the DNA of the chromosomes of anthrax, partially funded by the Department of Energy. NIH anticipates information derived from the genome-sequencing project to substantially aid in developing rapid diagnostic tests, as well as new vaccines and antibiotic therapies against mutant strains of anthrax.

NIAID research on smallpox emphasizes extending existing vaccine stock to increase the number of available doses and to develop new vaccines and treatments and new diagnostic tools to detect smallpox quickly. NIAID, DoD, CDC, and the Department of Energy have funded and planned research to (1) develop and evaluate at least three antiviral drugs with pre-clinical activity against smallpox and acceptable clinical safety, (2) extend the usefulness of the currently available stockpile of doses of older vaccine by conducting human studies to see whether they can stretch available stocks by diluting it, (3) help develop a safe, sterile smallpox vaccine grown in cell cultures using modern technology, (4) explore the development of a vaccine that can be used in all segments of the civilian population, and (5) increase basic knowledge of the genome of smallpox and related viruses.

In an echo of the pioneering work the New Orleans station in the 1880s to scientifically identify and test the effectiveness of various germicides that gradually spread to all other immigration-reception stations, in 2002, NIAID began clinical trials to evaluate the effectiveness of different strengths of vaccines to expand the now limited supply of smallpox vaccine. NIAID and the DoD's Advanced Research Projects fund collaborative efforts with four academic centers and with the CDC, USAMRIID, and the American Type Culture Collection that focus on designing and implementing an Orthopoxvirus Genomics and Bioinformatics Resource Center to conduct sequence and functional comparisons of genes to provide insights for the selection of targets for the design of antivirals and vaccines. As Henderson notes, this new center will design and maintain databases to store, display, annotate and query genome sequences, structural information, phenotypic data and bibliographic information and construct and maintain a website to facilitate the availability of such data for other researchers (10–13).

CONCLUSION

Unless lessons are learned from past battles with pandemic diseases, history will repeat itself. Although future epidemics involving newly emerging pathogens, or the mutated strain of an older, re-emergent biological enemy, may be inevitable, the pandemic spread of the disease need not be. The lessons learned and discussed here may enable planning for procedures, treatments, and anti-biological therapies that can substantially mitigate or contain a new epidemic. Though a new epidemic may be inevitable, its development into a global pandemic on the scale of the influenza pandemic of 1918–1919 might be avoidable. The threat of a future pandemic of that scale is serious and pressing. Considering today's far greater global population, and the evidence that human disease pathogens are developing that are increasingly drug-resistant to known antibacterial therapies, the lessons discussed here must be applied if we are to avoid a death rate in excess of 50 million lives. To effectively combat that threat, policymakers (both immigration-related and public health–related) must increasingly think locally but act globally (Drexler: 275–277).

Our increasingly complex society means that humankind and pathogens will cross paths more often. The emerging threat, be it a pandemic flu, inhalational anthrax, foodborne illness, or insectborne disease, requires keen surveillance and well-planned, rapid response. It necessitates a global web of health care workers, bacteriological laboratories, and an elaborate communication system that can identify an aberrant infection or novel disease quickly and at virtually any place around the globe. Public health policy and programs have been proven to be effective prevention against epidemics and pandemics. Public health, in essence, is a rational step-by-step process involving the application of the lessons learned in all previous outbreak investigations. It defines a problem, recognizes its true nature, finds out what causes or spreads it, and develops plans and programs to control or prevent it. Its global focus is increasingly necessary.

> Doctors and nurses around the world must be trained in the practical aspects
> of public health and be welcomed into an international network of health care

colleagues. Independent laboratories and timely electronic reporting systems must operate free of government interference. Meanwhile, researchers must keep tabs on conditions such as altered habitats or large population movements that give rise to emerging infections. How close are we to approaching such a system, a kind of global Epidemic Intelligence Service akin to the CDC's elite corps of disease detectives? According to one U.S. government estimate, at least ten years away. (Drexler: 277)

The medical pioneers of the late nineteenth century enabled great strides to be made against pandemic disease during the twentieth century. Now in the opening decades of the twenty-first century, medical scientists and public health planners today need to play a role as did those described here. Perhaps the lessons learned here will enable policymakers to avoid some of the unanticipated consequences of the past. It is to be hoped that the lessons learned will teach us to modify the customs of human behavior that contribute to the spread of pandemic disease—and that these lessons will inform public policy to better cope with pandemic disease during this newest age of mass migration.

GLOSSARY

Chain migration: friends and relatives of immigrants drawn to specific locations by their compatriots already living in the United States.

Chimera: a genetically engineered or altered virus.

Civil law: regulates the relations between or among persons and corporations and the government, as distinct from criminal law, offenses against which are usually considered misdemeanors, punishable by fines rather than incarceration.

Criminal law: regulates the relation between persons and the state, offenses against which may be misdemeanors or felonies, punished by fines and incarceration of determined length.

Earned legalization: proposal to allow unauthorized immigrants to change their status to that of legal permanent residents by paying fines and satisfying stipulated conditions akin to those satisfied by those who came as authorized permanent resident aliens.

Endemic: a disease common or native to a particular area, always present but under control.

Epidemic: outbreak of a disease produced by some special cause not generally present in the affected area, with higher than usual morbidity and mortality rates.

Epidemiology: the study of epidemic and pandemic diseases and their causes and spread.

Eugenics: the pseudoscience proposing proof of the inherent superiority or inferiority of certain racial groups.

Forty-Eighters: German immigrants who came to the United States after 1848 and until the early 1850s who fled after the failed revolution attempt in Germany in 1848.

Gateway states: the top seven or so immigrant receiving states to which immigrants first migrate before moving on to settle in other states.

Gentlemen's Agreement: 1907 executive order issued by President Theodore Roosevelt pressuring the government and prime minister of Japan to limit emigration to the United States from Japan and Korea, then a Japanese colony.

Germ theory: a theory of the causes of disease that led to bacteriology and the modern scientific approach to medicine.

Intermestic policy: blends inexorably laws or procedures of both national and international considerations.

Know-Nothing Party: a third political party operating in the United States from 1849 to 1856, was notably anti-Catholic and anti-immigrant.

National sovereignty: right and power of a country to control its land.

Open Door Era: the period 1820–1880, when the United States actively sought immigrants for permanent resettlement.

Padrone: the boss system employed by Greek immigrants from 1880 to the early 1900s.

Padroni: the boss system used by Italian immigrants from 1880 to the early 1900s.

Pandemic: epidemic that goes regional or even global in scope, with very high morbidity and mortality rates.

Pathogens: natural agents of disease.

Pogroms: outbreaks of violence against Jews, mostly in Russia and Poland, often condoned, or even sponsored, by the government.

Polonia: name used to refer to the Polish American community.

Push factors: events compelling large numbers of persons to emigrate.

Pull factors: aspects of a receiving nation that draw immigrants for resettlement.

Racial profiling: pattern of behavior of police officers based on racial appearance.

Restrictionism: social movement of the late nineteenth and early twentieth centuries that advocated outright banning of, or severe limits on, immigration.

Scandinavians: residents of Norway, Sweden, Denmark, Finland,

Sojourner: immigrant who comes to the United States intending to stay only temporarily.

The Spanish Flu: the great influenza pandemic of 1918.

Trafficking: transportation of persons for illegal purposes involving sexual or labor exploitation.

Tories: American colonists, also called Loyalists, who preferred staying united with Great Britain, subjects of the British crown.

Unauthorized immigrants: those who enter a country undocumented or who break or overstay the conditions of their visa, becoming illegal immigrants without the status of permanent resident aliens.

Unfunded mandates: requirements placed by the federal government on state or local government with no offsetting funding provided for their implementation.

Virgin population: a population having little or no immunity to a particular disease.

Vectors: carriers of diseases to humans.

Xenophobia: unwarranted or exaggerated fear of foreigners.

Yersinia pestis: the bacteria causing the plague (also known as the Black Death).

NOTES

CHAPTER 1: THE AGE OF MASS MIGRATION, 1820–1920

1. The strong German immigrant/Republican Party influence and connection are discussed by Louis Adamic, *Nation of Nations* (New York: Harper and Brothers, 1945), for example, at page 181; in Vincent Parrillo, *Strangers to These Shores* (Boston, MA: Houghton-Mifflin, 1980) at page 144; and in Richard Schaefer, *Racial and Ethnic Groups* (1998: 32–49. By contrast, LaVern Rippley, in his *The German Americans* (Chicago, IL: Claretian Press, 1973) notes that German Americans in the Midwest were loyal to the Democratic Party and not very enthusiastic supporters of the Civil War. He discusses rural counties in Wisconsin where their Democratic Party support was high and notes anti-draft riots among Germans of Milwaukee and nearby Ozaukee and Washington counties.

2. As to immigrants themselves arriving during this period, estimates of their numbers vary widely. Some sources estimate the number of Poles at over 1 million (for example, Dinnerstein and Reimers, 1988; Parrillo, 1985; and Dinnerstein and Jaher, 1977). Lopata (1976) estimates a maximum of 1,670,000 immigrating to the United States from 1885 to 1972. Levy and Kramer (1973) estimate the total Polish American group (including children born in the United States) to range from 6 million to 12 million.

3. See, for example, Thomas and Znanieki (1977), Parrillo (1988), Lopata (1976), and Dinnerstein and Reimers (1988). As with Italians and with other Slavic groups, Polish immigrants had difficulty adjusting to the Irish-dominated hierarchy of the Roman Catholic Church.

4. The "Jewish Ghetto" is elaborately described in Irving Howe, *World of Our Fathers* (1976): 518–551; and see also Dinnerstein and Reimers: 37–38.

5. See, for example, Pitkin: 46; M. Jones (1960): 260–265; Divine: 4; and LeMay (1987): 65–66. For a discussion of the laws and brief summarization of

laws and court decisions from 1820 to 1920, see LeMay and Barkan, eds. (1999), *U.S. Immigration and Naturalization Laws and Issues: A Documentary History,* (Westport, CT: Greenwood Press, parts 1 and 2: 1–125). This section draws from that source.

CHAPTER 2: THE PERIOD OF PANDEMICS

1. Primary documents of the U.S. M.H.S., files regarding yellow fever, are in the NARA archives, RG 90, Boxes 169–178. Boxes 170–175 contain files covering the 1903–1906 outbreak with numerous letters and telegrams about the service's efforts to places with major epidemic outbreaks, such as Eagle Pass, El Passo, Banquete, Galveston, and Laredo, Texas; Jacksonville, Florida; and Vicksburg, Mississippi. For the period 1924–1935, see the yellow fever files, 425–432, in Box 906. The general subject files for 1936–1944 have Box 534, File 425, on yellow fever during those years.

2. RG 90, Central File, 1897–1923, has five archive boxes in file class 2796 devoted to the U.S. M.H.S. (by then called the P.H.S.), records regarding small-pox. Subject files 1924–1935 and 1936–1944 include a separate file, 425, for smallpox-related correspondence.

3. There are extensive files on smallpox outbreaks and reports on vaccination campaigns in the United States and abroad in the National Archives and Records Administration (NARA) archives at College Park, Maryland, Record Group 90, Central Files, 1897–1923. File 2796, Smallpox, has folders in boxes 250–254 covering the years 1900–1923 with literally many hundreds of communications on outbreaks and reports on the vaccination campaign of the Public Health Service, reporting on the surgeon general's office. See also Ralph Williams, *The United States Health Service, 1798–1950.*

4. Rosenberg: 105. This section draws on his book. See also LeMay, 2006: 41.

5. There are extensive files on cholera in the NARA archives, RG 90, Central File, 1987–1923. See Files 375–397, Boxes 052–057. These files number thousand of pages of documents and were used to write this section. Hereafter, only file and box number will be given.

6. One cannot know for sure, of course, whether the plague first came by the initial visit and aboard his ship. Because we now understand the role that the rat played in the movement of the disease, it is entirely possible that other ships from China carried infected rats that debarked and entered Chinatown, transferring the infection to a colony of local rats and thence to the Chinese residents. Certainly by the time that the epidemic was notably entrenched in San Francisco, a large colony of rats had to have been infected. That process may have taken several months, so the initial infestation may well have come from an earlier ship.

7. The file for influenza is RG 90, Central File, 1897–1923, File 1622, Box 144. It contains many hundreds of pages of documents on the outbreak in the United States in 1918–1919. Also useful is File 3655, Box 363, which deals with licensing, acquisition of serums, and so on. It contains several documents pertaining to

the influenza epidemic in 1918. The most comprehensive and authoritative history of the 1918–1919 pandemic is John Barry, *The Great Influenza* (New York: Penguin Books, 2005), from which this section draws heavily. For a comprehensive discussion of influenza more generally, including the 1918–1919 pandemic, see Alfred Crosby Jr., *Epidemics and Peace, 1918* (Westport, CT: Greenwood Press, 1976).

8. See RG 90, Central Files 1897–1923, File 3655, Box 363. These files cover 1917–1923. Files are monthly by year and during outbreaks contain many requests by stations for vaccines and serums—for example, in 1918, Eagle Pass, Texas for typhoid vaccine, and El Paso, Texas for smallpox vaccine, and so on. Boxes 369–370, labeled special files, have folders regarding each disease vaccine. They report on manufacture, problems with quality of various laboratories and manufacturers, problems of adequate supply of sera during disease outbreaks, shipment problems to stations, and inspecting of civilian manufacturing plants.

CHAPTER 3: THE ANGEL ISLAND QUARANTINE/ IMMIGRATION STATION, 1891–1946

1. Because a fire in 1940 destroyed the Administration Building and most of the records, exact numbers of immigrants passing through Angel Island can only be estimated. Estimates range from about 300,000 to as high as 1 million. Immigration totals for the station at the INS headquarters, which were sent to the NARA archives in College Park, have not yet been found. The 300,000 estimate is based on 340,000 alien arrivals at the Port of San Francisco, 1910–1940, of whom 70 percent were detained at Angel Island, in data presented by Maria Sakovich, "Angel Island Immigration Station Reconsidered: Non-Asian Encounters with the Immigration Laws, 1910–1940" (MA thesis, Sonoma State University, 2002). Detention data are being posted on an online index, Early Arrivals Records Search (EARS), a project of the Institute of Business and Economic Research; University of California, Berkeley; and the National Archives and Records Administration. Currently, data up to 1915 have been processed and indexed, and data to 1921 will be available soon. The NARA–San Francisco files are the most comprehensive nationwide.

2. Barde, *Social Science History,* Table 5. Using anecdotal sources, Shah states that they were detained for weeks: 183–186.

3. Primary source documents for the plague outbreak in the United States, and especially on the 1900–1905, and the 1907–1908 epidemics in San Francisco, are in RG 90, Central File, 1897–1923, File 544, Boxes 065–067, NARA and in File 5608, Box 627, folders for the years 1900–1901. Kinyoun's papers at the National Library of Medicine, Box 1, Folders 10 and 11 are also useful primary source documents. The best secondary sources on the plague outbreaks, in which they are thoroughly and excellently discussed, are Marilyn Chase, *The Barbary Plague*, New York: Random House, 2003; and Nayan Shah, *Contagious Divides*, Berkeley: University of California Press, 2001.

4. The best primary sources for Dr. Joseph Kinyoun are in his personal papers, files 1–16 in Box 1, National Library of Medicine in Washington, D.C. Other useful primary documents are at the National Archives and Records Administration (NARA) at College Park, Maryland in Record Group 90, Central Files 1897–1923, especially files for the plague outbreak in San Francisco, File 544, Boxes 065–067; File 4605, Box 505; and File 5608, Box 627. A thorough biography is in Kelly and Burrage, 1971: 736–737. His role at the quarantine station in San Francisco and the plague outbreaks there in 1900–1902 is discussed in Chase, 2003: 70–90 and in Shah: 120–146. See also Mullan: 39–40.

5. Letter from JK to MHS, 10/09/1899; RG 90, File 4605, Box 505; Letter of JK to Kensington Engine Works, 9/30/1899, File 4605, Box 505.

6. Files of the INS, Arrival Inspection Files, Box 1211, 1884–1944; Report of Wilfred Kellogg, City of San Francisco, to Joseph Kinyoun, March, 1900; see also the discussion in Chase: 13–18.

7. Ibid.

8. See www.surgeongeneral.gov/library/history/bioblue.htm for a solid biography of Rupert Blue. His critically important role in San Francisco in 1902–1905 and in 1907–1908 is extensively covered throughout Chase, 2003 and in Shah: 145–157. A more critical view of Blue as surgeon general, and particularly in his role during the 1918–1919 influenza pandemic, is in John Barry: 178–179, and 300–312.

9. Letter of Blue to Wyman, 10/02/1901, RG 90, File 5608, Box 616.

10. RG 90, File 5608, Box 616, Letter to Surgeon General.

11. For the steam chamber devices and modifications to their design and their use and spread throughout the P.H.S. in the United States and abroad, the best primary source are documents in the Kinyoun papers, National Library of Medicine, Box 1, Folder 16; and in the NARA files, RG 90, Central File, 1897–1923, File 4605, "Sterilizing Machines," in Boxes 505–509.

CHAPTER 4: THE ELLIS ISLAND STATION

1. This chapter draws on Barbara Benton's pictorial history of Ellis Island, see pages 21, 36–37, 47–57, 74–81, 144–145.

2. www.americanparknetwork.com/parkinfo/sl/history/nation.html, and see summary in "Act of August 3, 1882: Regulation of Immigrants," 22 Stat. 214: 8 U.S.C., in LeMay and Barkan: 55–56.

3. Paranscandola: 3; and this section draws on a number of excellent sources discussing the hysteria of the period. See especially Goldstein: 55–78; Murray, 1955; Preston, 1963; and Pitkin: 121–128. How the hysteria contributed to the pandemic across the United States, as at Ellis Island, is thoroughly discussed in Barry, 2005 and Osborne, 1977.

4. 40 Stat. 542; 8 U.S.C. 388; for a summary of its many provisions, see LeMay and Barkan, Document 67: 116–118.

5. Howe: 278–282, discusses the pressures on him and his resistance to summarily deport them. His position was backed by the secretary of labor, whose department at that time had control over the service.

6. RG 90, File 227, Box 039; and reports from the U.S. Marine Hospital Service on foreign quarantine stations, as they were referred to, from major ports around the world, in Files 1004 and 1005.

7. See, for example, reports by George W. Stoner, J. G. Wilson, and J.W . Kerr to Washington, D.C. in RG 90, Files 1174–1190, Boxes 105 and 106.

8. Letters sent by President Theodore Roosevelt, dated 2/20/1906, to Secretary of State Elihu Root and Secretary of Commerce and Labor V. H. Metcalf, whose department was then the parent department of the immigration service, in RG 90, File 219, Box 036.

CHAPTER 5: THE NEW ORLEANS STATION

1. In the epilogue to her definitive book on the subject, Fenn concludes that more than 130,000 Native Americans died in the great smallpox pestilence of 1775–1782; see Fenn, *Pox Americana:* 250–275. For the U.S. M.H.S. efforts to cope with later and sporadic cases of smallpox at various immigration stations, see the smallpox records at RG 90, File 2796, Boxes 250–254. The authoritative source on the 1898–1903 smallpox epidemics is Michael Willrich, *Pox: An American History.* See also Amy Fairchild, *Science at the Borders: Immigrant Medical Inspection and the Shaping of the Modern Industrial Labor Force.*

2. See such reports of Dr. Holt as "Report of the Committee on Disinfectants of the American Public Health Association," Concorde Republican Press Association, 1887, and "An Epitomized Review of the Principles and Practices of Maritime Sanitation," New Orleans, 1892. See also his correspondence with Dr. George Miller Sternberg, in the George Miller Sternberg Papers, 1861–1912: MSC 100.

3. For reports and correspondence related to the various sera developed, see RC 90, File 3655, Boxes 363 and 369–370, which have special files labeled for each disease vaccine developed.

4. For the P.H.S. files on the 1918–1919 influenza epidemic, see RG 90, File 3655, Box 363, and File 1622, Box 144. Box 144 has copies of Blue's reports of November 9, 1918, and October 22, 1918.

5. See, for example, House Report 8061, 1907: "Havana Yellow Fever Commission Report," MSC 31; the Holt reports of 1887 and 1892, "Plague Cases in New Orleans," MSC 109; Walter Reed et al. 1900, Reports of the USMHS, Fiscal Year 1887; Sternberg Papers, MSC 100; PHS Report, "Marine Hospitals at New Orleans, 1914–1923," MSC 475; Charles H. White Papers, MS ACC 701; and the Joseph White Report, "Methods of Controlling Yellow Fever," MSC 210, 1921.

CHAPTER 6: TEN LESSONS LEARNED

1. Etheridge: 18–19. The role of mission complexity as it applies to the newly created Department of Homeland Security is discussed in Michael LeMay, *Public Administration, 2e.* 2006: 295. See also Kenneth Mitchell, "The Other Homeland

Security Threat: Bureaucratic Haggling," *The Public Manager*, 32(1) (Spring, 2003): 15–18 and Elisha Kraus, "Building a Bigger Bureaucracy," *The Public Manager*, 32(1) (spring 2003): 57–58.

2. This section on bioterrorism draws on D. A. Henderson, "The Science of Bioterrorism," www.house.gov/science/full/dec05/henderson.htm; Michael LeMay, *Guarding the Gates: Immigration and National Security* (Westport, CT: Praeger International Security, 2006); Mark Walters, 2003; Michael Oldstone, 1998; Frank Ryan, 1997; Madeline Drexler, 2003; Arno Karlen, 1995; and C. J. Peters and Mark Olshaker, 1997.

3. The concept of "gateway states" and the newly emerging pattern of far wider dispersal of illegal immigrants in the United States is thoroughly discussed in Zuniga and Henderson-Leon, eds., 2005; Chavez, 1992; Hammamoto and Torres, eds. 1997; and LeMay, *Illegal Immigration: A Reference Handbook*, 2007. For a discussion of the worldwide dispersal of immigration, both legal and illegal, see Thomas Faist, 2000; Hirschman, DeWind, and Kasinits, eds., 1999; Kraut, 1994; and Lynch and Simon, 2003.

BIBLIOGRAPHY

Adamic, Louis. *Nation of Nations*. New York: Harper Brothers, 1945.

Adams, Annmarie. *Medicine by Design: The Architect and the Modern Hospital, 1893–1943*. Minneapolis: University of Minnesota Press, 2008.

Alfano, Louis S. "The Immigration Experience—Ellis Island, 1892," "Castle Garden," www.members.tripod.com/.../alfano/castle.htm.

Alfano, Louis S. "The National Quarantine," 1998, www.fortunecity.com/little italy/amalfi/100/food.94.htm.

Allport, Alan, and John Ferguson, eds. *Immigration Policy*, 2nd ed. New York: Chelsea House/Facts on File, 2009.

Anderson, Stuart. *Immigration*. Westport, CT: Greenwood Press, 2010.

"Angel Island: Guardian of the Western Gates," *Prologue: Quarterly of the National Archives and Records Administration* 30, no. 2 (summer 1998).

"Angel Island Immigration Station." www.angelisland.org.

Angel Island Immigration Station Foundation. www.aiisf.org/about/history -mission. Accessed June 25, 2015.

Antin, Mary. *The Promised Land*. New York: Houghton-Mifflin, 1912.

Arnold, Kathleen R., ed. *Anti-Immigration in the United States: A Historical Encyclopedia*. Santa Barbara, CA: ABC-CLIO, 2011.

Arrival Inspection Files, Immigration and Naturalization Service, Box 1211, 1884–1944, National Archives and Records Administration (NARA).

Asian America. www.asianamerica.org/museum. Accessed June 25, 2015.

Bailey, Thomas H. *Voices of America*. New York: Free Press, 1976.

Bakken, Gordon M., and Alexandra Kindell. *Encyclopedia of Immigration and Migration in the American West*, 2 vols. Los Angeles: Sage Publications, 2006.

Barde, Robert. "Prelude to the Plague: Public Health and Politics in America's Pacific Gateway, 1899." *Journal of the History of Medicine* 58 (April 2003): 153–186.

Barde, Robert. *Immigration at the Golden Gate: Passenger Ships, Exclusiveness, and Angel Island*. Westport, CT: Praeger, 2008.

Barde, Robert, and Gustavo Bobonis. "Detention at Angel Island: First Empirical Evidence." *Social Science History* 30, no. 1 (spring 2006): 103–136.

Barry, John M. *The Great Influenza: The Epic Story of the Deadliest Plague in History*. New York: Penguin Books, 2005.

Barstram, David, Maritsa V. Poros, and Pierre Monfort. *Key Concepts in Migration*. Los Angeles: Sage Publications, 2014.

Bayor, Ronald. *Neighbors in Conflict*. Baltimore: The Johns Hopkins University Press, 1978.

Beals, Carleton. *Brass Knuckle Crusade*. New York: Hastings House, 1960.

Benton, Barbara. *Ellis Island: A Pictorial History*. New York: Facts on File Publications, 1998.

Berland, Rebecca, and Edward. *A True Picture of Emigration*. New York: The Citadel Press, 1968.

Bertolli, E. Robert, and Constantine Forkiotis. "Smallpox: Response team review." *The Forensic Examiner* 12, iss.11–12 (November–December 2003): 7–12.

Billington, Ray A. *The Origins of Nativism in the United States, 1800–1944*. New York: Arno Press, 1974.

Breslow, Lester. *Encyclopedia of Public Health*, vols. 1–4. New York: Macmillan Reference USA / Thomson Learning, 2002.

Brewer, Stewart. *Borders and Bridges: A History of U.S.–Latin American Relations*. Westport, CT: Praeger Securities International, 2006.

Brock, Thomas. *Robert Koch: A Life in Medicine*. Madison, WI: Science Tech Publications, 1988.

Bynum, W. F., and Helen Bynum, eds. *Dictionary of Medical Biography*. Westport, CT: Greenwood Press, 2007.

Carrigan, Jo Ann. "Yellow Fever in New Orleans: Abstractions and Realities." *Journal of Southern History* 25 (1959): 339–355.

Carter, Henry R. "Are Vessels Infected with Yellow Fever? Some Personal Observations," *Yellow Fever Institute Bulletin* no. 9. Washington, DC: Yellow Fever Institute, 1902.

"Castle Garden" (from a December 23, 1866, *New York Times* article). www .members.tripod.com/~L_Alfano/castle.htm.

Cecchine, Gary, and Melinda Moore. *Infectious Disease and National Security: Strategic Information Needs*. Santa Monica, CA: RAND Corporation, National Defense Research Institute, 2006.

Centers for Disease Control and Prevention. "Enterovirus D68." Washington, DC: Centers for Disease Control and Prevention, 2015. www.cdc.gov/non -polio-enterovirus/about/ev-d68.html.

Centers for Disease Control and Prevention. www.cdc.gov/agents/smallpox/ overview/disease-facts.asp. Accessed December 2014.

Chan, Sucheng, ed. *Entry Denied: The Exclusion of the Chinese Community in America, 1882–1943*. Philadelphia: Temple University Press, 1991.

Chartre, Christine. "La Disinfection Dans le Systeme quarantenaire maritime de Grosse-Ile: 1832–1937," Internal Research Report, Parks Canada, 1995.

Chase, Marilyn. *The Barbary Plague: The Black Death in Victorian San Francisco*. New York: Random House, 2004.

Cieslik, Thomas, David Felsen, and Akis Kalaitzidic. *Immigration: A Documentary and Reference Guide*. Westport, CT: Greenwood Press, 2008.

Conway, Alan. "New Orleans as a Port of Immigration, 1820–1860." M.A. thesis, University of London, 1949.

Cook, Robin. *Contagion*. New York: G. A. Putnam's Sons, 1995.

Cooke, J. J. "Ships Passenger Lists, Ireland to Louisiana, 1847–1871," J.J. Cooke, Shipping Agent, Londonderry to New Orleans, 1847–1871.

Craddock, Susan. *City of Plagues: Diseases, Poverty, and Deviance in San Francisco*. Minneapolis: University of Minnesota Press, 2000.

Crosby, Alfred W. *America's Forgotten Pandemic: The Influenza of 1918*. New York: Cambridge University Press, 1989.

Daniels, Roger. "No Lamps Were Lit for Them: Angel Island and the Historiography of Asian American Immigration." *Journal of American Ethnic History* 17, no. 1 (fall 1997): 3–26.

Daniels, Roger, and Harry Kitano. *American Racism*. Englewood Cliffs, NJ: Prentice- Hall, 1970.

Davies, Pete. *The Devil's Flu*. New York: Henry Holt and Company, 2000.

Davis, Jerome. *The Russian Immigrant*. New York: Arno Press, 1969.

Department of Commerce. *Statistical Abstract of the United States, 2002*.

Department of Homeland Security. *Yearbook of Immigration Statistics, 2010*.

Department of Justice. *Statistical Yearbook of the Immigration and Naturalization Service, 2001*.

Diddle, Albert W. "Medical Events in the History of Key West." *Bulletin of the History of Medicine* 15, no. 5 (1944): 14–37.

Dinnerstein, Leonard, and David Reimers. *Ethnic Americans*. New York: Harper and Row, 1975.

Divine, Robert A. *American Immigration Policy, 1924–1952*. New Haven, CT: Yale University Press, 1957.

"Docket of the Meeting of the International Board of Health, October 23, 1917, 'Report by Dr. William Crawford Gorgas,'" MS B 478. U.S. National Library of Medicine, National Institute of Health, Washington, DC.

Dong, Lorraine. "Island: Poetry and History of Chinese Immigrants on Angel Island, 1910–1940." *Journal of American Ethnic History* 14, no. 4 (summer 1995): 80–82.

Drexler, Madeline. *Secret Agents: The Menace of Emerging Infections*. New York: Penguin Books, 2002.

Duffy, John. *Epidemics in Colonial America*. Baton Rouge, LA: Louisiana State University Press, 1953.

Duffy, John. *A History of Public Health in New York City, 1866–1966*. New York: Russell Sage Foundation, 1974.

Engel, Johnathan. *The Epidemic: A Global History of Aids.* New York: Penguin Books, 2006.

Esslinger, Dean. "Immigration through the Port of Baltimore" (61–74). In M. Mark Stolarik, *Forgotten Doors: The Other Ports of Entry to the United States.* Philadelphia: The Balch Institute Press, 1988.

Essortment. www.scsc.essortment.com/edwardjennersm_rmfk.htm. Accessed June 25, 2015.

Estes, J. Worth. "Maritime Medicine." *New England Journal of History* 53, no. 1 (spring 1996): 2–13.

Etheridge, Elizabeth W. *Sentinel for Health: A History of the Centers for Disease Control.* Berkeley, CA: University of California Press, 1992.

Fairchild, Amy. *Science at the Borders: Immigrant Medical Inspection and the Shaping of the Modern Industrial Labor Force.* Baltimore, MD: The Johns Hopkins University Press, 2003.

Faist, Thomas. *The Volume and Dynamics of International Migration and Transnational Social Spaces.* New York: Oxford University Press, 2000.

Federal Writers Project. *The Italians of New York.* New York: Arno Press, 1969.

Fee, Elizabeth. *Disease and Discovery: A History of the Johns Hopkins School of Hygiene and Public Health, 1916–1939.* Baltimore: The Johns Hopkins University Press, 1987.

Fenn, Elizabeth A. *Pox Americana: The Great Smallpox Epidemic of 1775–1782.* New York: Hill and Wang, 2001.

Flanagan, Alice K. *Angel Island.* Minneapolis, MN: Compass Point Books, 2006.

Foner, Nancy. *From Ellis Island to J.F.K.: New York's Two Great Waves of Immigration.* New Haven, CT: Yale University Press, 2000.

Fox, Daniel M., Marcia Maldrum, and Ira Rezals, eds. *Nobel Laureates in Medicine or Physiology: A Biographical Dictionary.* New York: Garland, 1990.

Fox, Stephen. *Transatlantic.* New York: Harper and Collins, 2004.

Freedman, Benjamin, MD. "The Louisiana State Board of Health, Established 1855." *The American Journal of Public Health* 41 (October 1951): 1280–1284.

Friedenberg, Zachary B. *Medicine under Sail.* Annapolis, MD: Naval Institute Press, 2002.

French, Laurence Armand. *Running the Border Gauntlet: The Mexican Migrant Controversy.* Santa Barbara, CA: Praeger, 2010.

Fuchs, Lawrence H., ed. *American Ethnic Politics.* New York: Harper and Row, 1968.

Fuchs, Lawrence H. "Immigration through Boston" (17–25). In M. Mark Stolarik, *Forgotten Doors: The Other Ports of Entry to the United States.* Philadelphia: The Balch Institute Press, 1988.

Gans, Judith, Elaine M. Replogie, and Daniel J. Tic. *Debates on U.S. Immigration.* Los Angeles: Sage Publications, 2012.

Garraty, John A., and Mark C. Carnes. *American National Biography,* 12 vols. New York: Oxford University Press, 1999.

Gaston, J. McFadden, MD. "Present Status of Inoculation against Yellow Fever." *Journal of the American Medical Association* 29, no. 17 (1897): 847–849.

Getz, David. *Purple Death: The Mysterious Flu of 1918.* New York: Henry Holt and Company, 2000.

Goldstein, Robert J. "The Anarchist Scare of 1918: A Sign of Tensions in the Progressive Era." *American Studies* 15, no. 2 (1974): 55–78.

Google.org. Mission statement.

Gostin, Lawrence. *Public Health Law: Power, Duty, Restraints.* Berkeley, CA: University of California Press, 2000.

Grant, Madison. *The Passing of the Great Race.* New York: Arno Press, 1916.

Guillet, Edwin C. *The Great Migration.* Toronto: Thomas Nelson and Sons, 1937.

Hammamoto, Darrell, and Rodolfo Torres, eds. *New American Destinies: A Reader in Contemporary Asian and Latin Immigration.* New York: Routledge, 1997.

Handlin, Oscar, ed. *Immigration as a Factor in American History.* Englewood Cliffs, NJ: Prentice-Hall, 1959.

Haugen, David M. *Immigration.* Detroit: Greenhaven Press, 2009.

"Havana Yellow Fever Commission Reports, 1856–1879," MSC 31. U.S. National Library of Medicine, National Institute of Health, Washington, DC.

Hayes, J. N. *The Burden of Disease: Epidemics and Human Response in Western History.* New Brunswick, NJ: Rutgers University Press, 1998.

Hayes, Patrick J., ed. *The Making of Modern Immigration: An Encyclopedia of People and Ideas.* Santa Barbara, CA: ABC-CLIO, 2012.

Henderson, D. A. "The Science of Bio-terrorism." *Science* 282, no. 5406 (February 1999): 1279–1282.

Higham, John. *Send These to Me: Jews and Other Immigrants in Urban America.* New York: Atheneum, 1975.

Higham, John. *Strangers in the Land: Patterns of American Nativism, 1860–1925.* New Brunswick, NJ: Rutgers University Press, 1955.

Highsmith, Carol M., and Ted Landphair. *Ellis Island.* New York: Random House, 2000.

Hirschman, Charles, Joshua DeWind, and Philip Kasinitz, eds. *The Handbook of International Migration.* New York: Russell Sage, 1999.

Hirst, L. Fabian. *The Conquest of Plague: A Study of the Evolution of Epidemiology.* London: Oxford University Press, 1953.

Historical Statistics of the United States, vol. 1: *Population.* Cambridge, UK: Cambridge University Press, 2006.

History Central. www.historycentral.com/1812/NewOrleans.html. Accessed June 25, 2015.

Hofstadter, Richard, and Michael Wallace. *American Violence.* New York: Knopf, 1971.

Holt, Joseph, MD. "The Quarantine Station of Louisiana: Methods of Disinfection Practiced," Report of the Committee on Disinfectants, American Public Health Association. Memphis: Concorde Republican Press Association, November 1887.

Holt, Joseph. *An Epitomized Review of the Principals and Practices of Maritime Sanitation.* New Orleans: 1892.

Holt, Michael F. "The Politics of Impatience: The Origins of Know-Nothingism." *Journal of American History* 60, no. 2 (1973): 309–331.

Howe, Frederic C. *Confessions of a Reformer.* Kent, OH: Kent State University Press, 1988.

Howe, Irving. *World of Our Fathers.* New York: Simon and Schuster, 1976.

"Immigration Station at New Orleans, Louisiana," House Report 8061, OL 16094216M. Washington, DC: U.S. House of Representatives / U.S. Government Printing Office, 1907.

"Interrogation of Chinese Immigrants at Angel Island." www.freestudentessays .com/social_issues/chineseimmigrants.shtml.

Iorizzo, Luciano, and Salvatore Mondello. *The Italian Americans.* New York: Twayne Publishing, 1971.

John Hopkins University. Biography of Dr. Donald Henderson. http://www.jhsph .edu/faculty/directory/profile/3691/donald-henderson.

Jones, Maldwyn Allen. *American Immigration.* Chicago: University of Chicago Press, 1960.

Karlen, Arno. *Man and Microbes: Disease and Plagues in History and Modern Times.* New York: Touchstone Books, 1995.

Kaufman, Martin, Stuart Galishoff, Todd L. Savitts, eds. *Dictionary of American Medical Biography*, vol. 2. Westport, CT: Greenwood Press, 1984.

Kelly, Howard A., and Walter L. Burrage. *Dictionary of American Medical Biography.* Boston: Milford House, 1971.

Kelly, John. *The Great Mortality: An Intimate History of the Black Death, the Most Devastating Plague of All Time.* New York: Harper Collins, 2005.

Kendall, John. History of New Orleans. Chicago: Lewis Publishing, 1922.

Kettner, James H. *The Development of American Citizenship, 1608–1870.* Chapel Hill, NC: University of North Carolina Press, 1978.

Kinyoun Papers, National Library of Medicine, Box 1, Folders 1–16.

Kitano, Harry. *Japanese Americans: The Evolution of a Subculture.* Englewood Cliffs, NJ: Prentice-Hall, 1969.

Kivisto, Peter, and Thomas Faist. *Beyond a Border: Causes and Consequences of Contemporary Immigration.* Los Angeles: Sage Publications, 2010.

Kohn, George C. ed. *Encyclopedia of Plague and Pestilence.* New York: Facts on File, 1995.

Kolata, Gina. *Flu: The Story of the Great Influenza Pandemic of 1918 and the Search for the Virus That Caused It.* New York: Touchstone Books, 1999.

Kraus, Elishia. "Building a Bigger Bureaucracy." *The Public Manager* 32, no. 1 (spring 2003): 57–59.

Kraut, Alan. *Silent Travelers: Germs, Genes, and the "Immigrant Menace."* Baltimore: The Johns Hopkins University Press, 1994.

Lai, Him Mark, Genny Lim, and Judy Yung. *Island: Poetry and History of Chinese Immigrants on Angel Island, 1910–1940.* San Francisco: Hoc Doi, 1999.

Leavitt, Judith W. *Sickness and Health in America: Readings in the History of Medicine and Public Health*, 3rd ed. Madison, WI: University of Wisconsin Press, 1997.

Lee, Erika. "The Chinese Exclusion Example: Race, Immigration, and American Gatekeeping, 1882–1924." *Journal of American Ethnic History* 21 (2002): 36–62.

Lee, Erika, and Judy Young. *Angel Island: Immigrant Gateway to America*. New York: Oxford University Press, 2010.

LeMay, Michael C. *The Struggle for Influence*. Lanham, MD: University Press of America, 1985.

LeMay, Michael C. *From Open Door to Dutch Door: An Analysis of U.S. Immigration Policy since 1820*. New York: Praeger Publishers, 1987.

LeMay, Michael C., and Elliott Barkan, eds. *U.S. Immigration and Naturalization Laws and Issues*. Westport, CT: Greenwood Press, 1999.

LeMay, Michael C. *The Perennial Struggle*, 2nd ed. Upper Saddle River, NJ: Prentice-Hall, 2005.

LeMay, Michael C. *Guarding the Gates: Immigration and National Security*. Westport, CT: Praeger Press, 2006.

LeMay, Michael C. *Illegal Immigration: A Reference Handbook*. Santa Barbara, CA: ABC-CLIO, 2007.

LeMay, Michael C. "Overview of Immigration History and Issues: Founding to 1865." In Michael LeMay, ed., *The Making of a Nation of Nations: Immigration History and Issues*. Santa Barbara, CA: ABC-CLIO, 2013.

LeMay, Michael C., ed. *Transforming America: Perspectives on Immigration*, 3 vols. Santa Barbara, CA: Praeger/ABC-CLIO, 2013.

LeMay, Michael C. "Mushrooming Cities: The Beginnings of Urbanization in America." In Michael LeMay, ed., *The Making of a Nation of Nations: Immigration History and Issues*. Santa Barbara, CA: ABC-CLIO, 2013.

Leventman, Seymour. *The Ghetto and Beyond*. New York: Random House, 1969.

Levy, Mark, and Michael Kramer. *The Ethnic Factor*. New York: Simon and Schuster, 1972.

Lewis, Pierce. *New Orleans: The Making of an Urban Landscape*, 3rd ed. Charlottesville, VA: University of Virginia Press, 2003.

Lieberson, Stanley. *A Piece of the Pie*. Berkeley, CA: University of California Press, 1980.

Litt, Edgar. *Ethnic Politics in America*. Glenview, IL: Scott, Foresman, 1970.

Logsdon, Joseph. "Immigration through the Port of New Orleans" (105–124). In M. Mark Stolarik, ed. *Forgotten Doors: The Other Ports of Entry to the United States*. Philadelphia: The Balch Institute Press, 1988.

Lopata, Helena Znaniecki. *Polish Americans*. Englewood Cliffs, NJ: Prentice-Hall, 1976.

Loucky, James, Jeanne Armstrong, and Larry J. Estrada. *Immigration in America Today: An Encyclopedia*. Westport, CT: Greenwood Press, 2006.

Luckingham, Bradford. *Epidemics in the Southwest, 1918–1919*, Monograph No. 72. El Paso, TX: The University of Texas at El Paso, 1984.

Lucoccine, Luigi F. "The Public Health Service on Angel Island." *Public Health Reports* 3, no. 1 (January/February 1996): 92–95.

Lynch, James P., and Rita Simon. *Immigration the World Over: Statutes, Policies, and Practices.* Lanham, MD: Rowman and Littlefield, 2003.

Magill, Frank N., ed. *The Nobel Prize Winners: Physiology or Medicine,* vol. 1: *1901–1944.* Englewood Cliffs, NJ: Salem Press, 1991.

Markel, Howard. "'The Eyes Have It': Trachoma, the Perception of Disease, the United States Public Health Service, and the American Jewish Immigration Experience, 1897–1924." *Bulletin of the History of Medicine* 74 (2000): 525–560.

Matas, Rudolph. "A Yellow Fever Retrospect and Prospect." *Louisiana Historical Quarterly,* July 8, 1925: 455.

Mayo Clinic. "Diseases and Conditions: Measles." 2014. www.mayoclinic.org/diseases-conditions/measles/basics/prevention/con-20019675.

McClain, Charles. "Of Medicine, Race, and American Law: The Bubonic Plague Outbreak of 1900." *Law and Social Inquiry* 13, no. 3 (1988): 447–470.

McLemore, Dale S. *Racial and Ethnic Relations in America.* Boston: Allyn and Bacon, 1980.

McNeill, William H. *Plagues and People.* New York: Anchor Books, 1989.

Medscape. http://emedicine.medscape.com/article/1202088-overview. Accessed June 2015.

Merino, Noel. *Illegal Immigration.* Detroit: Greenhaven Press, 2012.

Millard Fillmore Papers, vol. 2. New York: Krause Reprint, 1970.

Miller, Debra A. *Immigration.* Detroit: Greenhaven Press, 2014.

Miller, Randall M. "Immigration through the Port of New Orleans: A Comment." In Stolarik, M. Mark, *Forgotten Doors: The Other Ports of Entry to the United States.* Philadelphia: The Balch Institute Press, 1988: 125–142.

Mitchell, Kenneth. "The Other Homeland Security Threat: Bureaucratic Haggling." *The Public Manager* 32, no. 1 (spring 2003): 15–18.

Moote, Lloyd A., and Dorothy G. Moote. *The Great Plague: The Story of London's Deadliest Year.* Baltimore: The Johns Hopkins University Press, 2004.

Moreno, Barry. "Castle Garden: The Forgotten Gateway." *Ancestry Magazine* 2 (March/April 2003). www.ancestry.com/Bain/library/article.aspx?article=7233.

Moreno, Barry. *Encyclopedia of Ellis Island.* Westport, CT: Greenwood Press, 2004.

Moskos, Charles C. *Greek Americans.* Englewood Cliffs, NJ: Prentice-Hall, 1980.

Mullan, Fitzhugh. *Plagues and Politics: The Story of the United States Public Health Service.* New York: Basic Books, 1989.

Murray, Robert K. *Red Scare: A Study in National Hysteria, 1919–1920.* New York: McGraw-Hill, 1955.

National Institute of Medicine at the National Institute of Health. www.nim.nigh.gov/hmd/manuscripts/nimarchives/sgi.html. Accessed December 2006.

National Institute of Medicine at the National Institute of Health. www.nim.nih.gov/medicineplus/ency/article/001486htm. Accessed December 2006.

"A Nation of Immigrants." www.americanparknetwork.com/parkinfo/si/history/nation.html.

Nelli, Humbert. *Italians in Chicago: 1830–1930.* New York: Oxford University Press, 1970.

Nevins, Allan. *Ordeal in the Union: A House Dividing.* New York: Charles Scribners Sons, 1947.

Niehaus, Earl. *The Irish in New Orleans, 1800–1860.* New York: Arno Press, 1976.

Nobel Organizations. www.nobelprize.org/medicine/laureates/1905/koch-bio.html. Accessed June 25, 2015.

Nohl, Johannes. *A Chronicle of the Plague.* Yardley, PA: Westholme Publishing, 1960.

Novak, William J. *The People's Welfare: Law and Regulation in Nineteenth Century America.* Chapel Hill, NC: University of North Carolina Press, 1996.

Novotny, Ann. *Strangers at the Door: Ellis Island, Castle Garden, and the Great Migration to America.* Riverside, CT: The Chatham Press, 1971.

Nugent, Walter T. K. *Crossings: The Great Transatlantic Migration, 1875–1914.* Bloomington, IN: Indiana University Press, 1995.

Nuland, Sherwin. *Doctors: The Illustrated History of Medical Pioneers.* New York: Black Dog and Leventhal, Publishers, 1988.

Office of the Surgeon General of the United States. ww.surgeongeneral.gov/library/hsitory/bioblue.htm. Accessed June 25, 2015.

O'Grady, Joseph D. *How the Irish Became Americans.* New York: Twayne, 1973.

Oldstone, Michael B. *Viruses, Plagues and History.* New York: Oxford University Press, 1998.

Omran, Abdel. "Epidemiology Transition in the U.S.: The Health Factor in Population Change." *Population Bulletin* 32, no. 2 (May 1977; Washington, DC: The Population Bureau).

"Operations of the United States Public Health and Marine Hospital Service." Washington, DC: U.S. Government Printing Office, 1903.

Osborn, June E., ed. *Influenza in America, 1918–1976.* New York: Prodist, 1977.

Overdyke, S. Darrell. *The Know-Nothing Party in the South.* Gloucester, MA: Peter Smith Publishers, Inc., 1968.

Parascandola, John. "Doctors at the Gates: PHS at Ellis Island." *Public Health Reports* 113, no. 1 (January/February 1998): 83–86.

Parrillo, Vincent. *Strangers to These Shores.* Boston: Houghton-Mifflin Co., 1980.

Passel, Jeffrey S., D'Vera Cohn, Jens Manuel Krogstad, and Ana Gonzalez-Barrera. "As Growth Stalls, Unauthorized Immigrant Population Becomes More Settled." Pew Research Center, 2014. www.pewhispanic.org/2014/09/03/as-growth-stalls-unauthorized-immigrant-population-becomes-more-settled/.

Payan, Tony. *The Three U.S.–Mexico Border Wars: Drugs, Immigration, and Homeland Security.* Westport, CT: Praeger Securities International, 2006.

Peters, C. J., and Mark Olshaker. *Virus Hunter: Thirty Years of Battling Hot Viruses Around the World*. New York: Anchor Books/Doubleday, 1997.

Peterson, Paul M. *Swedish Chicago: Images of America*. Chicago: Arcadia Publishing, 2003.

Pitkin, Thomas M. *Keepers of the Gates: A History of Ellis Island*. New York: New York University Press, 1975.

"Plague Cases in New Orleans," MS C 109. U.S. National Library of Medicine, National Institute of Health, Washington, DC: U.S. Government Printing, 1915.

Porter, Roy. *The Greatest Benefit to Mankind: A Medical History of Humanity*. New York: Harper Collins Ltd., 1999.

Powell, John. *Encyclopedia of North American Immigration*. New York: Facts on File, 2005.

Power, J. Gerard, and Theresa Byrd. *U.S.–Mexico Border Health: Issues for Regional and Migrant Populations*. Los Angeles: Sage Publications, 1996.

Preston, Richard. *The Hot Zone*. New York: Anchor Books, 1994.

Preston, Richard. *The Cobra Event*. New York: Ballantine Books, 1997.

Preston, William Jr. *Aliens and Dissenters, Federal Suppression of Radicals, 1903–1933*. Cambridge, MA: Harvard University Press, 1963.

Public Health Reports 30, iss. 14–26. New Orleans, LA: U.S. Public Health Service, Washington, DC, 1914.

Rauch, John H., MD. "Report of an Inspection of the Atlantic and Gulf Quarantines between the St. Lawrence and Rio Grande." Illinois State Board of Health, Springfield, IL, 1896. From the files of John Rauch, MD.

Ravenel, Mayzyk, ed. *A Half Century of Public Health*. New York: American Public Health Association, 1921.

Record Group (RG) 90, Central File, 1897–1923, File 219 (Ellis Island), Box 38, National Archives and Records Administration (hereafter, NARA).

RG 90, Central File, 1897–1923, Files 375–397 (Cholera), Boxes 052–057, NARA.

RG 90, Central File, 1897–1923, Files 537 to File 544 (Plague), Boxes 065–067, NARA.

RG 90, Central File, 1897–1923, File 1622 (Influenza), Box 144. NARA.

RG 90, Central File, 1897–1923, File 2796 (Smallpox), Boxes 250–254, NARA.

RG 90, Central File, 1897–1923, File 2796 (Yellow Fever), Boxes 169–178.

RG 90, Central File, 1897–1923, File 3655, (Serums/Vaccines) Boxes 363, 369–370, NARA.

RG 90, Central File, 1897–1923, File 4605, (Sterilizing Machines), Boxes 505–509.

RG 90, Central File, 1897–1923, File 5608, Box 627 (Plague, San Francisco).

RG 90, General Subject File, 1924–1935, Files 425–432 (Diseases), Box 906 (Yellow Fever).

RG 90, General Subject File, 1924–1935, Files 425–432 (Diseases), Box 904 (Smallpox).

RG 90, General Subject File, 1936–1944, File 425, Box 906 (Diseases).

RG 90, General Subject File, 1936–1944, File 425 (Diseases), Box 534 (Yellow Fever).

RG 90, General Subject File, 1936–1944, Domestic Stations, Boxes 52–55.

RG 90, General Correspondence With Quarantine Stations, 1927–1934, Boxes 13–14 (New Orleans).

RG 90, Inspections and Investigations, 1919–1941, Boxes 206–212 (New Orleans).

RG 90, Reports and Correspondence Relating to Stations, 1923–1936, Boxes 115–124 (New Orleans).

Records of the INS, District 28 (New Orleans), 85.5.13, Passenger Lists for New Orleans, 1903–1945 (189 Rolls).

Reed, Walter, et al. "The Etiology of Yellow Fever: A Preliminary Note." *Philadelphia Medical Journal* 6 (October 27, 1900): 790–796.

Reeves, Pamela. *Ellis Island: Gateway to the American Dream*. New York: Barnes and Noble, 1998.

"Report of the United States Marine Hospital Service for Fiscal Year, 1887." Washington, DC: U.S. Government Printing Office, 1888.

Riis, Jacob. *How the Other Half Lives*. New York: Courier Dover, 1971.

Ringer, Benjamin. *We the People and Others*. New York: Travistock, 1983.

Ripley, William. *The Races of Europe*. New York: Appleton and Company, 1899.

Rippley, LaVern T. *The German Americans*. Chicago: Claretian Press, 1973.

Rosenau, Milton J. *Disinfection and Disinfectants*. Philadelphia: P. Blakiston, 1902.

Rosenberg, Charles E. *The Cholera Years: The United States in 1832, 1849, and 1866*. Chicago: University of Chicago Press, 1987.

Rosenberg, Charles E. *Explaining Epidemics and Other Studies in the History of Medicine*. New York: Cambridge University Press, 1992.

Rosenberg, Charles E., and Janet Golden. *Framing Disease: Studies in Cultural History*. New Brunswick, NJ: Rutgers University Press, 1992.

Rosner, David, ed. *Hives of Sickness: Public Health and Epidemics in New York City*. New Brunswick, NJ: Rutgers University Press, 1995.

Ryan, Frank, MD. *Virus X: Tracking the New Killer Plagues*. Boston: Little, Brown and Company, 1997.

Sakovich, Maria. "Angel Island Immigration Station Reconsidered: Non-Asian Encounters with the Immigration Laws, 1910–1940." MA thesis, Sonoma State University, 2002.

Samuel, Joseph. *Jewish Immigration to the United States, 1881–1910*. New York: Arno Press, 1969.

Satcher, David. "The History of the Public Health Service and the Surgeon General's Priorities." Paper presented at the 42nd Annual Educational Conference, Washington, DC, December 16–17, reprinted in *Food and Drug Law Journal* 54 (1998): 13–19.

Schaefer, Richard. *Racial and Ethnic Groups*, 7th ed. New York: HarperCollins, 1998.

Sevigny, Andre. *Report to the Historic Sites and Monuments Board*. Quebec City: Parcs Canada, Quebec Service Center, 1995a.

Sevigny, Andre. 1995b. *Internal Research Report.* "Quarantine and Public Health: The Changing Role of Grosse Ile." http://parcscanada.risqc.ca/grosseile/history/html.

Shah, Nayan. *Contagious Divides: Epidemics and Race in San Francisco's Chinatown.* Berkeley, CA: University of California Press, 2001.

Shilts, Randy. *And the Band Played On: Politics, People and the AIDS Epidemic.* New York: St. Martin's Press, 1987/2007.

Shrady, George F., and Thomas L. Stedman, eds. *Medical Record* 62 (1902).

Shumsky, Neil L. *The Evolution of Political Protest and the Workingmen's Party of California.* Columbus, OH: Ohio State University Press, 1991.

Smith, Geddes. *Plague on US.* New York: Oxford University Press, 1946.

Smith, James M. *Freedom's Fetters: Alien and Sedition Laws.* Ithaca, NY: Cornell University Press, 1956.

Smith, Marian. "The Creation and Destruction of Ellis Island Immigration Manifests." *Prologue: Quarterly of the National Archives and Records Administration* 18 (1996): 340–345.

Soennichsen, John. *Miwoks to Missiles: A History of Angel Island.* Tiburon, CA: Angel Island Association, 2001.

Soloutos, Theodore. *The Greeks in the United States.* Cambridge, MA: Harvard University Press, 1964.

Soulé, Leon C. *The Know Nothing Party in Louisiana: A Reappraisal.* Baton Rouge, LA: Louisiana State University Press, 1961.

Spletsfoser, Frederick Marcel. "Back Door to the Land of Plenty, 1820–1860," Ph.D. dissertation, Louisiana State University, 1978.

Steiner, Edward A. *On the Trail of the Immigrant.* New York: Revell, 1906.

Sternberg, George Miller. "George Miller Sternberg Papers, 1861–1912," MS C 100. U.S. National Library of Medicine, National Institute of Health, Washington, DC.

St. Louis Medical Review, August 26, 1905: 182.

Stolarik, M. Mark, ed. *Forgotten Doors: The Other Ports of Entry to the United States.* Philadelphia: Balch Institute Press, 1988.

Taylor, Philip. *Distant Magnet: European Emigration to the United States.* New York: Harper and Row, 1971.

Tetrault, Martin. "Frederick Montizambert et la quarantine de Grosse-Ile, 1869–1899." *Scientia Canadensis* 19 (1995): 5–28.

Thernstrom, Stephen. *Harvard Encyclopedia of American Ethnic Groups.* Cambridge, MA: Harvard University Press, 1980.

Thomas, William, and Florian Znanicki. "The Polish American Community." In Leonard Dinnerstein and Frederick Jaher, eds. *Uncertain Americans.* New York: Oxford University Press, 1977.

Time. *The Science of Epidemics: Inside the Fight against Deadly Diseases, from Ebola to AIDS.* New York: Time, Inc., 2014.

Tomes, Nancy. *The Gospel of Germs: Men, Women, and the Microbe in American Life.* Cambridge, MA: Harvard University Press, 1998.

Train, Harry D. II, Admiral, U.S. Navy. *American Naval Fight Ships*, vol. 5. Washington, DC: U.S. Government Printing Office, 1979.

Trask, Benjamin H. "The World of 'Septic Vapours,' Yellow Fever and United States Shipping, 1798–1905." *The Northern Mariner* 15, no. 2 (April 2005): 1–18.

U.S. Bureau of the Census. *Population of States and Counties, 1780–1990.* Washington, DC: Bureau of the Census, U.S. Government Printing Office, 1996.

U.S. Bureau of the Census. *Statistical Abstract of the United States, 2002.* Washington, DC: Bureau of the Census, U.S. Government Printing Office, 2003.

U.S. Bureau of the Census. *The Foreign Born Population in the United States.* Washington, DC, 2001

U.S. Marine Hospital Service. "Marine Hospital at New Orleans, 1914–1923." MSC 475, U.S. National Library of Medicine, National Institute of Health, Washington, DC.

United States National Archives. Records of the Immigration and Naturalization Service, San Francisco District. Arrival Investigation Case Files, 1884–1944. Box 1211, December 1917.

Vecoli, Rudolph, and Joy K. Lintelman. *A Century of American Immigration, 1884–1984.* Minneapolis: University of Minnesota, Continuing Education and Extension, 1984.

Walters, Mark Jerome. *Six Modern Plagues and How We Are Causing Them.* Washington, DC: Island Press, 2004.

Warner, Judith Ann. *Battleground Immigration*, 2 vols. Westport, CT: Greenwood Press, 2008.

Warner, Judith Ann. *U.S. Border Security: A Reference Handbook.* Santa Barbara, CA: ABC-CLIO, 2010.

Weber, Gustavis A. *The Food, Drug, and Insecticide Administration.* Baltimore: The Johns Hopkins University Press, 1928.

Weinberg, Daniel E. "Ethnic Identity in Industrial Cleveland, 1900–1920." *Ohio History* 86, no. 13 (summer 1971).

Weiser, Marjorie P. *Ethnic America.* New York: H.W. Wilson Co., 1978.

White, Dr. Charles B. "C. B. White Papers, 1864–1867," MS ACC 701. U.S. Library of Medicine, National Institute of Health, Washington, DC.

White, Dr. Joseph Hill. "Methods Used in Controlling the 1905 Yellow Fever Epidemic in New Orleans," MS C 210, 1921 Report. U.S. National Library of Medicine, National Institute of Health, Washington, DC.

Williams, Ralph C. *The United States Public Health Service, 1798–1950.* Washington, DC: Shepperson, 1951.

Willrich, Michael. *Pox: An American History.* New York: Penguin Press, 2011.

Winslow, Charles E. *The Evolution and Significance of the Modern Public Health Campaign.* New Haven, CT: Yale University Press, 1923.

Winslow, Charles E. *The Conquest of Epidemic Disease: A Chapter in the History of Ideas.* Madison: University of Wisconsin Press, 1971.

Wood, Andrew Grant, ed. *The Borderlands: An Encyclopedia of Culture and Politics on the U.S.–Mexico Divide.* Westport, CT: Greenwood Press, 2008.

Yam, Philip. *The Pathological Protein: Mad Cow, Chronic Wasting, and Other Deadly Prion Diseases.* New York: Copernicus Books, 2003.

Zolberg, Aristide R. *A Nation by Design: Immigration Policy and the Fashioning of America.* New York: Russell Sage / Harvard University Press, 2006.

Zuniga, Victor, and Ruben Hernandez-Leon, eds. *New Destination: Mexican Immigration to the United States.* New York: Russell Sage, 2005.

INDEX

About the Author

Dr. Michael C. LeMay is professor emeritus at California State University–San Bernardino, where he served as director of the national securities studies M.A. program and as chair of the Department of Political Science. He served three years as assistant dean at the College of Social and Behavioral Science. He has frequently written and presented papers at professional conferences and has written a number of journal articles and book reviews. His writing has been published in the *International Migration Review*, *In Defense of the Aliens*, *Journal of American Ethnic History*, *Southeastern Political Science Review*, *Teaching Political Science*, and the *National Civic Review*. Author of more than 20 academic volumes, his prior books on the topic of immigration history and policy include the following: author, contributor, and series editor, *Transforming America: Perspectives on Immigration*, 3 vols., 2013, ABC-CLIO; *The Perennial Struggle*, 3rd ed., 2009, Prentice-Hall; *Illegal Immigration: A Reference Handbook*, 2007, ABC-CLIO; *Guarding the Gates: Immigration and National Security*, 2006, Praeger Security International; *U.S. Immigration: A Reference Handbook*, 2004, ABC-CLIO; *Immigration and Naturalization Laws and Issues*, 1999, edited with Elliott Barkan, by Greenwood Press; *Anatomy of a Public Policy: The Reform of Contemporary Immigration Policy*, 1994, Praeger Press; *The Gatekeepers: Comparative Immigration Policy*, 1989, Praeger Press; and *From Open Door to Dutch Door: An Analysis of U.S. Immigration Policy since 1820*, 1987, Praeger Press. He has also written a public administration textbook with Wadsworth Press that features considerable discussion of immigration policy: *Public Administration: Clashing Values in the Administration of Public Policy*, 2nd ed., 2006.